1989
YEAR BOOK OF
CARDIOLOGY®

The 1989 Year Book® Series

Year Book of Anesthesia®: Drs. Miller, Kirby, Ostheimer, Roizen, and Stoelting

Year Book of Cardiology®: Drs. Schlant, Collins, Engle, Frye, Kaplan, and O'Rourke

Year Book of Critical Care Medicine®: Drs. Rogers and Parrillo

Year Book of Dentistry®: Drs. Rose, Hendler, Johnson, Jordan, Moyers, and Silverman

Year Book of Dermatology®: Drs. Sober and Fitzpatrick

Year Book of Diagnostic Radiology®: Drs. Bragg, Hendee, Keats, Kirkpatrick, Miller, Osborn, and Thompson

Year Book of Digestive Diseases®: Drs. Greenberger and Moody

Year Book of Drug Therapy®: Drs. Hollister and Lasagna

Year Book of Emergency Medicine®: Dr. Wagner

Year Book of Endocrinology®: Drs. Bagdade, Braverman, Halter, Horton, Korenman, Kornel, Metz, Molitch, Morley, Rogol, Ryan, Sherwin, and Vaitukaitis

Year Book of Family Practice®: Drs. Rakel, Avant, Driscoll, Prichard, and Smith

Year Book of Geriatrics and Gerontology: Drs. Beck, Abrass, Burton, Cummings, Makinodan, and Small

Year Book of Hand Surgery®: Drs. Dobyns, Chase, and Amadio

Year Book of Hematology®: Drs. Spivak, Bell, Ness, Quesenberry, and Wiernik

Year Book of Infectious Diseases®: Drs. Wolff, Barza, Keusch, Klempner, and Snydman

Year Book of Infertility: Drs. Mishell, Lobo, and Paulsen

Year Book of Medicine®: Drs. Rogers, Des Prez, Cline, Braunwald, Greenberger, Wilson, Epstein, and Malawista

Year Book of Neurology and Neurosurgery®: Drs. DeJong, Currier, and Crowell

Year Book of Nuclear Medicine®: Drs. Hoffer, Gore, Gottschalk, Sostman, Zaret, and Zubal

Year Book of Obstetrics and Gynecology®: Drs. Mishell, Kirschbaum, and Morrow

Year Book of Oncology®: Drs. Young, Coleman, Longo, Ozols, Simone, and Steele

Year Book of Ophthalmology®: Dr. Laibson

Year Book of Orthopedics®: Dr. Sledge

Year Book of Otolaryngology—Head and Neck Surgery: Drs. Bailey and Paparella

Year Book of Pathology and Clinical Pathology®: Drs. Brinkhous, Dalldorf, Grisham, Langdell, and McLendon

Year Book of Pediatrics®: Drs. Oski and Stockman

Year Book of Perinatal/Neonatal Medicine: Drs. Klaus and Fanaroff

Year Book of Plastic, Reconstructive, and Aesthetic Surgery: Drs. Miller, Bennett, Haynes, Hoehn, McKinney, and Whitaker

Year Book of Podiatric Medicine and Surgery®: Dr. Jay

Year Book of Psychiatry and Applied Mental Health®: Drs. Talbott, Frances, Freedman, Meltzer, Schowalter, and Weiner

Year Book of Pulmonary Disease®: Drs. Green, Ball, Michael, Peters, Terry, Tockman, and Wise

Year Book of Rehabilitation®: Drs. Kaplan, Frank, Gordon, Lieberman, Magnuson, Molnar, Payton, and Sarno

Year Book of Sports Medicine®: Drs. Shephard, Sutton, and Torg, Col. Anderson, and Mr. George

Year Book of Surgery®: Drs. Schwartz, Jonasson, Peacock, Shires, Spencer, and Thompson

Year Book of Urology®: Drs. Gillenwater and Howards

Year Book of Vascular Surgery®: Drs. Bergan and Yao

Editor-in-Chief

Robert C. Schlant, M.D.

Professor of Medicine (Cardiology), Department of Medicine, Division of Cardiology, Emory University School of Medicine, Atlanta, Georgia

Editors

John J. Collins, Jr., M.D.

Professor of Surgery, Harvard Medical School; Vice Chairman, Department of Surgery, Director, Sub-Department of Thoracic and Cardiac Surgery, Brigham and Women's Hospital, Boston, Massachusetts

Mary Allen Engle, M.D.

Stavros S. Niarchos Professor of Pediatric Cardiology, Director of Pediatric Cardiology, The New York Hospital—Cornell Medical Center, New York, New York

Robert L. Frye, M.D.

Chairman, Department of Medicine, Rose M. and Maurice Eisenberg Professor, Mayo Clinic, Rochester, Minnesota

Norman M. Kaplan, M.D.

Professor of Internal Medicine, Hypertension Division, University of Texas Southwestern Medical Center, Dallas, Texas

Robert A. O'Rourke, M.D.

Charles Conrad Brown Distinguished Professorship in Cardiovascular Disease, Director of Cardiology, The University of Texas Health Sciences Center, San Antonio, Texas

1989

The Year Book of CARDIOLOGY®

Editor-in-Chief
Robert C. Schlant, M.D.

Editors
John J. Collins, Jr., M.D.
Mary Allen Engle, M.D.
Robert L. Frye, M.D.
Norman M. Kaplan, M.D.
Robert A. O'Rourke, M.D.

Year Book Medical Publishers, Inc.
Chicago • London • Boca Raton

International Standard Book Number: 0-8151-7775-5

International Standard Serial Number: 0145-4145

Editor-in-Chief, Year Book Publishing: Nancy Gorham
Sponsoring Editor: Cathy Dombai
Manager, Medical Information Services: Laura J. Shedore
Assistant Director, Manuscript Services: Frances M. Perveiler
Assistant Managing Editor, Year Book Editing Services: Wayne Larsen
Production Coordinator: Max F. Perez
Proofroom Manager: Shirley E. Taylor

Table of Contents

The material covered in this volume represents literature reviewed through November 1988.

Journals Represented

Year Book Medical Publishers subscribes to and surveys nearly 850 U.S. and foreign medical and allied health journals. From these journals, the Editors select the articles to be abstracted. Journals represented in this YEAR BOOK are listed below.

American Heart Journal
American Journal of Cardiology
American Journal of Epidemiology
American Journal of Hypertension
American Journal of Medicine
American Journal of Obstetrics and Gynecology
American Journal of Physiology
American Journal of Public Health
American Journal of Roentgenology
Anesthesiology
Annals of Internal Medicine
Annals of Surgery
Annals of Thoracic Surgery
Archives of Internal Medicine
Archives of Surgery
British Heart Journal
British Medical Journal
Canadian Journal of Cardiology
Cardiovascular Research
Chest
Circulation
Circulation Research
Clinical Nuclear Medicine
Clinical Science
Current Problems in Cardiology
European Heart Journal
European Journal of Clinical Pharmacology
Hypertension
International Journal of Cardiology
Journal of the American College of Cardiology
Journal of the American Society of Echocardiography
Journal of the Applied Physiology
Journal of Cardiac Surgery
Journal of Clinical Investigation
Journal of Electrocardiology
Journal of Hypertension
Journal of Internal Medicine
Journal of Nuclear Medicine
Journal of Pediatrics
Journal of Pharmacology and Experimental Therapeutics
Journal of Thoracic and Cardiovascular Surgery
Journal of Trauma
Kidney International
Lancet
Mayo Clinic Proceedings
New England Journal of Medicine

Pediatric Cardiology
Pediatric Research
Psychosomatic Medicine
Radiology

Introduction

This 1989 YEAR BOOK OF CARDIOLOGY, which is the 29th in the series, continues the objectives and format of its predecessors. In addition to containing detailed abstracts and comments on 301 highly selective, clinically relevant cardiology articles, the volume contains 165 other references to articles that were used by the section editors in their comments and that provide additional current information on the topic.

All of the section editors again thank the staff at Year Book Medical Publishers for their assistance, patience, and understanding. In particular, we are indebted to Ms. Nancy Gorham and Ms. Cathy Dombai.

Robert C. Schlant, M.D.

1 Normal and Altered Cardiovascular Function

Introduction

In this section of the YEAR BOOK OF CARDIOLOGY, 50 recently published articles and many additional references providing clinically relevant information concerning cardiovascular physiology, myocardial metabolism, commonly used noninvasive techniques and newer diagnostic and therapeutic methods are reviewed. Both experimental animal and clinical studies are abstracted and discussed, with additional references provided at the end of various subsections.

In the first subsection on atrial natriuretic peptide (ANP), 3 articles concerning ANP release and its effect on cardiac human dynamics and coronary artery vasomotor tone are discussed. The dose-related coronary artery vasodilatation produced by these atrial peptins is of particular interest and may have relevance for patients with ischemic heart disease in whom congestive heart failure develops.

In the subsection on exercise and exercise training, 4 recently published manuscripts are abstracted and discussed and 4 additional references are provided. The first study describes the effects of altering β_2 adrenergic and α-adrenergic blockade on coronary blood flow velocity during exercise in the conscious preinstrumented dog. Theoretically, this study supports the use of β_1 specific adrenergic blockers or coronary vasodilator drugs such as the calcium blockers in patients with exercise-induced angina. Two additional abstracted studies indicate that the effects of exercise training are modified to some extent by the chronic administration of propranolol and that the baroreflex control of heart rate and sympathetic nerve activity is attenuated by endurance exercise training. The final study describes the usefulness of exercise Doppler echocardiography to evaluate cardiac drugs such as propranolol and verapamil on indices of aortic velocity and acceleration.

The third subsection includes 4 abstracts on ventricular hypertrophy and an additional 7 references from the recent literature. These abstracts provide information on left ventricular systolic and diastolic function during atrial pacing, the effect of age on myocardial adaptation to a volume overload, the production of volume overload hypertrophy in an animal model of chronic mitral regurgitation and the development of collagen remodeling in scar formation in nonhuman primates with pressure-overload left ventricular hypertrophy of slow onset.

Seven abstracted articles and 8 additional references are included in the

1

subsection (subsection 4) on ventricular function. The first 2 describe the effects of asynchronous left ventricular wall motion on myocardial relaxation and the relationship between systolic pressure and isovolumic relaxation in the right ventricle. The subsequent 2 discuss the usefulness and limitations of Doppler echocardiography for evaluating left ventricular diastolic function. This subsection also contains information on the effect of afterload resistance on the end-systolic pressure-thickness relationship and the effects of cocaine on cardiovascular function in the experimental animal.

The fifth subsection on electrophysiology includes 4 abstracted articles and 4 additional references. The first 2 abstracts provide information concerning the potential mechanisms for the development of ventricular tachycardia and atrial fibrillation. Subsequent articles provide clinically relevant information concerning the presence of electrical alternans as related to ventricular tachyarrhythmias and the arrhythmogenic effects of hypokalemia in the presence of myocardial infarction.

In the subsection on coronary artery vasomotor tone (subsection 6) 4 abstracts and 7 additional references provide useful data concerning the effects of atherosclerotic lesions and oxygen free radicals on endothelium-dependent dilatation of the coronary arteries, the production of coronary artery spasm by a nonselective inflammatory cell stimulant, and the improvement of coronary artery collateral blood flow by glyceryl trinitrate.

Twelve abstracted articles and 9 additional references are included in the extensive subsection on experimental myocardial ischemia/infarction indicating the extensive amount of basic and clinical investigation being performed in this area of interest. These articles provide interesting facts concerning various coronary artery receptors in myocardial ischemia, markers of myocyte viability in ischemic reperfused myocardium, the role of the inflammatory response in the extent of myocardial tissue injury after coronary artery occlusion, and the use of various interventions for reducing the extent of myocardial injury after coronary artery reperfusion and for improving left ventricular function after the myocardial infarction.

Subsection number 8, on noninvasive testing, contains 5 abstracted articles and 10 additional references from the recent literature. The first abstract describes potential limitations in the assessment of the severity of mitral stenosis by Doppler echocardiography in patients with coincident aortic regurgitation, whereas the second reviews the usefulness of transesophageal echocardiography. Two abstracts provide up-to-date information concerning the usefulness and further development of nuclear magnetic resonance imaging for use in patients with cardiovascular disease. The final abstract in this section compares SPEC imaging with thallium to PET imaging with ammonia in the detection of myocardial ischemia.

In subsection 9, concerning newer diagnostic and therapeutic techniques, 4 abstracted articles are presented and 7 additional references are listed. The first 2 abstracts concern the use of isonitrile technetium analogues for the detection and quantitation of ischemic heart disease. The third report concerns the usefulness and limitations of indium-labeled platelet scintigraphy and 2-dimensional echocardiography for detection of left atrial thrombi in an animal model, and the fourth concerns the quantitative assessment of regional left ventricular function using densitometric analysis of ventriculograms.

The tenth and final subsection concerns sudden death and cardiopulmonary resuscitation. The first abstract indicates that the risk of sudden cardiac death in postinfarction patients increases when either a depressed baroreflex sensitivity is present or reduced heart rate variability exists. The second suggests that the benefit of epinephrine during attempted cardiopulmonary resuscitation is due to factors other than improved myocardial oxygenation, and the final study indicates that the end-tidal CO_2 concentration during precordial impression may be a useful clinical indicator of prognosis.

Robert A. O'Rourke, M.D.

Atrial Natriuretic Peptide

Atrial Natriuretic Factor Gene Expression in Ventricles of Rats With Spontaneous Biventricular Hypertrophy
Lee RT, Bloch KD, Pfeffer JM, Pfeffer MA, Neer EJ, Seidman CE (Brigham and Women's Hosp, Boston; Harvard Univ)
J Clin Invest 81:431–434, February 1988   1–1

Atrial natriuretic factor (ANF) is a natriuretic and vasorelaxant cardiac hormone. Increased synthesis of ANF by the ventricle has been detected in animal models of cardiac hypertrophy. To examine this phenomenon, ANF production was evaluated in a subset of Wistar-Kyoto rats that have spontaneous and gradual development of biventricular hypertrophy (BVH).

Normal rats had low levels of ANF messenger (m)RNA in the left ventricle and barely detectable levels of mRNA in the right ventricle by Northern analysis. In contrast, the rats with biventricular hypertrophy had 6 times more ANF mRNA in their left ventricles and an equal amount in their right ventricles.

In this natural model of biventricular hypertrophy both left and right ventricles increase their ANF gene expression. These results may lead to further understanding of the factors leading to cardiac hypertrophy.

▶ In 1981, deBolt and associates (*Life Sci* 28:89, 1981) reported that the injection of crude atrial homogenates into rats produced a rapid and profound diuresis and natriuresis. In the subsequent 9 years considerable research has focused on a family of amino acid peptides, isolated initially from mammalian atria, which have various humoral effects on the cardiovascular and renal systems of intact animals. These atriopeptins have both a diuretic and natriuretic effect, suggesting that the kidney is a principal site of action. More recently, they have also been shown to relax both vascular and nonvascular smooth muscle; their effect on myocardial contractility remains controversial. Atrial natriuretic peptide (ANP) release has been related to an increase in right and left atrial pressures and the role of ANP in hypertension, congestive heart failure, and regulation of blood volumes has and is being investigated intensively.

Although ANP was initially shown to be synthesized and secreted predominantly by the atria in healthy adult mammals, small quantities have been detected in the ventricles. Increased ANF gene expression in the ventricle has been shown in animal models producing cardiac hypertrophy.

The above study in subsets of Wistar-Kyoto rats indicates that both left and right ventricles can concomitantly respond to hypertrophy and increased ANF transcription. Further studies in biventricular hypertrophic rats, a naturally occurring model of spontaneous hypertrophy, may provide important knowledge of the ANF's function in various physiologic and pathologic states.—R.A. O'Rourke, M.D.

Effects of Atrial Natriuretic Peptide in the Canine Coronary Circulation
Bache RJ, Dai X-Z, Schwartz JS, Chen DG (Univ of Minnesota)
Circ Res 62:178–183, January 1988   1–2

Atriopeptin II, an atrial natriuretic peptide (ANP), has been reported to cause coronary vasoconstriction in the isolated, perfused guinea pig and canine hearts. To examine the mechanisms of this effect, human ANP was injected as a bolus dose into the coronary circulation of 16 mongrel dogs.

Intracoronary administration of ANP produced dose-related coronary vasodilation with a threshold range of 2 ng/kg of body weight; a dosage of 2 μg/kg of body weight caused a 27% decrease in coronary vascular resistance. Coronary vasodilation was not inhibited by propranolol, (1 mg/kg of body weight), 8-phenyltheophylline (5 mg/kg of body weight), or indomethacin (5 mg/kg of body weight).

Administration of ANP to the coronary circulation resulted in coronary vasodilation. This vasodilation did not occur by adenosine-dependent or prostaglandin-dependent mechanisms.

► These studies show that intracoronary ANP produced a dose-dependent coronary artery vasodilation that was not altered by either β-adrenergic receptor blockade, blockade of adenosine receptors, or cyclooxygenase inhibition in the anesthetized, perfused dog heart. Whether or not such vasodilation of the coronary arteries is mediated by ANP at the plasma concentrations usually present in normal subjects or in patients with congestive heart failure remains to be defined.—R.A. O'Rourke, M.D.

Effects of Atrial Natriuretic Peptide on Coronary Vascular Resistance in the Intact Awake Dog
Laxson DD, Dai X-Z, Schwartz JS, Bache RJ (Univ of Minnesota)
J Am Coll Cardiol 11:624–629, March 1988   1–3

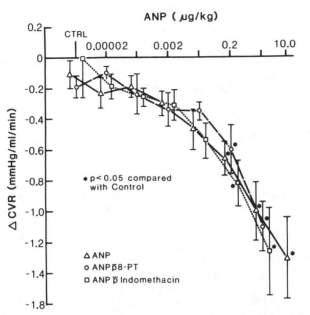

Fig 1—1.—Change in mean coronary vascular resistance *(ΔCVR)* in response to graded doses of human atrial natriuretic peptide *(ANP)* during control *(CTRL)* conditions, after adenosine receptor blockade with 8-phenyltheophylline (8-PT) and after cyclooxygenase inhibition with indomethacin. Values are mean ± SEM. (Courtesy of Laxson DD, Dai X-Z, Schwartz JS, et al: *J Am Coll Cardiol* 11:624–629, March 1988.)

Past studies of the effects of atrial natriuretic peptide (ANP) on the coronary vasculature have given conflicting results. The effects of human ANP and rat atriopeptin II on the coronary circulation in awake, unsedated dogs were compared to obviate the effects of general anesthesia and acute surgical trauma. Varying doses of ANP were injected into a coronary artery catheter before and after adenosine receptor blockade with 8-phenyltheophylline. Indomethacin was used to determine whether vasodilation from ANP involved prostaglandin-dependent mechanisms.

Diastolic coronary resistance was significantly reduced, and coronary flow was increased by human ANP in doses of 0.2 μg/kg and higher (Fig 1–1). Both effects were dose-related. Neither 8-phenyltheophylline nor indomethacin altered the response to ANP. Rat atriopeptin II also produced a dose-related decrease in coronary resistance and increased coronary blood flow. Neither peptide significantly altered left ventricular pressures, left ventricular dP/dt, or heart rate.

Both human ANP and rat atriopeptin caused transient coronary vasodilation in intact, awake dogs in this study. Coronary vasoconstriction did not occur. However, vasodilation occurred only with pharmacologic doses producing plasma levels higher than those present under physiologic conditions. The findings fail to support an important role for ANP in controlling coronary blood flow.

▶ This study by Laxson and associates showed a coronary vasodilation effect of atrial natriuretic peptide (ANP) in *unanesthetized* dogs with normal left ventricular (LV) function and without LV hypertrophy but only in doses that produced plasma levels far above those reported in normal humans and in patients with chronic congestive heart failure. The dose-dependent coronary vasodilation (as in the prior report) was not altered by either adenosine receptor blockade or cyclooxygenase inhibition. Interestingly, no changes in cardiovascular hemodynamics or left ventricular function (dP/dt) were observed with any dose of intracoronary ANP.—R.A. O'Rourke, M.D.

Additional important recent articles on atrial natriuretic peptide are as follows:

1. Goetz KL: Physiology and pathophysiology of atrial peptides. *Am J Physiol* 254:E−1, 1988.
2. Edwards BS, Ackermann DM, Lee ME, et al: Identification of atrial natriuretic factor within ventricular tissue in hamsters and humans with congestive heart failure. *J Clin Invest* 81:82−86, 1988.
3. Franch HA, Dixon RAF, Blaine EH, et al: Ventricular atrial natriuretic factor in the cardiomyopathic hamster model of congestive heart failure. *Circ Res* 62:31−36, 1988.
4. Gisbert M-P, Fischmeister R: Atrial natriuretic factor regulates the calcium current in frog isolated cardiac cells. *Circ Res* 62:660−667, 1988.
5. Springall DR, Bhatnagar M, Wharton J, et al: Expression of atrial natriuretic peptide gene in the cardiac muscle of rat extrapulmonary and intrapulmonary veins. *Thorax* 43:44−52, 1988.
6. Yasue H, Obata K, Okumura K, et al: Increased secretion of atrial natriuretic polypeptide from the left ventricle in patients with dilated cardiomyopathy. *J Clin Invest* 83:46−51, 1989.
7. Ishikura F, Nagata S, Hirato Y, et al: Rapid reduction of plasma atrial natriuretic peptide levels during percutaneous transvenous mitral commissurotomy in patients with mitral stenosis. *Circulation* 29:1−7, 1989.

Exercise and Exercise Training

Role of β_2-Adrenergic Receptors on Coronary Resistance During Exercise
DiCarlo SE, Blair RW, Bishop VS, Stone HL (Univ of Texas, San Antonio; Univ of Oklahoma, Oklahoma City)
J Appl Physiol 64:2287−2293, June 1988   1−4

The role of β-adrenergic receptors in controlling the coronary circulation during exercise remains to be precisely determined. The effects of regional α- and β_2-receptor blockade on the coronary flow response to exercise was studied in conscious dogs. Responses to 4 weeks of daily exercise also were studied. Specific β_2-receptor blockade was produced with ICI 118.551, and α-adrenergic receptor blockade, with phentolamine.

β_2-Adrenergic receptor blockade reduced coronary blood flow velocity (Fig 1−2) and increased late diastolic coronary resistance by blocking vasodilator tone. α-Adrenergic receptor blockade significantly increased coronary flow volume and decreased late diastolic coronary resistance by blocking sympathetically mediated vasoconstrictor tone. Daily exercise and left stellate ganglionectomy prevented phentolamine-induced vasodilation, but not ICI 118.551-induced vasoconstriction.

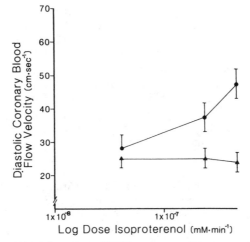

Fig 1–2.—Coronary blood flow velocity (CBFV) responses to intracoronary infusion of isoproterenol (circle) and isoproterenol after specific β₂-adrenergic receptor blockade with ICI 118.551 (triangle). Note that increase in CBFV induced by an isoproterenol challenge independent of altering factors that influence myocardial metabolism was completely blocked by ICI 118.551. (Courtesy of DiCarlo SE, Blair RW, Bishop VS, et al: *J Appl Physiol* 64:2287–2293, June 1988.)

Both α- and β₂-adrenergic receptors have a significant role in influencing coronary flow volume and coronary resistance during exercise. Daily exercise appears to reduce sympathetic vasoconstrictor tone without affecting β₂-adrenergic receptors, and this may be an important protective adaptation.

▶ Coronary artery vasoconstriction is an important factor in the causation of myocardial ischemia in many patients with chronic exertional angina as well as being the predominant factor in patients with variant angina. In the above study, regional β₂-adrenergic blockade during exercise decreased coronary blood flow velocity (CBFV) by attenuating β₂-receptor vasodilator tone independently of α-receptor mediated tone and independently of altering myocardial metabolism, whereas α-adrenergic blockade increased CBFV by blocking sympathetically mediated vasoconstrictor tone. These findings have important significance for those prescribing antianginal drugs that might be expected to augment or prevent coronary vasodilation during exercise.— R.A. O'Rourke, M.D.

Effects of Chronic β-Adrenergic Blockade on Exercise Training in Dogs

Wolfel EE, Lindenfeld J, Smoak J, Horwitz LD (Univ of Colorado, Denver)
J Appl Physiol 64:1960–1967, May 1988   1–5

The effects of β-adrenergic blockade on exercise training have not been made clear by previous studies, whether of animals or humans. A trial was designed to evaluate the effects of propranolol on treadmill training in dogs. Six dogs were trained on an exercise treadmill for 8 weeks and were treated with daily oral doses of propranolol at 10 mg/kg/day. Seven dogs underwent the same program without medication. A control group of 5 dogs remained sedentary during the 8-week period.

The dogs were tested at rest and at both submaximal and peak exercise. Heart rate responses were monitored weekly. Lactate analysis and blood volume were among the measurements taken.

During training, the heart rates in treated dogs were 11% lower than those of untreated dogs; in high-intensity exercise, the rate was 12% lower. Submaximal exercise caused a significant lowering of resting heart rate and mean heart rate scores in both groups. At peak exercise, the heart rate was unchanged in the treated group and decreased in the untreated group. The control group showed no significant changes in heart rate.

Resting blood volume in propranolol-treated and untreated animals was similar, indicating that this response to training may not be influenced by β-adrenergic mechanisms. Arterial lactate levels decreased during submaximal exercise in both groups. In both groups the treadmill time to lactate threshold was significantly greater after training, showing that more work was performed before lactate accumulation in arterial blood. The untreated dogs had both a greater reduction in peak exercise lactate and a greater increase in lactate threshold.

In dogs, exercise training effects are not prevented by propranolol, although the intensity of cardiovascular work is diminished.

▶ Controversy persists as to whether treatment with β-blocking drugs attenuates the effects of exercise training in normal subjects or in patients with coronary heart disease. In the above studies definite training effects occurred in normal mongrel dogs during submaximal exercise despite the administration of propranolol during training. However, β-adrenergic blockade appeared to interfere with training-induced alteration in sympathetic control at peak exercise, thus preventing the full development of peripheral training effects. Additional studies are needed to determine whether similar alterations occur in patients with and without ischemic heart disease.—R.A. O'Rourke, M.D.

Exercise Training Attenuates Baroreflex Regulation of Nerve Activity in Rabbits
DiCarlo SE, Bishop VS (Univ of Texas, San Antonio)
Am J Physiol 255:H974–H979, 1988   1–6

Endurance training appears to alter the baroreflex control of the cardiovascular system. A longitudinal study was conducted to assess the effects of endurance exercise training on control of the heart rate and renal sympathetic nerve activity in conscious rabbits. The animals underwent 8 weeks of treadmill endurance training, and an effect was discerned from exercise-induced bradycardia.

Resting and exercise heart rates were lower after endurance training. The mean arterial pressure decreased at similar rates before and after training, but reflex increases in the heart rate and renal sympathetic nerve activity were significantly attenuated after training. The slope as well as the range of baroreflex control of these responses also was attenuated after the animals exercised.

Endurance exercise training significantly attenuates the baroreflex control of the heart rate and renal sympathetic nerve activity in the conscious rabbit. An increase in the tonic inhibitory influence of the cardiopulmonary baroreflex could be responsible for the change.

▶ This study is consistent with most investigations of the effect of endurance exercise training on blood pressure control mechanisms with attenuated control mechanisms reported in trained individuals and animals. Importantly, this report quantitated the reduction in baroreflex control of heart rate and renal sympathetic nerve activity resulting from endurance exercise training.—R.A. O'Rourke, M.D.

Use of Exercise Doppler Echocardiography to Evaluate Cardiac Drugs: Effects of Propranolol and Verapamil on Aortic Blood Flow Velocity and Acceleration
Harrison MR, Smith MD, Nissen SE, Grayburn PA, DeMaria AN (Univ of Kentucky; VA Med Ctrs, Lexington, Ky)
J Am Coll Cardiol 11:1002–1009, May 1988   1–7

Doppler echocardiography can be used to reliably measure blood flow velocity and acceleration in the ascending aorta. The technique has been used successfully for assessing changes in ventricular function induced by vigorous exercise. Because the influence of cardiac drugs on cardiocirculatory function during exertion has not been well studied, a study was done to determine whether exercise Doppler echocardiography could be used to identify changes in ventricular performance associated with the administration of cardiac drugs.

The subjects were 6 women and 14 men aged 22–42 years (mean age, 30 years) who were all in good health but varied in cardiovascular conditioning from sedentary to well trained. Each underwent continuous wave Doppler echocardiographic testing from the suprasternal notch at rest, during the final 90 seconds of each exercise stage of a Bruce protocol, and immediately after exercise. On completion of the control exercise test, each subject immediately received 60–80 mg of propranolol or 120 mg of verapamil orally, and the same exercise protocol was repeated 90 minutes later. On another day, under similar conditions, the control and exercise Doppler studies were repeated with the same volunteers, but with each subject receiving the alternate drug.

During the control test, peak modal velocity, peak acceleration, and flow velocity integral were increased significantly with exercise. Flow velocity and acceleration increased progressively with increasing levels of exertion. During the propranolol test, the heart rates at rest and at maximal exercise were significantly depressed compared with control values. Peak modal velocities at baseline and at maximal exercise were significantly lower after propranolol administration. The effect of propranolol on acceleration was even greater, with blunting of both baseline and exertional acceleration. The flow velocity integral at rest was not altered by propranolol but was significantly increased at maximal exercise. Verapamil did not affect any of the Doppler-measured parameters of aortic blood flow.

Propranolol profoundly alters the Doppler-measured hemodynamic exercise response in young healthy subjects, whereas exercise-induced hemodynamic changes are not affected by verapamil administration.

▶ Because of its ability to measure blood flow velocity and acceleration in the ascending aorta at rest and during exercise, Doppler echocardiography is being used with increasing frequency for the noninvasive assessment of left ventricular function before and after various interventions, including drug therapy. However, its sensitivity and accuracy as compared with other noninvasive methods for evaluating left ventricular performance (e.g., radionuclide and 2-D echo ejection fraction) needs further evaluation.

In this study the effects of 2 antianginal drugs on Doppler echocardiographic indices of velocity and acceleration were evaluated in 20 normal subjects with different hemodynamic responses to exercise demonstrated with the propranolol as compared with verapamil.—R.A. O'Rourke, M.D.

Four additional references of interest concerning exercise are as follows:

1. Sullivan MJ, Higginbotham MB, Cobb FR: Exercise training in patients with severe left ventricular dysfunction: Hemodynamic and metabolic effects. *Circulation* 78:506–515, 1988.
2. Victor RG, Bertucci LD, Pryor SL, et al: Sympathetic nerve discharge is coupled to muscle cell pH during exercise in humans. *J Clin Invest* 82:1301–1305, 1988.
3. Hopper MK, Coggan AR, Coyle EF: Exercise stroke volume relative to plasma-volume expansion. *J Appl Physiol* 64:404–408, 1988.
4. Gwirtz PA, Mass HJ, Strader JR, et al: Coronary and cardiac responses to exercise after chronic ventricular sympathectomy. *Med Sci Sports Exer* 20:126–135, 1988.

Ventricular Hypertrophy

Systolic and Diastolic Dysfunction During Atrial Pacing in Conscious Dogs With Left Ventricular Hypertrophy
Fujii AM, Gelpi RJ, Mirsky I, Vatner SF (Harvard Univ)
Circ Res 62:462–470, March 1988   1–8

Decreased myocardial perfusion reserve may help explain deteriorating left ventricular (LV) function in pressure overload LV hypertrophy, and the eventual development of irreversible heart failure. The authors studied the effects of chronotropic stress from atrial pacing on both systolic and diastolic LV function in the conscious dog with severe LV hypertrophy, produced by a Teflon band about the ascending aorta.

The ratio of LV free wall to body weight was 70% greater in dogs with LV hypertrophy than in sham-operated animals. Baseline LV systolic wall stress was similar in the 2 groups, but on atrial pacing, systolic LV function declined in the dogs with LV hypertrophy (Fig 1–3). Diastolic dysfunction also was observed in dogs with LV hypertrophy, during atrial pacing at 240 beats/minute. Left ventricular end-diastolic pressure increased, along with end-diastolic stress and the stiffness constant. The endocardial-to-epicardial blood flow ratio decreased from 1.07 to 0.85 on rapid atrial pacing.

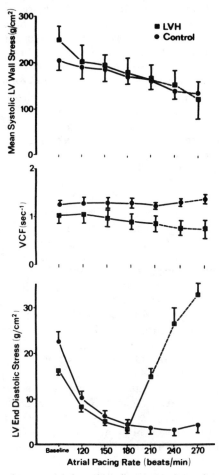

Fig 1–3.—Responses of average global systolic wall stress *(upper panel)* and end-diastolic wall stress *(lower panel)* and mean left ventricular *(LV)* velocity of circumferential fiber shortening *(VCF) (middle panel)*. In both control dogs and in dogs with LV hypertrophy, there is rate-related decrease in average global LV systolic wall stress. In dogs with LV hypertrophy, VCF decreases with increasing atrial pacing rates, whereas VCF remains relatively constant in control dogs. There is rate-related decrease in end-diastolic wall stress with atrial pacing rates of 120–180 beats/minute in both groups of animals. At atrial pacing rates ≥210 beats/minute, end-diastolic wall stress increases with increasing pacing rates in dogs with LV hypertrophy, but it remains low in control animals. (Courtesy of Fujii AM, Gelpi RJ, Mirsky I, et al: *Circ Res* 62:462–470, March 1988.)

In conscious dogs with severe compensated pressure overload LV hypertrophy, the ability to respond to chronotropic stress is compromised. Both systolic and diastolic LV dysfunction are observed in hypertrophied hearts at rapid atrial pacing rates. Relative subendocardial hypoperfusion was observed in response to pacing in dogs with LV hypertrophy.

▶ These investigators demonstrated both a decrease in ejection phase indexes of left ventricular systolic function and an increase in diastolic myocardial stiffness during rapid atrial pacing in dogs with pressure overload hypertrophy as compared with sham-operated littermates. As in studies by others, they also showed relative subendocardial hypoperfusion during atrial pacing in the dogs with hypertrophy. The exact cause-and-effect relationship between diastolic function and myocardial perfusion requires further study. Diminished myocardial perfusion reserve may be the reason for the eventual development of irreversible heart failure in animals and man when severe pressure overload left ventricular hypertrophy is not reversed.— R.A. O'Rourke, M.D.

Effect of Age on Myocardial Adaptation to Volume Overload in the Rat
Isoyama S, Grossman W, Wei JY (Charles A Dana Research Inst, Boston; Beth Israel Hosp, Boston; Harvard Univ)
J Clin Invest 81:1850–1857, June 1988   1–9

The same degree of stress is more likely to cause heart failure in older than in younger individuals. This may be related to the aging heart's lessened ability for a hypertrophic response. Investigators tested this hypothesis by creating arterial insufficiency in old and young rats and comparing the cardiac response with volume overload.

The rats were tested for aortic and left ventricle pressures and aortic flow before, immediately after, and 2 and 4 weeks after arterial insufficiency was induced. Body and heart weights were also recorded. The older rats had a higher death rate (57%) than the younger rats (37%). Rats with arterial insufficiency had a higher rate (56%) than control rats of similar age (35%). Although control rats in both age groups gained weight during the 4 weeks, old rats with arterial insufficiency lost weight.

In both age groups with arterial insufficiency, the left ventricular end-diastolic wall stress was greater than that recorded in controls. The older rats with arterial insufficiency had higher readings than young rats with arterial insufficiency. The young rats with arterial insufficiency adapted to this change, with their left ventricular end-diastolic pressure decreasing toward normal levels by 2 weeks. The decrease indicates that volume overload hypertrophy develops in response to such stress. The old rats did not experience this decrease in pressure and would be unlikely to do so, even after 4 weeks.

Thus, in rats, the aging cardiovascular system is less tolerant of volume overload than a younger cardiovascular system. This may be applied to human patients as well, and helps to explain why heart failure is much more common in old age.

▶ Such studies concerning the capacity for left ventricular hypertrophy in response to a volume overload in older as compared with younger animals are increasingly important, considering the aging of our patient population. A recent American College of Cardiology Bethesda Conference addressed the subject of "Cardiovascular Disease in the Elderly" (Wenger N, Marcus FI, O'Rourke RA: *J Am Coll Cardiol* 10:7A–87A, 1987). Aging itself results in cardiac hypertrophy as part of the physiologic adaptation, and volume overload appears to be less tolerated by the senescent heart.—R.A. O'Rourke, M.D.

Volume Overload Hypertrophy in a Closed-Chest Model of Mitral Regurgitation
Kleaveland JP, Kussmaul WG, Vinciguerra T, Diters R, Carabello BA (Univ of Pennsylvania, Temple Univ)
Am J Physiol 254:H1034–H1041, June 1988   1–10

Left ventricular volume overload, as in mitral regurgitation, eventually leads to ventricular dysfunction, but the mechanisms involved are uncertain. A canine model of volume overload hypertrophy produced by mitral regurgitation was used to make longitudinal observations. An arterially placed forceps was used to disrupt mitral chordae or the leaflets without performing a thoracotomy.

Weighed left ventricular mass correlated well with angiographically derived mass (Fig 1–4). In 11 dogs with severe regurgitation that lived for

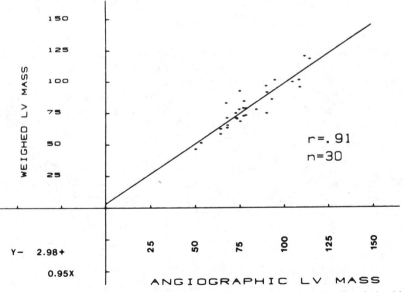

Fig 1–4.—Relationship between weighed left ventricular mass and angiographically calculated left ventricular mass for 16 dogs with mitral regurgitation and 14 control dogs. There is excellent correlation ($r = 0.91$) calculated with least-squares linear regression analysis. (Courtesy of Kleaveland JP, Kussmaul WG, Vinciguerra T, et al: *Am J Physiol* 254:H1034–H1041, June 1988.)

at least 3 months, end-diastolic volume increased from 48 to 85 ml, and left ventricular mass rose from 71 to 90 gm. Left ventricular end-diastolic pressure increased from 9 to 19 mm Hg, whereas cardiac output decreased from 2.3 to 1.8 L/minute. The mass-to-volume ratio decreased from 1.44 to 1.09 in animals with marked regurgitation. Relative wall thickness decreased significantly.

This closed-chest model of chronic mitral regurgitation should prove useful in studying the long-term effects of volume overload on the left ventricle, as well as ventricular mechanics in mitral regurgitation.

▶ When to recommend valve replacement or repair for patients with chronic severe mitral regurgitation remains controversial. Once preoperative measurements of left ventricular (LV) function are reduced, the clinical results of technically successful amelioration of mitral regurgitation are often suboptimal. Postoperative LV performance is frequently worse, particularly because the regurgitant flow into the low-resistance left atrium is no longer present. There has been great need for an animal model of chronic mitral regurgitation with progression to LV decompensation as described above. Studies in such models should provide important, clinically relevant information.—R.A. O'Rourke, M.D.

Collagen Remodeling of the Pressure-Overloaded, Hypertrophied Nonhuman Primate Myocardium

Weber KT, Janicki JS, Shroff SG, Pick R, Chen RM, Bashey RI (Univ of Chicago, Univ of Pennsylvania)
Circ Res 62:757–765, April 1988   1–11

Heart muscle is tethered within a fibrillar collagen matrix that maximizes force generation when the muscle contracts. Collagen is increased in the pressure-overloaded, hypertrophied human left ventricle, but the relation of collagen remodeling to cell necrosis and altered myocardial mechanisms is not understood. Systemic hypertension was produced in the long-tailed adult macaque by wrapping 1 kidney in cellophane. Hypertensive animals were killed after 4, 35, or 88 weeks.

Increased collagen was noted at 4 weeks, and the proportion of type III collagen was increased. At 35 weeks, collagen septas were thick and dense, but proportions of types I and III were similar to those in control animals. Necrosis was observed at 88 weeks. The systolic stress-strain relation of the myocardium was altered in relation to structural remodeling of collagen and scar formation, whereas diastolic myocardial stiffness was unchanged at all intervals. The slope of the systolic stress-strain relation was lowest in hearts with scarring.

Reactive fibrosis and collagen remodeling occur early in the course of left ventricular hypertrophy in this hypertensive model, in the absence of necrosis. Later reparative fibrosis is observed. It remains to be established whether the altered collagen composition of hypertrophied myocardium is responsible for altered mechanical behavior during systole or diastole.

▶ Abnormal left ventricular diastolic function frequently precedes impaired systolic function in patients and research animals with pressure overload, hypertrophied myocardium. In the adult heart, left ventricular hypertrophy is primarily the result of myocyte growth, but the concentration of collagen is also increased. Because collagen represents a relatively nonelastic element, it could be responsible for abnormalities in diastolic function that occur with left ventricular hypertrophy.

In this study of nonhuman primates with slow-onset, pressure-overload left ventricular hypertrophy, reactive fibrosis and collagen remodeling occurred early in left ventricular hypertrophy without necrosis (4 and 35 weeks), whereas reparative fibrosis was present at 88 weeks. Although the systolic stress-strain relationship was favorably or unfavorably altered in relation to collagen remodeling and scar formation, diastolic muscle stiffness was unchanged early and late. The latter result differs from that found in studies of other animal species with pressure-overload hypertrophy.

Because hypertension is present in a large number of patients, including a large percentage of those older than 65 years, and is a common predisposing factor for the development of pulmonary nervous hypertension and eventually left heart failure, further studies of the cause and effect relationship between collagen composition of hypertrophied ventricles and altered mechanical properties are indicated.—R.A. O'Rourke, M.D.

Other important recent articles on left ventricular hypertrophy are as follows:

1. Longabaugh JP, Vatner DE, Vatner SF, et al: Decreased stimulatory guanosine triphosphate binding protein in dogs with pressure-overload left ventricular failure. *J Clin Invest* 81:420–424, 1988.
2. Friberg P: Diastolic characteristics and cardiac energetics of isolated hearts exposed to volume and pressure overload. *Cardiovasc Res* 22:329–339, 1988.
3. Kromer EP, Riegger GAJ: Effects of long-term angiotensin converting enzyme inhibition on myocardial hypertrophy in experimental aortic stenosis in the rat. *Am J Cardiol* 1:161–163, 1988.
4. Kurabayashi M, Tsuchimochi H, Komuro I, et al: Molecular cloning and characterization of human cardiac and form myosin heavy chain complementary DNA clones. Regulation of expression during development and pressure overload in human atrium. *J Clin Invest* 82:524–531, 1988.
5. Iimoto DS, Covell JW, Harper E: Increase in cross-linking of type I and type III collagens associated with volume-overload hypertrophy. *Circ Res* 63:399–408, 1988.
6. Boheler KR, Dillmann WH: Cardiac response to pressure overload in the rat: The selective alteration of in vitro directed RNA translation products. *Circ Res* 63:448–456, 1988.
7. Delcayre C, Samuel J-L, Marotte SF, et al: Synthesis of stress proteins in rat cardiac myocytes 2–4 days after imposition of hemodynamic overload. *J Clin Invest* 82:460–468, 1988.

Ventricular Function

Effects of Asynchrony on Myocardial Relaxation at Rest and During Exercise in Conscious Dogs

Heyndrickx GR, Vantrimpont PJ, Rousseau MF, Pouleur H (State Univ of Ghent, Belgium; Univ of Louvain, Brussels)
Am J Physiol 254:H817–H822, May 1988   1–12

The effect of delayed or incomplete relaxation on diastolic cardiac function is accentuated when the duration of diastolie is reduced. The adaptation of left ventricular relaxation during marked exercise in the conscious dog was studied when the heart rate was increased and the diastolic filling time was reduced. The effect of ventricular asynchrony, induced by right ventricular pacing, on left ventricular relaxation was also studied.

Increasing the heart rate at rest by atrial pacing lowered left ventricular end-diastolic pressure and increased left circumflex coronary blood flow. Mean arterial pressure did not change significantly. The left ventricular maximum and minimum rates of pressure development increased, but the maximum rate decreased when heart rate was increased by ventricular pacing. During exercise with the heart rate kept constant by atrial pacing, both the maximum and minimum rates increased. Relaxation slowed during exercise with right ventricular pacing, as reflected by an increase in the relaxation constant.

In the presence of abnormal ventricular activation induced by right ventricular pacing, myocardial relaxation is slowed significantly. Asynchrony affects contraction and relaxation differently, depending on whether sympathetic stimulation is enhanced. In patients with hypertrophic cardiomyopathy, improved synchronicity of left ventricular contraction and relaxation during verapamil therapy has been associated with an increased left ventricular peak filling rate.

▶ The altered sequence of electrical activation significantly changed contraction as well as relaxation as a result primarily of the asynchrony rather than the changes in inotropy or loading condition. Importantly, during exercise in the presence of abnormal excitation relaxation was significantly prolonged. These findings may be relevant to the therapy of patients with left ventricular diastolic dysfunction. Improved synchronicity may improve left ventricular diastolic filling.—R.A. O'Rourke, M.D.

Determinants of the Relation Between Systolic Pressure and Duration of Isovolumic Relaxation in the Right Ventricle

Triffon D, Groves BM, Reeves JT, Ditchey RV (Univ of Colorado, Denver)
J Am Coll Cardiol 11:322–329, February 1988   1–13

Previous studies have indicated that right ventricular systolic pressure can be estimated from the interval between pulmonary valve closure and tricuspid valve opening. To examine the basis for this relationship, phonocardiograms and high fidelity right atrial and ventricular pressures were measured in 29 patients with right ventricular systolic pressures from 20 to 149 mm Hg.

In 22 patients with normal right arterial pressure, the time interval and the magnitude of pressure decrease were linearly related to systolic pressure. Early pulmonary valve closure contributed to the isovolumic pressure decrease at high systolic pressures. Correction for this factor did not eliminate the relationship between systolic pressure and the closure/opening interval. When patients with right coronary artery disease were excluded, the time constant for isovolumic pressure decrease also lengthened as a function of systolic pressure. The mean rate of pressure decrease was greater in patients with high pressure. The interval was predictive of systolic pressure in patients with right coronary artery disease, but was too short for patients with elevated mean right arterial pressure.

The amount of the isovolumic pressure decrease is the major determinant of the pulmonary valve closure—tricuspid valve opening interval. Pulmonary hypertension increases this interval by increasing the magnitude and time constant for the pressure decrease. Factors other than systolic pressure can affect this interval and are potential limitations on the use of this technique in predicting right ventricular systolic pressure.

▶ The noninvasive measurement of the right ventricular systolic pressure and pulmonary vascular resistance is an important objective, particularly considering patients who are candidates for isolated cardiac transplantation. A markedly elevated pulmonary vascular resistance is a contraindication to this therapeutic approach. In 1967, Burstin (*Br Heart J* 26:396–404) suggested that the pulmonary artery systolic pressure can be predicted from noninvasive estimates of the interval between pulmonary valve closure and tricuspid valve opening. More recently, Doppler echocardiographic methods to detect tricuspid valve opening have confirmed this relation.

The sophisticated clinical study described above confirms a linear relation between right ventricular systolic pressure and the duration of isovolumic relaxation. However, pulmonary hypertension and diseases or interventions that alter the rate of right ventricular relaxation, right atrial pressure, or pulmonary artery hang-out time may affect the duration of isovolumic relaxation independent of systolic pressure.—R.A. O'Rourke, M.D.

Doppler Echocardiography for Assessing Left Ventricular Diastolic Function
Spirito P, Maron BJ (Natl Insts of Health, Bethesda, Md)
Ann Intern Med 109:122–126, July 15, 1988   1–14

Recognition of left ventricular diastolic impairment has important clinical implications; however, assessing diastolic function is difficult. Doppler echocardiography could be used for diagnostic assessment of diastolic function and might have some advantages over other techniques.

The technique is noninvasive and relatively simple. The study of diastolic function by Doppler is based on measurement of the blood flow velocity through the mitral valve during left ventricular filling. The pulsed, or range gated, mode is usually used, but continuous wave Doppler is capable of measuring higher velocities.

The contour of the transmitral flow-velocity waveform is similar to that of the mitral valve echogram. When the mitral valve opens, the velocity of blood flow across the anulus peaks rapidly and then descends quickly to 0 baseline. The duration of diastasis is strongly correlated with cycle length.

Visually inspecting the Doppler waveform may be sufficient in some patients; however, it is not adequate for characterizing and comparing the pattern of diastolic flow-velocity in groups of patients. Therefore, most investigators use quantitative terms to describe the diastolic waveform. In an attempt to use Doppler to measure left ventricular filling volume, formulas have been derived which multiply the diastolic flow-velocity integral by the mitral valve cross-sectional areas. Results were correlated with the filling rate as measured by contrast angiography. However, these calculations make a number of theoretical assumptions.

These data suggest that Doppler echocardiography can be important in the assessment of left ventricular patterns in patients with cardiac disease. However, because ventricular filling is a complex phenomenon, the ultimate clinical value of the technique will depend on improved understanding of the determinants of Doppler diastolic waveform and the circumstances under which abnormal findings truly reflect intrinsic abnormalities of left ventricular diastolic function.

▶ Transmitral flow velocity is determined by the relative difference between left atrial and left ventricular (LV) pressure. Accordingly, Doppler transmitral flow-velocity waveform and indices of diastolic function are affected by many variables, including LV end-diastolic pressure, LV systolic load and function, age, heart rate, atrioventricular interval, and the respiratory cycle. Therefore, alterations in transmitral flow velocity may or may not reflect intrinsic abnormalities of diastolic LV function in specific patients.—R.A. O'Rourke, M.D.

Relation of Transmitral Flow Velocity Patterns to Left Ventricular Diastolic Function: New Insights From a Combined Hemodynamic and Doppler Echocardiographic Study
Appleton CP, Hatle LK, Popp RL (Stanford Univ)
J Am Coll Cardiol 12:426–440, August 1988   1–15

Left ventricular (LV) filling rate and the pattern of mitral flow velocity both are affected by factors other than the rate of LV relaxation. The mitral flow velocity patterns were correlated with hemodynamics in 70 patients having cardiac catheterization for reasons other than mitral stenosis. The goal was to determine what useful information on LV diastolic function can be inferred from noninvasive Doppler echocardiography. A

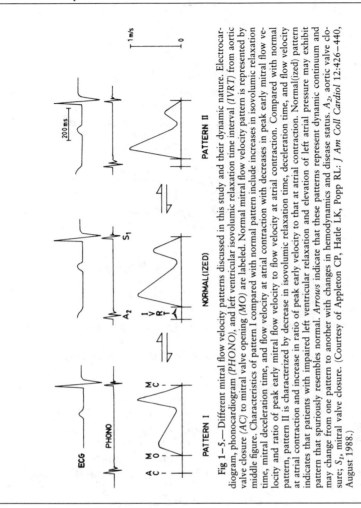

Fig 1–5.—Different mitral flow velocity patterns discussed in this study and their dynamic nature. Electrocardiogram, phonocardiogram (*PHONO*), and left ventricular isovolumic relaxation time interval (*IVRT*) from aortic valve closure (*AC*) to mitral valve opening (*MO*) are labeled. Normal mitral flow velocity pattern is represented by middle figure. Characteristics of pattern I compared with normal pattern include increases in isovolumic relaxation time, mitral deceleration time, and flow velocity at atrial contraction with decreases in peak early mitral flow velocity and ratio of peak early mitral flow velocity to flow velocity at atrial contraction. Compared with normal pattern, pattern II is characterized by decrease in isovolumic relaxation time, deceleration time, and flow velocity at atrial contraction and increase in ratio of peak early velocity to that at atrial contraction. Normal(ized) pattern indicates that patients with impaired left ventricular relaxation and elevation of left atrial pressure may exhibit pattern that spuriously resembles normal. *Arrows* indicate that these patterns represent dynamic continuum and may change from one pattern to another with changes in hemodynamics and disease status. A_2, aortic valve closure; S_1, mitral valve closure. (Courtesy of Appleton CP, Hatle LK, Popp RL: *J Am Coll Cardiol* 12:426–440, August 1988.)

majority of the patterns had coronary disease or idiopathic congestive cardiomyopathy; 14 had restrictive myocardial disease.

Most patients had 1 of 2 mitral flow velocity patterns (Fig 1–5). Patients with pattern I had a prolonged LV isovolumic relaxation time, a decreased peak early mitral flow velocity but normal or increased flow velocity at atrial contraction, a reduced ratio of peak early mitral flow velocity to later velocity, a prolonged mitral deceleration time, or a combination of these. Patients with pattern II tended to be more symptomatic and to have higher filling pressures. Their findings included a short LV isovolumic relaxation time, a normal or raised peak mitral flow velocity in early diastole, normal or reduced velocity at atrial contraction, an increased ratio of early to late mitral flow velocity, a short mitral deceleration time, or a combination of these. The flow velocity pattern was related more to myocardial function and hemodynamics than to type of disease. Increased left atrial pressure could "normalize" an abnormal mitral flow velocity pattern, or "mask" abnormal LV relaxation.

Mitral flow velocity recordings would seem to have some clinical value in assessing left ventricular diastolic function. Some patients may have reduced LV relaxation rates but accept volume without an abnormal rise in LV pressure later in diastole, after relaxation is complete. Others with abnormal LV relaxation have an abnormal increase in ventricular pressure with atrial contraction, possibly because of a coexisting decrease in myocardial or chamber compliance.

▶ Two abnormal mitral flow velocity patterns were defined. Pattern I was most frequent in patients with ischemic heart disease, a lower left atrial pressure, and impaired left ventricular relaxation, whereas pattern II appeared to indicate increased LV filling pressures, increased LV rapidly filling wave, and a "restrictive" LV filling pattern. However, the specificity and sensitivity reflect certain limitations. As indicated by the preceding abstract, the ultimate clinical role of Doppler echocardiography as a noninvasive test for determining diastolic function has not yet been defined.—R.A. O'Rourke, M.D.

Effect of Afterload Resistance on End-Systolic Pressure-Thickness Relationship

Aversano T, Maughan WL, Sunagawa K, Becker LC (Johns Hopkins School of Medicine; Kyushu Univ, Fukuoka, Japan)
Am J Physiol 254:H658–H663, April 1988   1–16

The end-systolic pressure-thickness relationship (ESPTR) and the end-systolic pressure-length relationship vary predictably with changes in global and regional inotropic state and with ischemia. The ESPTR is measured during a brief occlusion of the inferior vena cava without baroreceptor-mediated reflex changes in regional contractile state. The effect of afterload resistance on the ESPTR was studied in isolated canine left ventricles made to eject into a simulated arterial system.

An increase in simulated peripheral resistance led to a modest shift of the ESPTR up and to the right, indicating augmented contractile performance. Increased wall thickening impaired end-systolic performance, whereas decreased wall thickening enhanced performance.

Changes in resistance in the isolated canine heart result in modest but significant shifts of the ESPTR. The dependence of end-systolic performance on wall thickening is consistent with shortening deactivation, and this explains at least in part the observed shift in the ESPTR with altered afterload resistance.

▶ Prior studies in isolated hearts and in intact animals have shown that the end-systolic pressure-volume relationship may be affected by afterload resistance. The results of the above study indicate a modest but detectable influence of afterload resistance on the end-systolic pressure-thickness relationship (ESPTR) in the isolated heart. Therefore, if wall thickening changes during the perturbation in loading conditions necessary to measure ESPTR, then the

ESPTR will have been measured while the contractile performance was actually changing. This is a potential limitation to this technique for assessing regional function.— R.A. O'Rourke, M.D.

Cocaine and Cardiovascular Function in Dogs: Effects on Heart and Peripheral Circulation
Bedotto JB, Lee RW, Lancaster LD, Olajos M, Goldman S (Univ of Arizona; VA Med Ctr, Tucson, Ariz)
J Am Coll Cardiol 11:1337–1342, June 1988   1–17

There are an alarming number of reports of cardiovascular collapse related to cocaine abuse, and cocaine is reported to cause hypertension, myocardial infarction, myocarditis, and stroke. The physiologic effects of intravenous cocaine administration were studied in mongrel dogs. Continuous ECG monitoring was used to study the potential role of ventricular arrhythmias in cocaine-associated deaths. Cocaine was infused at a rate of 0.5 mg/kg per minute.

Cocaine caused vasoconstriction with elevations in left ventricular (LV) systolic pressure and systemic vascular resistance. The cardiac output, ejection fraction, and stroke volume declined, and the LV end-diastolic pressure increased. Arterial compliance decreased by about one third after cocaine. Mean circulatory filling pressure increased 28%. Resistance to venous return increased 42%. Coronary artery diameters did not change significantly after cocaine infusion. All dogs had sinus tachycardia and supraventricular tachycardia, but ventricular premature beats developed in only 2 of 6 dogs.

It is difficult to correlate these findings with clinical reports of cocaine-associated deaths. Ventricular irritability remains a potential mechanism of cardiovascular collapse in this setting. High serum levels of cocaine were achieved in this study, but the recent use of very pure forms of the drug is associated with a rapidly increasing plasma concentration.

▶ Cocaine abuse has been implicated as a predisposing factor for an increasing number of cardiac deaths. It has been reported to cause hypertension, aortic rupture, myocarditis, myocardial infarction, pulmonary edema, ventricular arrhythmias, and sudden death. In the above study, intravenous cocaine produced systemic arterial and venous vasoconstriction in anesthetized dogs. The increase in left ventricular afterload was associated with a reduced cardiac index, stroke volume, ejection fraction, and rate of isovolumic relaxation. There was no evidence of coronary vasoconstriction or ventricular tachyarrhythmias. However, direct measurements of coronary blood flow, coronary arterial resistance, and myocardial oxygen demands were not made.— R.A. O'Rourke, M.D.

Cardiovascular Effects of Cocaine in Conscious Dogs: Importance of Fully Functional Autonomic and Central Nervous Systems
Wilkerson RD (Med College of Ohio, Toledo)
J Pharmacol Exp Ther 246:466–471, August 1988   1–18

Cocaine has been related to myocardial ischemia/infarction in patients with preexisting coronary disease. In addition, cocaine may lead to coronary vasospasm and cardiac ischemia in patients with anatomically normal coronary arteries. The cardiovascular effects of intravenous cocaine in conscious dogs were studied using doses ranging from 0.06 mg/kg to 8 mg/kg. Tolerance was avoided by administering each dose on a separate day.

All doses of cocaine significantly increased systolic and diastolic blood pressure. Heart rate responses were considerably more variable. Arrhythmia occurred only with the highest dose of cocaine. The rate-pressure product more than doubled after 2 mg/kg of cocaine and increased nearly four-fold after 8 mg/kg. The blood pressure response was attenuated by pretreatment with hexamethonium and by anesthesia with pentobarbital.

The cardiovascular effects of cocaine involve a significant CNS component. The full effects are expressed only when the integrated CNS and peripheral actions of cocaine are unmodified by anesthesia or autonomic antagonists.

▶ The authors determined the dose response curve for the cardiovascular effects of cocaine in conscious, trained dogs. Intravenous cocaine-induced increments in mean arterial blood pressure, heart rate, and heart rate–systolic blood pressure product (an indirect determinant of myocardial oxygen demand) were dose-dependent at doses of 0.25 mg/kg and greater. The attenuation of the pressor response by pretreatment with hexamethonium or pentobarbital anesthesia indicates an important central nervous system component to cocaine's cardiovascular effects.—R.A. O'Rourke, M.D.

Additional important recent references concerning left ventricular systolic and diastolic performance include the following:

1. Negroni JA, Lascano EC, Pichel RH: A computer study of the relation between chamber mechanical properties and mean pressure-mean flow of the left ventricle. *Circ Res* 62:1121–1133, 1988.
2. Damiano RJ Jr, Asano T, Smith PK, et al: Hemodynamic consequences of right ventricular isolation: The contribution of the right ventricular free wall to cardiac performance. *Ann Thorac Surg* 46:324–330, 1988.
3. Raizada V, Sahn DJ, Covell JW: Factors influencing late night ventricular ejection. *Cardiovasc Res* 22:244–248, 1988.
4. Miller WP, Flygenring BP, Nellis SH: Effects of load alteration and coronary perfusion pressure on regional end-systolic relations. *Circulation* 78:1299–1309, 1988.
5. Santamore WP, Papa L: Alterations in diastolic ventricular interdependence due to myocardial infarction. *Cardiovasc Res* 22:726–731, 1988.
6. Courtois MA, Kovacs SJ Jr, Ludbrook PA: Transmitral pressure-flow velocity relation. Importance of regional pressure gradients in the left ventricle during diastole. *Circulation* 78:661–671, 1988.
7. Friberg P: Diastolic characteristics and cardiac energetics of isolated hearts exposed to volume and pressure overload. *Cardiovasc Res* 22:329–339, 1988.

8. Perlini S, Soffiantino F, Farilla C, et al: Load dependence of isovolumic relaxation in intact heart: Facts or artifacts. *Cardiovasc Res* 22:47–54, 1988.

Electrophysiology

Incidence of Reentry with an Excitable Gap in Ventricular Tachycardia: A Prospective Evaluation Utilizing Transient Entrainment
Kay GN, Epstein AE, Plumb VJ (Univ of Alabama in Birmingham)
J Am Coll Cardiol 11:530–538, March 1988   1–19

Transient entrainment of a tachycardia by rapid pacing is taken as evidence of reentry where an excitable gap exists between the advancing wave of depolarization and the receding trail of refractoriness. Transient entrainment has been demonstrated for several tachyarrhythmias, including ventricular tachycardia (VT). Invasive electrophysiologic testing was performed in 27 patients with sustained VT, including 25 with coronary disease and 2 with primary dilated cardiomyopathy.

Eight patients collapsed or had spontaneous termination of VT before rapid pacing was possible. In the 19 other patients, rapid pacing ended 21 of 25 episodes of VT. The mean effective rate was 139% of the spontaneous rate. Four episodes required direct current cardioversion after pacing accelerated the tachycardia. Transient entrainment was demonstrated in 15 of these 19 patients and in 76% of the 25 episodes of VT. The site of rapid pacing was important for demonstrating transient entrainment. The location of the recording electrodes also was important.

Sustained VT induced by programmed electrical stimulation can be transiently entrained by rapid pacing in most patients. This suggests that reentry incorporating an excitable gap is the most likely mechanism. The pacing site most likely to demonstrate transient entrainment is the right ventricular apex or outflow tract in VTs with a right bundle branch block configuration, and the left or right ventricular outflow tract in those with a left bundle branch block configuration. The best recording site is close to the area of earliest endocardial activation.

▶ From previous studies of atrial flutter and atrioventricular reentrant tachycardia, 3 criteria were developed to identify the presence of transient entrainment. In this prospective study of consecutive patients, transient entrainment was identified in 79% of 19 patients with sustained ventricular tachycardia (VT) induced by programmed electrical stimulation, suggesting that inducible VT is usually based on reentry incorporating an excitable gap.—R.A. O'Rourke, M.D.

Contraction-Excitation Feedback in the Atria: A Cause of Changes in Refractoriness
Kaseda S, Zipes DP (Indiana Univ)
J Am Coll Cardiol 11:1327–1336, June 1988   1–20

There appears to be feedback relating hemodynamic changes and electrical properties, but its nature is uncertain. The effects of altered atrial pressure on atrial excitability were studied in an in situ canine heart preparation. Atrial pressure was varied by changing the time delay from the atrial pacing stimulus to ventricular stimulus during atrioventricular (AV) segmental pacing at a constant pacing cycle length in dogs with complete AV block. The AV interval ranged from 0 to 280 msec in 20-msec steps.

Mean left atrial pressure was lowest at an AV interval of 47 msec when the refractory period was 135.5 msec. It was highest at an AV interval of 147 msec when the refractory period was 137.9 msec. Left atrial diameter increased at the higher AV interval, and mean aortic pressure declined. Similar relationships existed between right atrial pressure and refractory period, and between left atrial pressure and the refractory period of the interatrial septum.

Increased atrial pressure lengthens the refractory period of both atrial and the interatrial septum. A contraction-excitation feedback mechanism occurs during the AV relation simulating AV reentrant tachycardia. If the pressure increase differs in the 2 atria and the degree of stretch differs, a dispersion of refractoriness may result, disposing to arrhythmias.

▶ In patients with myocardial infarction or congestive heart failure, the initiation of atrial arrhythmias has been attributed to the increased left ventricular filling pressure and probable atrial stretch. While it is likely that several variables interact in a complex manner to cause atrial fibrillation, a contraction-excitation feedback loop in the atrium may be an important factor in the origination of atrial fibrillation during AV entry. This concept is supported by the above study.— R.A. O'Rourke, M.D.

Electrical Alternans and Cardiac Electrical Instability
Smith JM, Clancy EA, Valeri CR, Ruskin JN, Cohen RJ (Harvard-MIT Division of Health Sciences and Technology, Cambridge, Mass; Boston Univ School of Medicine; Massachusetts General Hosp, Brigham and Women's Hosp, Boston)
Circulation 77:110–121, January 1988   1–21

Electrical alternans has been related to many cardiac disorders as well as to electrolyte imbalances, exercise testing, and intoxications. The relationship between electrical alternans and cardiac electrical stability was studied in both dogs and human beings. Electrical alternans was detected in the QRS complex and the ST-T wave using a new multidimensional spectral technique. Electrical stability was tested by ventricular fibrillation threshold estimates in the dog and by programmed stimulation in human beings.

In dogs, systemic hypothermia decreased the ventricular fibrillation threshold 60% and significantly increased the magnitude of alternation, as expressed by the alternating ECG morphology index in parts per million of waveform energy. Transient coronary artery ligation had similar effects of the fibrillation threshold and alternating ECG morphology index of both the QRS and the ST-T wave.

In a pilot study of 19 patients, alternation in waveform morphology identified inducible patients with a sensitivity of 92%. Electrophysiologic testing was used as an independent measure of cardiac electrical stability. The study was 50% specific and had a positive predictive value of 70%. Only 1 of 13 patients with inducible tachycardia/fibrillation failed to be identified.

This relationship between electrical alternans and cardiac electrical stability is consistent with predictions from finite-element models of cardiac contraction and with predictions based on nonlinear dynamics. New forms of chaos theory may be required to describe the stability of cardiac electrical activation and the transition from stable sinus rhythm to ventricular fibrillation.

▶ Electrical alternation in morphology of the ECG complex has been associated with multiple conditions (e.g., hypothermia) besides pericardial effusion. Clinical observations suggest an increased incidence of electrical alternans and spontaneous ventricular fibrillation in patients with prolonged QT intervals and in patients with variant angina.

In the animal studies described above, a multidimensional spectral technique showed a significant increase in QRS and ST wave alternation when the ventricular fibrillation threshold was reduced by systemic hypothermia or transient coronary artery ligation. In a parallel clinical study of 19 patients an alternation in waveform morphology identified patients with electrophysiologic inducible ventricular tachycardia with a sensitivity of 92% and specificity at 50%. Although additional larger clinical studies are necessary before reaching firm conclusions, sophisticated analysis for electrical alternans of the QRS complex and ST-T wave may provide an important noninvasive method for assessing the likelihood of cardiac electrical stability.

Alternations of the action potential duration in ventricular muscle fibers is thought to result in the alternans of the T wave. An interesting in vitro study on alternans of action potential duration in dog Purkinje's and ventricular muscle fibers was recently published (Saitoh H et al: *Circ Res* 62:1027–1040, 1988).

A recent article on analysis of signal-averaging ECG for identifying patients with the substrate for ventricular tachycardia which compares 2 methods of analysis is: Machac J, Weiss A, Winters SL, et al: A comparative study of frequency domain and time domain analysis of signal-averaged electrocardiograms in patients with ventricular tachycardia.*J Am Coll Cardiol* 11:284–296, 1988.—R.A. O'Rourke, M.D.

The Effect of Potassium Ion Depletion on Postinfection Canine Cardiac Arrhythmias
Garan H, McGovern BA, Canzanello VJ, McCauley J, Bodvarsson M, Harrington JT, Madias NE, Newell JB, Ruskin JN (Harvard Med School)
Circulation 77:696–704, March 1988   1–22

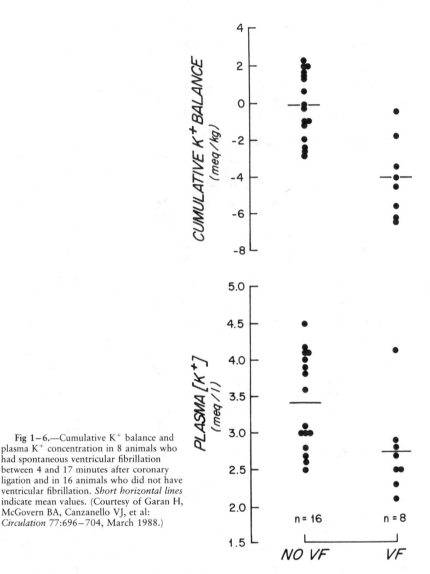

Fig 1–6.—Cumulative K⁺ balance and plasma K⁺ concentration in 8 animals who had spontaneous ventricular fibrillation between 4 and 17 minutes after coronary ligation and in 16 animals who did not have ventricular fibrillation. *Short horizontal lines* indicate mean values. (Courtesy of Garan H, McGovern BA, Canzanello VJ, et al: *Circulation* 77:696–704, March 1988.)

Hypokalemia is associated with a greater risk of ventricular arrhythmias during acute myocardial infarction, but it might be only a secondary marker of other arrhythmogenic factors. Varying degrees of potassium ion depletion was studied in a canine model of myocardial infarction produced by ligating the proximal left anterior descending coronary artery. Study animals were given a very low potassium diet for 15 days, and some of them received 4 doses of 50-mg hydrochlorothiazide in addition.

About one third of animals had spontaneous ventricular fibrillation during acute infarction. Cumulative potassium ion balance was −4.0 mEq/kg in animals with ventricular fibrillation and −0.1 mEq/kg in the others (Fig 1–6). There also was a significant difference in plasma K^+ concentrations at the time of coronary ligation and 1 hour afterward. The only independent predictors of spontaneous fibrillation were cumulative K^+ balance and the size of the infarct.

The degree of potassium ion deficit was an independent predictor of spontaneous ventricular fibrillation in acute myocardial infarction in dogs. The degree of deficit also correlated with fibrillation induced by programmed cardiac stimulation. The ionic and electrophysiologic mechanisms underlying this relationship remain to be determined.

▶ This important study examined the arrhythmogenic effects of graded K^+ deficit over an extended period of dietary K^+ deprivation in animals subsequently undergoing acute coronary artery ligation. Interestingly, the significant association between K^+ deficit and spontaneous ventricular fibrillation was independent of infarct size in this study. This study confirms the hypothesis that prior K^+ depletion is an independent factor that enhances ventricular arrhythmogenesis during spontaneous myocardial infarction.

Although not directly transferable to the clinical situation, this study suggests that factors which predispose to K^+ deficiency (e.g., diuretics, alkalosis) should be avoided in patients with severe myocardial ischemia such as occurs with acute coronary syndrome.— R.A. O'Rourke, M.D.

Below are listed some additional publications of interest on electrophysiology:

1. Franz MR, Swerdlow CD, Liem LB, et al: Cycle length dependence of human action potential duration in vivo. Effects of single extrastimuli, sudden sustained rate acceleration and deceleration, and different steady-state frequencies. *J Clin Invest* 82:972–979, 1988.
2. Nishimura M, Habuchi Y, Hiromasa S, et al: Ionic basis of depressed automaticity and conduction by acetylcholine in rabbit AV node. *Am J Physiol* 255:H7–H14, 1988.
3. Veenstra RD, DeHaan RL: Cardiac gap junction channel activity in embryonic chick ventricle cells. *Am J Physiol* 254:H170–H180, 1988.
4. Denniss AR, Richards DA, Waywood JA, et al: Electrophysiological and anatomic differences between canine hearts with inducible ventricular tachycardia and fibrillation associated with chronic myocardial infarction. *Circ Res* 64:155–166, 1989.

Coronary Artery Vasomotor Tone

Selective Attenuation of Endothelium-Mediated Vasodilation in Atherosclerotic Human Coronary Arteries
Förstermann U, Mügge A, Alheid U, Haverich A, Frölich JC (Hannover Med School, Hannover, West Germany)
Circ Res 62:185–190, February 1988   1–23

Previous clinical and arteriographic studies have shown that atherosclerotic human coronary arteries may be predisposed to spontaneous vasospasm. It has also been shown that a potent vasodilator substance, called endothelium-derived relaxing factor, mediates vascular relaxations induced by vasodilators such as acetylcholine, substance P, bradykinin, and the calcium ion ionophore, A23187.

The purpose of this in vitro study was to compare the effect of these 4 endothelium-dependent vasodilators on intact and atherosclerotic human coronary arteries. The effects of the vasodilators isoprenaline and glyceryl trinitrate whose activity is not mediated by the endothelium were also studied.

Epicardial coronary arteries were obtained from 17 hearts of cardiac transplantation patients, including 6 patients aged 14−25 years with end-stage congestive cardiomyopathy, and 11 patients aged 42−55 years with coronary heart disease.

Atherosclerotic lesions lead to a selective attenuation of endothelium-dependent vasodilation in human coronary arteries. This defect was observed for all 4 endothelium-dependent vasodilators tested. In contrast, relaxations by isoprenaline were unchanged, and relaxations by glyceryl nitrate were attenuated only at its lowest concentration.

The attenuation of relaxations mediated by endothelium-derived relaxing factor observed in this study may be one of the reasons why patients with atherosclerosis experience an increased incidence of coronary vasospasm. Thus, impairment of this potent vasodilator mechanism may well promote coronary vasospasm and ultimately cause myocardial ischemia.

▶ The above study shows that atherosclerotic lesions result in a selective attenuation of *endothelium-dependent* but not endothelium-independent vasodilation in human coronary arteries. Whether this is due to decreased ability of the endothelium to produce endothelium-derived relaxing factor (EDRF), impaired diffusion of EDRF, a blunted response of vascular smooth muscle, or some combination of these remains to be defined.— R.A. O'Rourke, M.D.

Free Radicals Inhibit Endothelium-Dependent Dilation in the Coronary Resistance Bed
Stewart DJ, Pohl U, Bassenge E (Univ of Freiburg, West Germany; McGill Univ)
Am J Physiol 255:H765−H769, 1988   1−24

Oxygen free radicals appear to contribute to myocardial reperfusion injury. Such injury is associated with depressed endothelium-dependent dilation of large coronary arterial rings in canine studies. The effects of reactive oxygen products on coronary resistance vessels in the isolated rabbit heart were studied. Reactive products were generated by electrolysis of the saline perfusate.

Contractile function declined with electrolysis. Responses to the endothelium-independent vasodilators adenosine and papaverine were increased 1.5- to 2-fold, but responses to the endothelium-dependent agents acetylcholine and serotonin were markedly depressed. Catalase, superoxide dismutase, and desferrioxamine, which inhibits hydroxyl radical production, all conferred protection against increased perfusion pressure and inhibition of endothelium-dependent dilation.

Inhibition of endothelium-dependent dilation results from exposure of coronary resistance vessels to reactive oxygen products. This, combined with an increase in vessel tone, could limit the recovery of myocardial perfusion after ischemia. Further research in this area might lead to interventions that optimize myocardial salvage during the postischemic period.

▶ The importance of oxygen free radicals in reperfusion injury in vivo has been demonstrated in several studies using various selective scavengers of free radicals. Prior studies have also shown that endothelium-derived relaxing factor is rapidly inactivated in the presence of oxygen free radicals. This study suggests that the oxygen free radical-reduced increase in coronary resistance vessel tone may limit the recovery of myocardial perfusion after ischemia.—R.A. O'Rourke, M.D.

---

fMLP Provokes Coronary Vasoconstriction and Myocardial Ischemia in Rabbits

Gillespie MN, Booth DC, Friedman BJ, Cunningham MR, Jay M, DeMaria AN (Univ of Kentucky)

Am J Physiol 254:H481–H486, March 1988   1–25

Coronary arteries from patients with suspected coronary spasm exhibit increased intramural inflammatory cells, which presumably release vasoactive chemical mediators. Coronary angiography was performed in anesthetized rabbits to determine the coronary vasoactivity of N-formyl-L-methionyl-L-leucyl-L-phenylalanine (fMLP), a nonselective inflammatory cell stimulant.

Intracoronary injection of fMLP evoked marked coronary narrowing, accompanied by ST segment deviation and dysrhythmias. Scintigraphy showed hypoperfusion of the left ventricular free wall and septum supplied by the spastic vessel. Vasoconstriction, the ischemic ECG changes, and the perfusion defect were reversed by intravenously given nitroglycerin. Studies in isolated rabbit hearts perfused with salt solution showed that fMLP failed to exert a direct coronary vasoconstrictor effect.

A nonselective inflammatory cell stimulant produces coronary spasm with myocardial hypoperfusion and ischemic ECG changes in the anesthetized rabbit. The effect is not attributable to a direct action of fMLP on arterial smooth muscle. This model may prove useful for studying the role of inflammatory cells in the development of coronary spasm and myocardial ischemia.

▶ In this study fMLP, a nonselective inflammatory cell stimulant, induced profound epicardial coronary vasoconstriction and myocardial ischemia after intracoronary injection. The coronary artery spasm and evidence of myocardial ischemia was reversed by intravenous nitroglycerin. This interesting rabbit model of coronary spasm may permit better pharmacologic studies of drugs developed for preventing recurrent episodes of myocardial ischemia resulting from coronary vasoconstriction.—R.A. O'Rourke, M.D.

Effects of Glyceryl Trinitrate on Functionally Regressed Newly Developed Collateral Vessels in Conscious Dogs
Fujita M, McKown DP, McKown MD, Franklin D (Univ of Missouri–Columbia)
Cardiovasc Res 22:639–647, September 1988   1–26

The effects of glyceryl trinitrate on the relationship between collateral blood flow and myocardial oxygen demand in the collateral-dependent zone during transient coronary occlusion were studied. Collateral growth was promoted by repeated brief occlusions of the left circumflex coronary artery. Glyceryl trinitrate was given just before a 2-minute occlusion in 10 conscious dogs with well-developed collaterals. A dose of 5 μg/kg was given intravenously 1 minute before coronary occlusion.

Collateral blood flow velocity increased after pretreatment with glyceryl trinitrate. Systolic subendocardial segment shortening in the collateral-dependent zone increased from 7.8% to 12.6% after 2 minutes of occlusion. The blood flow debt repayment after release of occlusion decreased from 122% to 68%.

In conscious dogs with regressed new collateral vessels, glyceryl trinitrate acts predominantly through dilating collateral vessels. Lessening of myocardial functional depression during coronary occlusion can be ascribed to a drug-induced increase in collateral blood flow.

► The authors studied the effects of glyceryl trinitrate (TNG) in dogs with newly developed collateral vessels 5 to 7 days after cessation of coronary artery occlusion. In these animals with preexisting but regressed coronary collateral function, pretreatment with TNG increased collateral flow and improved segmental myocardial dysfunction during occlusion, after the systemic effects of TNG pretreatment had disappeared. This provides important information concerning the favorable anti-ischemic effects of TNG that likely are due in part to improved collateral coronary blood flow.—R.A. O'Rourke, M.D.

Seven recent publications related to this important subject are listed as follows:

1. Inoue T, Tomoike H, Hisano K, et al: Endothelium determines flow-dependent dilation of the epicardial coronary artery in dog. *J Am Coll Cardiol* 11:187–191, 1988.
2. Nichols WW, Mehta JL, Thompson L, et al: Synergistic effects of LTC$_4$ and TxA$_2$ on coronary flow and myocardial function. *Am J Physiol* 255:H153–H159, 1988.
3. Roth DM, White FC, Bloor CM: Altered minimal coronary resistance to antegrade reflow after chronic coronary artery occlusion in swine. *Circ Res* 63:330–339, 1988.
4. Schwartz JS, Bache RJ: Combined effects of calcium antagonists and ni-

troglycerin on large coronary artery diameter. *Am Heart J* 115:964, 1988.

5. Munzel T, Holtz J, Mulsch A, et al: Nitrate tolerance in epicardial arteries or in the venous system is not reversed by N-acetylcysteine in vivo, but tolerance-independent interactions exist. *Circulation* 79:188–197, 1989.

6. Bennett BM, Schroder H, Hayward LD, et al: Effect of in vitro organic nitrate tolerance on relaxation, cyclic GMP accumulation, and guanylate cyclase activation by glyceryl trinitrate and the enantiomers of isoidide dinitrate. *Circ Res* 63:693–701, 1988.

7. Canty JM Jr: Coronary pressure-function and steady-state pressure-flow relations during autoregulation in the unanesthetized dog. *Circ Res* 63:821–836, 1988.

Experimental Myocardial Ischemia/Infarction

Cardioprotective Actions of Thromboxane Receptor Antagonism in Ischemic Atherosclerotic Rabbits

Osborne JA, Lefer AM (Jefferson Med College, Philadelphia)
Am J Physiol 255:H318–H324, 1988   1–27

Because thromboxane A_2 (TxA_2) is implicated in myocardial ischemia and ischemic heart disease, a specific thromboxane receptor antagonist, BM 13505, was evaluated in rabbits with induced atherosclerosis. Disease was produced in the rabbits by feeding them a 0.5% cholesterol-enriched chow for 10 to 12 weeks. Myocardial ischemia was produced at this time by ligating the left anterior descending coronary artery.

Myocardial creatine kinase activity was maintained in ischemic myocardium in BM 13505-treated animals. Loss of free amino nitrogen-containing compounds from the myocardium was reduced, and the plasma increase in creatine kinase was blunted in treated animals. The effects could not be ascribed to differences in myocardial oxygen demand among the experimental and control groups. In addition, BM 13505 reduced the deposition of cholesterol in the aortic wall and retarded plaque formation in coronary vessels. Plasma cholesterol was not lowered by the TxA_2 antagonist.

A thromboxane receptor antagonist appears to prevent plaque formation and resultant coronary stenosis in this model by inhibiting platelet activation leading to cholesterol-rich deposits. In addition, it may reduce cell injury during acute infarction by inhibiting platelet aggregation and vasoconstriction from the release of TxA_2.

▶ The thromboxane breakdown product TxB_2 increases significantly during acute myocardial infarction, indicating that activation of platelets readily occurs in coronary artery disease. Coronary vasospasm and platelet aggregation likely contribute to myocardial infarction or propagate myocardial ischemic damage once ischemia is initiated. In the above study, a thromboxane receptor antagonist given chronically appeared to prevent initial plaque formation and resulting coronary artery stenosis in hypercholesterolemic rabbits. Also, prior treatment with the thromboxane antagonist decreased the extent of myocardial damage following acute coronary ligation in a rabbit infarct model. Appropriate patient studies of thromboxane receptor antagonism efficacy appear indicated.— R.A. O'Rourke, M.D.

Intracoronary α_2-Adrenergic Receptor Blockade Attenuates Ischemia in Conscious Dogs During Exercise
Seitelberger R, Guth BD, Heusch G, Lee J-D, Katayama K, Ross J Jr (Univ of California, San Diego, La Jolla)
Circ Res 62:436–442, March 1988   1–28

There is evidence that, in the presence of coronary stenosis, sympathetic coronary vasoconstriction can aggravate myocardial ischemia. Because direct nerve stimulation may not be analogous to physiologic autonomic activation, the authors determined whether α_2-adrenergic receptor-induced coronary vasoconstriction can limit myocardial flow and contractility in a regionally ischemic zone during treadmill exercise. Systolic wall thickening was estimated regionally by sonomicrometry in the anterior and posterior left ventricular walls of the conscious dog. The circumflex coronary artery was constricted with a hydraulic cuff.

In the presence of acute coronary artery stenosis, posterior wall thickening increased when idazoxan, a selective α_2-blocker, was infused into the coronary artery. Blood flow to the endocardium and midmyocardium

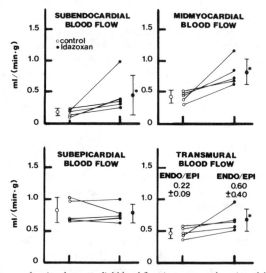

Fig 1–7.—Summary of regional myocardial blood flow in transmural sections following acute stenosis of left circumflex coronary artery during exercise (O, left-hand data set) and after administration of idazoxan (●, right-hand data set). Mean values with standard deviations are shown adjacent to individual data points. Transmural blood flow is average of 3 transmural sections in presented with transmural blood flow (endo/epi). *$P < .05$, n = 5. (Courtesy of Seitelberger R, Guth BD, Heusch G, et al: *Circ Res* 62:436–442, March 1988.)

of the posterior wall improved markedly (Fig 1–7). In control animals regional wall thickening in systole continued to deteriorate.

In exercising dogs under β-adrenergic blockade, significant postjunctional α_2-adrenergic receptor-mediated coronary vasoconstriction was observed, even during marked ischemia. Regional α_2-adrenergic receptor blockade in this setting can reduce regional ischemia and improve contractile function by reducing exercise-induced sympathetic vasoconstriction.

▶ In contradiction to the widely accepted concept that maximal coronary vasodilation occurs during ischemia, recent studies suggest that sympathetic coronary vasoconstriction can overcome local metabolic vasodilation and worsen myocardial ischemia; this effect is mediated by α_2-adrenergic receptors. The results of the above study demonstrate neurally or humorally mediated sympathetic vasoconstriction or both in acutely ischemic myocardium during exercise in the awake animal with acute coronary stenosis. Relevant clinical studies have suggested an important role of α-adrenergic-mediated coronary vasoconstriction in patients with exercise-induced angina pectoris (Berkenboom GM et al: *Am J Cardiol* 57:195, 1986).—R.A. O'Rourke, M.D.

Fatty Acid Analogue Accumulation: A Marker of Myocyte Viability in Ischemic-Reperfused Myocardium
Miller DD, Gill JB, Livni E, Elmaleh DR, Aretz T, Boucher CA, Strauss HW (Massachusetts Gen Hosp, Boston)
Circ Res 63:681–692, October 1988   1–29

A sensitive, noninvasive marker of myocardial viability would help in the evaluation of interventional measures against evolving myocardial infarction. 15-(Para-iodophenyl)-3-methyl pentadecanoic acid, a 3-methyl-substituted radioiodinated long chain fatty acid analogue, was assessed for noninvasively detecting altered fatty acid uptake in reperfused, post-ischemic myocardium. Dogs received the analogue intravenously at 3 hours of reperfusion after 15 minutes or 1 hour of left anterior descending coronary artery occlusion. Myocardial blood flow was measured using labeled microspheres, and regional left ventricular function was examined using subendocardial ultrasonic crystals.

Myocardial segments that stained with triphenyltetrazolium chloride (TTC) had greater fatty acid analogue activity than TTC-negative segments. The ratio of analogue activity to reperfusion blood flow was 27% greater in TTC-positive segments. Electron microscopy confirmed the presence of reversible changes in TTC-positive regions. Excessive ^{123}I-analogue activity over flow when compared with perfusion (as measured with ^{201}Tl) also was observed in an occlusion model adapted for in vivo single photon emission computed tomography (Fig 1–8).

Accumulation of this analogue can be used noninvasively to identify zones of discordance between fatty acid and flow distribution, characteristic of ischemically "stunned" but viable tissue. Single photon emission

Short-Axis   Long Axis

Border Zone   Mid LV

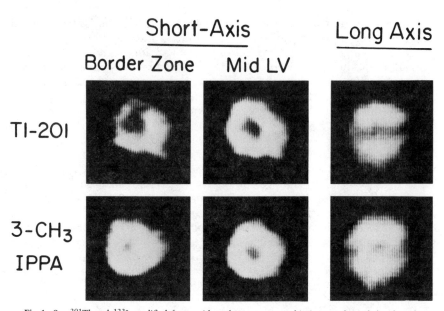

TI-201

3-CH₃
IPPA

Fig 1–8.—^{201}Tl and ^{123}I modified fatty acid analogue tomographic images through border of anteroapical perfusion defect (**left**) and midventricle (**right**). Oblique (short axis) coronal reconstructions have been made from raw data set using identical coordinates. Animals were secured to prevent motion artifacts. Note that there is no change in diameter of left ventricle on ^{201}Tl and ^{123}I images. Clear excess of fatty acid activity is apparent in border zone, whereas ^{201}Tl and fatty acid activity are well matched in midventricle. On long axis reconstructions, neither ^{201}Tl nor ^{123}I fatty acid analogue activity was seen at center of apical infarction. (Courtesy of Miller DD, Gill JB, Livni E, et al: *Circ Res* 63:681–692, October 1988.)

computed tomography imaging may prove to be a widely applicable method of identifying viable ischemic myocardium early in the course of reperfusion.

▶ The accumulation of this non-beta-oxidized fatty acid noninvasively identified zones of myocardium with abnormal segmental systolic shortening but reversible ischemic ultrastructural changes despite a marked reduction in regional myocardial blood flow. Such areas of discordance between fatty acid and flow distribution are characteristic of ischemically "stunned" but viable myocardium. In this important animal study, single photon emission computed tomography (SPECT) was used for "metabolic" imaging rather than the less frequently available and more costly positron emission tomography (PET), which is being used to assess the viability of myocardium by "metabolic" (18FDG) and myocardial perfusion imaging (^{13}NH3) in patients with coronary artery stenoses (see also Tamaki N et al: *J Nucl Med* 29:1181–1188, 1988, for a comparison of SPECT vs. PET imaging).—R.A. O'Rourke, M.D.

Myocardial Oxygen Consumption, Oxygen Supply/Demand Heterogeneity, and Microvascular Patency in Regionally Stunned Myocardium

Stahl LD, Weiss HR, Becker LC (Johns Hopkins Univ; Robert Wood Johnson Med School, Piscateaway, NJ)
Circulation 77:865–872, April 1988   1–30

Prolonged ventricular dysfunction, without necrosis, occurring after a brief episode of myocardial ischemia with reperfusion has been termed *myocardial stunning*. Although myocardial oxygen consumption closely parallels energy production and mechanical work in the normal heart, previous studies have found that the stunned myocardium may have normal or even above normal oxygen utilization despite depressed function.

In this study with mongrel dogs, microspectrophotometry was used to compare oxygen extraction and consumption in stunned and normal myocardium. Stunning was produced by 5-minute periods of occlusion alternating with 10-minute periods of reflow, which were followed by a 90-minute recovery period. In 10 dogs, quick-frozen biopsy samples were removed from regionally stunned and normal myocardial regions. Oxygen saturation of blood was measured in small arteries and veins less than 100 μm in diameter. In 5 dogs, patency of the microvasculature in stunned and normal myocardium was assessed by microscopic analysis of hearts infused in situ with Microfil or drafting ink.

Regional myocardial blood flow and mean arteriolar oxygen saturation were similar in stunned and normal regions. However, mean venous oxygen saturation in the stunned region was lower than that in the normal region, indicating increased oxygen extraction and consumption. Furthermore, there was greater vein-to-vein heterogeneity of oxygen saturation in the stunned region than in the normal region, with an excess of veins in the stunned region having low oxygen saturations. Assessment of patency of the microvasculature showed fillings of more than 95% in the arterioles and of 85% in the capillaries of stunned regions. Similar values were found for the normal myocardial regions.

The results of this study suggest an inefficient transfer of energy into myocyte contraction or an increased use of energy for noncontractile activities in the stunned myocardium. The finding of increased heterogeneity of oxygen extraction further suggests that injury to stunned myocardium may not be uniform to all contractile elements but that the injury may be focally and irregularly distributed.

▶ In this study regionally "stunned" myocardium exhibited higher mean oxygen extraction and consumption in the presence of normal mean myocardial blood flow. These interesting results provide new mechanistic information concerning postischemic regionally stunned myocardium in a dog model of myocardial infarction.—R.A. O'Rourke, M.D.

Beneficial Effects of Iloprost in the Stunned Canine Myocardium
Farber NE, Pieper GM, Thomas JP, Gross GJ (Med College of Wisconsin)
Circ Res 62:204–215, February 1988   1–31

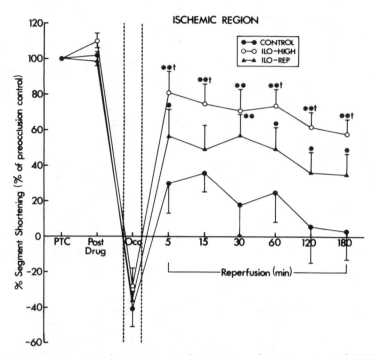

Fig 1–9.—Percent segment shortening expressed as percentage of pretreatment control *(PTC)* value in ischemic-reperfused area at 10 minutes postdrug *(Post Drug)* or saline, 12 minutes after occlusion *(Occ),* and at various times of reperfusion. Significant differences from control group are indicated by *P <.05 and **P <.01 and from ILO-REP are depicted by †P <.05. Mean PTC %SS was 20.8 for controls, 21.4 for ILO-HIGH, and 18.6 for ILO-REP. (Courtesy of Farber NE, Pieper GM, Thomas JP, et al: *Circ Res* 62:204–215, February 1988.)

Iloprost is a chemically stable analogue of prostacyclin. The effect of iloprost on reversibly damaged myocardium was examined in dogs that were subjected to 15 minutes of coronary artery occlusion followed by 3 hours of reperfusion.

Iloprost, 0.05 µg/kg/minute, (ILO-LOW), or 0.1 µg/kg/minute (ILO-HIGH), was infused for 15 minutes before occlusion and then was continued during occlusion or was infused before reperfusion at the higher level (ILO-REP). Another set of dogs (controls) received saline. The percentage of myocardial segment shortening (%SS) was measured by sonomicrometry.

At 3 hours of reperfusion, the %SS in the previously ischemic region had recovered to only 3% of pretreatment values in the control group. In the iloprost groups the %SS was enhanced at all time points, and by 3 hours of reperfusion the %SS was 43% of pretreatment value in the ILO-LOW group, 58% in the ILO-HIGH group, and 35% in the ILO-REP group (Fig 1–9).

Infusion of iloprost had a greater effect when it was carried out before occlusion (HIGH or LOW) rather than immediately before reperfusion. Iloprost did not effect collateral blood flow in the ischemic region or myocardial content of high-energy phosphate.

When sodium nitroprusside was administered before occlusion, there was no significant effect on postischemic recovery after 5 minutes, suggesting that the hypotensive action of iloprost did not play a significant role in ischemic recovery. However, in vitro experiments indicated that iloprost decreased the superoxide burst of stimulated neutrophils.

Iloprost ameliorates postischemic dysfunction in the stunned myocardium in a dose-dependent manner. This effect does not appear to be mediated by changes in blood flow or content of adenine nucleotides but by inhibition of oxygen-derived free radicals.

▶ In this study the prostacyclin analogue iloprost caused a dose-dependent increase in the recovery of regional myocardial function after coronary artery occlusion and several hours of reperfusion that was greatest when iloprost was administered before occlusion. The in vitro experiments suggested that the responsible mechanism was inhibition of oxygen-derived free radicals (see Abstracts 1–24 and 1–32).—R.A. O'Rourke, M.D.

Influence of Risk Area Size and Location on Native Collateral Resistance and Ischemic Zone Perfusion
Gumm DC, Cooper SM, Thompson SB, Marcus ML, Harrison DG (Univ of Iowa; VA Hosp, Iowa City)
Am J Physiol 254:H473–H480, March 1988   1–32

There is evidence that the perfusion of ischemic myocardium is affected by the size of the perfusion field of the occluded vessel, and this may be related in turn to differences in resistance of collateral vessels. The effects of risk area size on collateral resistance and perfusion of the ischemic region were investigated in dogs having occlusion of the left anterior descending or circumflex coronary artery at different sites. Risk areas ranged from 13% to 43% of left ventricular mass.

Total collateral flow was greatest in the largest-risk areas, but collateral flow per unit ischemic myocardium was much greater in the small-risk regions than the large ones. Collateral resistance was significantly lower in small-risk areas. In comparing small-risk areas at different sites, collateral flow per unit of ischemic myocardium was higher at the apex than at the base, and transcollateral resistance was lower.

The size of the risk area, its location, and variation between animals all are important determinants of collateral resistance. Because the survival of ischemic myocardium is dependent on collateral perfusion, these factors may be of importance in the clinical manifestations of myocardial ischemia. The findings of more collateral flow in small-risk areas may explain why such regions often do not become infarcted after coronary occlusion.

▶ These experimental studies provide further important information in an area of continuing investigation concerning the role of collateral coronary circulation and the factors that influence it in myocardial ischemia and infarction.—R.A. O'Rourke, M.D.

Reduction of Experimental Canine Myocardial Reperfusion Injury by a Monoclonal Antibody (Anti-Mo1, Anti-CD11b) That Inhibits Leukocyte Adhesion

Simpson PJ, Todd RF III, Fantone JC, Mickelson JK, Griffin JD, Lucchesi BR
(Univ of Michigan, Harvard Med School)

J Clin Invest 81:624–629, February 1988

1–33

A monoclonal antibody that binds to a leukocyte adhesion-promoting glycoprotein was administered to open-chest anesthetized dogs 45 minutes after induction of regional myocardial ischemia by occluding the circumflex coronary artery. After a 90-minute occlusion, reperfusion continued for 6 hours. Antibody was infused in a dose of 1 mg/kg over 10 minutes. Control animals received the vehicle, 0.5%, or 5% human serum albumin.

Administration of the monoclonal antibody lowered myocardial infarct size by 46% (Fig 1–10). The area at risk of infarction was similar in the study and control groups. There were no significant differences in arterial pressure, circumflex blood flow, or circulating neutrophil counts. The reduction in infarct size was independent of the severity of ischemia, as es-

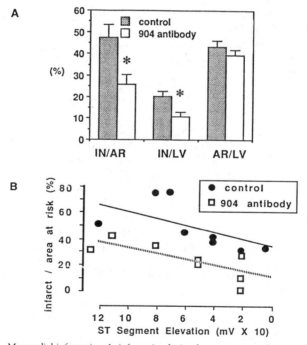

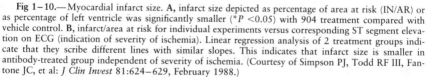

Fig 1–10.—Myocardial infarct size. **A,** infarct size depicted as percentage of area at risk (IN/AR) or as percentage of left ventricle was significantly smaller (*P <0.05) with 904 treatment compared with vehicle control. **B,** infarct/area at risk for individual experiments versus corresponding ST segment elevation on ECG (indication of severity of ischemia). Linear regression analysis of 2 treatment groups indicate that they scribe different lines with similar slopes. This indicates that infarct size is smaller in antibody-treated group independent of severity of ischemia. (Courtesy of Simpson PJ, Todd RF III, Fantone JC, et al: *J Clin Invest* 81:624–629, February 1988.)

timated from ST-segment elevation. A control monoclonal antibody of the same subtype, murine immunoglobulin G, had no effect on infarct size. Histologic study showed that the active antibody attenuated accumulation of neutrophils within the myocardium.

A specific neutrophil suppressive agent lowered myocardial infarct size in this model of acute infarction. This method could be used in patients with evolving infarction who are candidates for reperfusion by thrombolysis or mechanical means. The treatment may lack serious side effects.

▶ In a study relevant to the prior selection, a neutrophil suppressive agent with great selectivity and specificity and with a known mechanism of action was shown to inhibit tissue injury in dogs with acute myocardial infarction. Whereas other experimental therapies (neutrophil depletion, prostacyclin and its analogues) may suppress neutrophil function, each has serious side effects or is unfeasible for use in patients. However, the use of monoclonal antibodies may develop as an important therapeutic approach to patients with early myocardial infarction who are candidates for reperfusion by thrombolytic agents, percutaneous transluminal coronary angioplasty, or bypass surgery.—R.A. O'Rourke, M.D.

Therapy to Reduce Free Radicals During Early Reperfusion Does Not Limit the Size of Myocardial Infarcts Caused by 90 Minutes of Ischemia in Dogs
Richard VJ, Murry CE, Jennings RB, Reimer KA (Duke Univ)
Circulation 78:473–480, August 1988   1–34

Reperfusion is widely used in treating acute myocardial infarction, but oxen-centered free radicals produced on reperfusion may themselves lead to myocyte death. Previous studies suggest that anti-free radical treatment does not limit infarct size after 40 minutes of ischemia and 4 days of reperfusion in dogs. Infarcts produced by 90 minutes of ischemia now have been studied. Dogs received a 1-hour infusion of superoxide dismutase and catalase starting 25 minutes before reperfusion, or a single injection of the xanthine oxidase inhibitor oxypurinol. Reperfusion after circumflex coronary occlusion lasted 4 days.

Infarct size as a proportion of the area at risk was not significantly altered by either superoxide dismutase-catalase treatment or oxypurinol administration. Infract size was inversely related to collateral blood flow in control dogs, and neither treatment altered this relationship.

Treatment with superoxide dismutase-catalase or oxypurinol did not limit infarct size after a 90-minute period of coronary occlusion and 4 days of reperfusion in this study. Apparently, free radicals do not cause substantial myocyte death in this model. Differing results of trials of anti-free radical measures cannot be ascribed to differences in the duration of ischemia before reperfusion.

▶ Treatment with neither superoxide dismutase nor oxypurinol limited infarct size when infarcts were caused by 90 minutes of coronary occlusion followed by 4 days of reperfusion in dogs. Studies by others have suggested infarct size limitation by similar therapy against free radical production after 60 to 90 minutes of ischemia. Thus, controversy persists. Important considerations include the difference in methods for measuring infarct size and its baseline predictors, the need to consider both areas at risk and collateral blood flow, and the dosage of the drugs used and the technique of reperfusion plus its duration. Both positive and negative reports of anti-free radical therapy continue with its efficacy still in question.— R.A. O'Rourke, M.D.

Hormonal and Cardiac Effects of Converting Enzyme Inhibition in Rat Myocardial Infarction
Michel J-B, Lattion A-L, Salzmann J-L, de Lourdes Cerol M, Philippe M, Camilleri J-P, Corvol P (Hôpital Broussais, Paris; Centre Hospitalier Universitaire, Lausanne, Switzerland)
Circ Res 62:641–650, April 1988   1–35

An experimental rat model of left ventricular myocardial infarction has previously been used to demonstrate that treatment with a converting enzyme inhibitor (CEI) can improve the hemodynamic pumping ability of the heart and increase survival curves in these animals. However, the effect of CEI on markers of structure and function of the peripheral circulation and the structures of the heart itself has not yet been studied.

In an effort to better understand how inhibition of the renin-angiotensin system may improve the prognosis of myocardial infarction, and using the same experimental rat model, the authors measured changes in blood pressure, plasma hormones involved in cardiovascular homeostasis, isoenzyme profile of left ventricular myosin, volume density of collagen within the viable myocardium, and changes in atrial natriuretic factor messenger RNA after treatment for 2 months with a new CEI, S9490–3. A group of rats in which myocardial infarction was not treated and a control group of sham-operated rats were also studied.

Induction of myocardial infarction led to an immediate, significant, but transient decrease in systolic blood pressure in all the infarcted rats. Treatment for 2 months with S9490–3 reversed all the quantitative and qualitative baseline variables measured in the heart but did not totally normalize these variables when compared with those in the sham-operated controls. The S9490–3 reversed the cardiac increase in mass, the isoenzyme profile of cardiac myosin, and the collagen content in the left ventricle and decreased the atrial natriuretic factor gene expression in the 4 parts of the myocardium. However, the CEI did not completely normalize heart variables other than collagen.

In this experimental rat model, myocardial infarction profoundly modified several variables of peripheral circulation and quantitative and qualitative myocardial protein expression. Although treatment with a CEI largely reversed these changes, the CEI did not entirely normalize the measured variables.

▶ Since the initial studies by Pfeffer and associates (*Circ Res* 57:84–95, 1985), there has been considerable interest in the usefulness of chronic therapy with angiotensin converting enzyme inhibits to favorably affect ventricular geometry and function as well as survival post myocardial infarction. In the above study converting enzyme inhibition (CEI) did not alter infarct size but decreased left ventricular afterload and partially reversed abnormalities of myocardial protein expression. Nevertheless, the clinical usefulness of CEI agents in patients with recent myocardial infarction remains to be demonstrated.—R.A. O'Rourke, M.D.

Acceleration of the Wavefront of Myocardial Necrosis by Chronic Hypertension and Left Ventricular Hypertrophy in Dogs
Dellsperger KC, Clothier JL, Hartnett JA, Haun LM, Marcus ML (Univ of Iowa)
Circ Res 63:87–96, July 1988   1–36

Recent laboratory studies in dogs have shown that chronic hypertension and left ventricular hypertrophy (HT-LVH) increase the size of the completed myocardial infarction resulting from occlusion of a single vessel. These findings suggest that accelerated atherosclerosis is not the only explanation for the increase in infarction size when coronary occlusion occurs in the presence of HT-LVH. Several investigators have described a wavefront phenomenon of myocardial necrosis from the subendocardium to the subepicardium. The hypothesis that the wavefront of ischemic cell necrosis is accelerated in dogs with chronic arterial HT-LVH when compared with controls was tested.

Hypertension and left ventricular hypertrophy were induced in 42 dogs using a single-kidney, single-clip model; 17 dogs served as controls. One hour of circumflex coronary artery occlusion was followed by 4 hours of reperfusion, and 3 hours of circumflex coronary artery occlusion by 90 minutes of reperfusion in 2 control groups and 2 HT-LVH groups. In another HT-LVH group, nitroprusside was infused to reduce mean arterial pressure to 100 mm Hg, starting 1 hour after occlusion, and continued for the duration of the reperfusion period.

Fifteen (88%) of the 17 control animals, but only 17 (40%) of the 42 HT-LVH animals, survived coronary occlusion. After 1 hour of circumflex coronary artery occlusion, more than twice as much midwall and epicardium was infarcted in the HT-LVH group than in the control group. After 3 hours of circumflex coronary artery occlusion, significantly more endocardium, midwall, and epicardium were infarcted in the HT-LVH group than in the control group. However, the size of the infarcts in the nitroprusside-treated HT-LVH animals was similar to that in the control animals.

The findings confirm that the wavefront of ischemic cell necrosis is accelerated in dogs with chronic arterial HT-LVH when compared with controls, resulting in greater mortality. Early nitroprusside infusion appeared to retard this wavefront of infarction.

▶ This study indicates that an enhanced wave front of ischemic cell necrosis occurs following coronary artery occlusion in animals with preocclusion hypertension and left ventricular hypertrophy (LVH), and the accelerated coronary atherosclerosis is not the only factor adversely affecting morbidity and mortality in patients with chronic hypertension undergoing myocardial infarction. The data presented also suggest that the time window for effective reperfusion therapy may be shortened by the presence of chronic hypertension and LVH.—R.A. O'Rourke, M.D.

Mediation of Reocclusion by Thromboxane A$_2$ and Serotonin after Thrombolysis with Tissue-Type Plasminogen Activator in a Canine Preparation of Coronary Thrombosis
Golino P, Ashton JH, Glas-Greenwalt P, McNatt J, Buja LM, Willerson JT (Univ of Texas, Dallas; Univ of Cincinnati)
Circulation 77:678–684, March 1988   1–37

Despite frequent reperfusion after treatment with recombinant tissue-type plasminogen activator (rt-PA), many patients have acute coronary reocclusion. Intracoronary platelet activation may lead to reocclusion despite adequate anticoagulant therapy. Examination was made of the role of thromboxane A$_2$ and serotonin in mediating reocclusion in open-chest dogs having a copper coil placed in the left anterior descending coronary artery. Reperfusion by rt-PA was followed by heparin treatment, repeated cycles of gradual occlusion, and finally persistent occlusion.

Heparin alone did not prevent cyclic flow variations in the coronary artery; reocclusion occurred in a mean of 25 minutes. Flow variations were abolished by an intravenous bolus of SQ29548, a thromboxane A$_2$/prostaglandin H$_2$-receptor antagonist, and a bolus of ketanserin, a serotonin receptor antagonist. Reocclusion time exceeded 158 minutes. A maintenance infusion of both types of agent prevented reocclusion throughout the study period.

Reocclusion after thrombolysis is at least partly mediated by thromboxane A$_2$ and serotonin in this model of coronary thrombosis. The use of both thromboxane A$_2$ and serotonin receptor antagonists prevents or markedly delays reocclusion after thrombolysis. The findings may have important clinical implications.

▶ Intracoronary platelet activation after thrombolysis often results in reocclusion in spite of adequate therapy with heparin. The results of the above study are consistent with reports showing positive synergistic effects of serotonin and thromboxane A$_2$ receptor antagonists as antiplatelet agents and in blocking coronary artery cyclic flow variations. These experimental results may be clinically important considering the relatively high rate of early reocclusion (>20%)

following successful thrombolytic therapy of patients with acute myocardial infarction.—R.A. O'Rourke, M.D.

Mechanism of Complement Activation After Coronary Artery Occlusion: Evidence That Myocardial Ischemia in Dogs Causes Release of Constituents of Myocardial Subcellular Origin That Complex With Human C1q In Vivo

Rosen RD, Michael LH, Kagiyama A, Savage HE, Hanson G, Reisberg MA, Moake JN, Kim SH, Self D, Weakley S, Giannini E, Entman ML (Baylor College of Medicine, Houston)

Circ Res 62:572–584, March 1988   1–38

Myocardium subjected to prolonged ischemia often exhibits inflammatory cell infiltration, and this may contribute to ischemic injury. It appears that complement fixed by ischemic myocardium generates C5a, followed by leukocyte infiltration and inflammation and the release of lysozomal enzymes and oxygen radicals into the microenvironment, augmenting anoxic tissue damage. Spread of inflammation might result from the release of subcellular constituents that activate the complement cascade in extracellular fluid.

In the first group of studies, cardiac lymph, collected after reperfusion of ischemic tissue in dogs with infarction due to circumflex coronary occlusion, was found to contain molecules of cardiac subcellular origin, bound to C1q. Radiolabeled human C1q was injected intravenously before coronary occlusion. Rabbit antisera against substances precipitated from postreperfusion cardiac lymph by anti-human C1q reacted with specific constituents of isolated cardiac sarcoplasmic reticulum and mitochondria. A protein arising from mitrochondria was identified as one of the subcellular constituents activating the complement cascade.

In a second group of studies to assess clinical relevancy, sera from 12 of 15 patients with myocardial infarction was shown to contain large amounts of substances forming macromolecular complexes with C1q. Only 5 of 38 suspect patients without infarction had C1q-binding substances. In patients with infarction, high levels of C1q-binding activity were associated temporally with depressed C4, C3, or both, levels.

These findings provide further evidence that myocardial ischemia leads to the release of subcellular constituents of cardiac muscle that bind C1q and may activate the complement cascade. Leukotactic anaphylatoxins then are released that stimulate infiltration by inflammatory cells and subsequent worsening of myocardial tissue injury.

▶ During the past 10 years, there has developed an increased interest in the role of the inflammatory response in determining the extent of myocardial tissue injury after coronary artery occlusion. This study and several previous reports implicate complement activation within the ischemic tissue as the trigger for release of leukotactic anaphylotoxins and infiltration of inflammatory cells. The dog and patient studies described above suggest that C1q-binding substances released from ischemic myocardium initiate the response.

Others have shown that inactivation of the complement cascade (Pinckard RN et al: *J Clin Invest* 66:1050, 1980), precoronary occlusion induced neutropenia (Romson JL et al: *Circulation* 67:1016, 1983), or free radical scavenging systems (Jolly SR et al: *Circ Res* 54:277, 1984) can reduce myocardial damage early after coronary artery occlusion. The clinical relevance of these findings for patients with acute myocardial infarction is currently undergoing intensive investigation.—R.A. O'Rourke, M.D.

Additional recent references of clinical relevance in this area of intensive research study are listed as follows:

1. Hagestad EL, Verrier RL: Delayed myocardial ischemia following the cessation of sympathetic stimulation. *Am Heart J* 115:45–52, 1988.
2. Liedtke JA, DeMaison L, Eggleston AM, et al: Changes in substrate metabolism and effects of excess fatty acids in reperfused myocardium. *Circ Res* 62:535–542, 1988.
3. Yasuda T, Gold HK, Fallon JT, et al: Monoclonal antibody against the platlet glycoprotein (GP) 11b/111a receptor prevents coronary artery reocclusion after reperfusion with recombinant tissue-type plasminogen activator in dogs. *J Clin Invest* 81:1284–1291, 1988.
4. Kitakaze M, Weisfeldt ML, Marban E: Acidosis during early reperfusion prevents myocardial stunning in perfused ferret hearts. *J Clin Invest* 82:920–927, 1988.
5. Simpson PJ, Mickelson J, Fantone JC, et al: Reduction of experimental canine myocardial infarct size with prostaglandin E_1: Inhibition of neutrophil migration and activation. *J Pharmacol Exp Ther* 244:619–624, 1988.
6. Van Der Giessen WJ, Verdouw PD, Ten Cate FJ, et al: In vitro cyclic AMP induced phosphorylation of phospholamban: An early marker of long-term recovery of function following reperfusion of ischaemic myocardium? *Cardiovasc Res* 22:714–718, 1988.
7. Miller DD, Gill JB, Livni E, et al: Fatty acid analogue accumulation: A marker of myocyte viability in ischemic-reperfused myocardium. *Circ Res* 63:681–692, 1988.
8. Force T, Kemper A, Leavitt M, et al: Acute reduction in functional infarct expansion with late coronary reperfusion: Assessment with quantitative two-dimensional echocardiography. *J Am Coll Cardiol* 11:192–200, 1988.
9. Kawaguchi H, Yasuda H: Effect of various plasminogen activators on prostacyclin synthesis in cultured vascular cells. *Circ Res* 63:1029–1035, 1988.

Noninvasive Testing

Value and Limitations of Doppler Echocardiography in the Quantification of Stenotic Mitral Valve Area: Comparison of the Pressure Half-Time and the Continuity Equation Methods
Nakatani S, Masuyama T, Kodama K, Kitabatake A, Fujii K, Kamada T (Osaka Univ; Osaka Police Hosp, Osaka, Japan)
Circulation 77:78–85, January 1988

Two Doppler methods, the pressure half-time method and one based on the equation of continuity, were used to estimate stenotic mitral valve area noninvasively in 41 patients with mitral stenosis, 20 of whom had associated aortic regurgitation. The mean mitral valve area on cardiac catheterization was 1.29 cm². Using the equation of continuity, mitral valve area was estimated as a product of aortic or pulmonic annular cross-sectional area and the ratio of the time velocity integral of aortic or pulmonic flow to that of the mitral stenotic jet. Using the pressure half-time method, valve area was 220/pressure half-time, the time from the peak transmitral velocity to half the square root of the peak velocity on the continuous-wave Doppler-determined transmitral flow velocity pattern.

Mitral valve area using the pressure half-time method was correlated with catheterization estimates with a coefficient of .69, or .90 when patients with aortic regurgitation were excluded. Overestimates were often made in patients with regurgitation. Valve area estimated by the continuity equation method was correlated with catheterization measurements at a coefficient of .91, regardless of whether or not aortic regurgitation was present.

The continuity equation method of estimating stenotic mitral valve area is more accurate than the pressure half-time method, particularly in patients with moderate to severe aortic regurgitation.

▶ Doppler echocardiography is being used with increasing frequency as the noninvasive method of choice for determining the severity of mitral stenosis, and in many medical centers appropriate patients with severe mitral stenosis are sent to surgery without cardiac catheterization. This study shows that the Doppler measurement most commonly used, the pressure half-time method, is less accurate (underestimating the extent of stenosis) than the Doppler equation of continuity method for quantitating the severity of mitral stenosis in patients with coincident aortic regurgitation.—R.A. O'Rourke, M.D.

Transesophageal Echocardiography
Mitchell MM, Sutherland GR, Gussenhoven EJ, Taams MA, Roelandt JRTC (Univ of California, San Diego; Erasmus Univ, Rotterdam, the Netherlands; Interuniversity Cardiology Inst of the Netherlands, Rotterdam)
J Am Soc Echo 1:362–377, September–October 1988   1–40

Transesophageal echocardiography (TEE) can provide much clinically useful diagnostic information. Image quality often is as good as or better than that obtained with epicardial echocardiography during thoracotomy. It may be done in either the anesthetized or the conscious patient. A 4-chamber view is obtained by rotating the probe at 30–35 cm. If the probe tip is pulled back, the aortic valve appears. Deeper probing provides an oblique cross section through the left and right ventricles. The descending aorta is readily visualized.

Transesophageal echocardiography is a sensitive means of detecting mitral valve regurgitation from either valve disease or a prosthesis. It is better than precordial echocardiography in examining the left atrium and detecting thrombus or tumor and also is helpful in distinguishing among fibromuscular ring, left ventricular outflow tract tunnel, and localized septal hypertrophy. Aortic aneurysm formation and dissection may be evident on TEE. For visualizing the left main coronary artery and its proximal branches TEE is better than precordial study. Left heart vegetations from endocarditis may be visualized. Some aspects of congenital heart disease may be amenable to the transesophageal approach.

Monitoring with TEE is applicable to older patients having major surgery who are at risk of perioperative infarction. The probe should be placed as soon as possible after endotracheal intubation. Transesophageal echocardiography appears to be a safe modality, but it should be used only in an appropriately staffed environment.

▶ Transesophageal echocardiography is being used with increased frequency as an intraoperative technique for monitoring left ventricular function, for guidance and assessment of surgical intervention, and for assessment of anesthetic intervention. It also has been particularly useful for imaging patients with an inadequate precordial study and for defining disease of the thoracic aorta, for detecting left atrial vegetations and thrombi, and for assessing prosthetic valve function. The indications for and results of transesophageal echocardiography require further definition, but the reported complications have been negligible (Geibel A et al: *Am J Cardiol* 62:337–339, 1988).—R.A. O'Rourke, M.D.

MR of the Heart: Anatomy, Physiology, and Metabolism
Higgins CB (Univ of California, San Francisco)
AJR 151:239–248, August 1988   1–41

The techniques used in magnetic resonance imaging (MRI) of the heart are dependent on the purpose of the procedure. The capability of MRI to show anatomical features of various cardiovascular diseases is reviewed, and the current capability and future outlook of MRI in the evaluation and monitoring of cardiac physiology and myocardial metabolism are discussed.

When the primary goal is evaluation of anatomical abnormalities, the use of the electrocardiographic-gated spin-echo technique produces static images with high signal-to-noise ratios. Cine MRI is important in assessment of cardiac contractile function. The imaging plane is also dependent on the purpose of the study. If purely anatomical information is desired, imaging should be in a transverse, sagittal, or coronal plane. Imaging in planes along the cardiac axis is indicated when measurements of cardiac dimensions are required.

Magnetic resonance imaging is effective for showing a variety of pericardial diseases. The accuracy of MRI has been favorably compared with that of angiography for the evaluation of complex ventricular abnormalities. Thoracic aortic disease is best evaluated with MRI.

Previously, MRI was used primarily to display normal and abnormal cardiac anatomy. Recent technologic advances have now made it possible to evaluate cardiac physiology. Fast imaging techniques now make it possible to quantitate cardiac function through images with essentially high temporal resolution. The use of proton and P-31 magnetic resonance spectroscopy adds information to enable sequential monitoring of both cardiac function and metabolism.

▶ The ultimate clinical utility of nuclear magnetic resonance imaging will depend on the development of specific application such as noninvasive imaging of the coronary arteries; noninvasive, high-resolution assessment of regional myocardial blood flow distribution; the ability to evaluate regional metabolism; and the capability of characterizing myocardial disease using proton T_1 and T_2 alterations. An important reference is: Magnetic Resonance Imaging Panel, Council on Scientific Affairs: *JAMA* 259:253–259, 1988.—R.A. O'Rourke, M.D.

Left Ventricular Volume Measured Rapidly by Oblique Magnetic Resonance Imaging
Underwood SR, Gill CRW, Firmin DN, Klipstein RH, Mohiaddin RH, Rees RSO, Longmore DB (Natl Heart and Chest Hosps, London; Bank of England, London)
Br Heart J 60:188–195, September 1988   1–42

The ability to obtain left ventricular magnetic resonance images in oblique planes allows more rapid measurements from images containing the long axis of the ventricle. Volume then may be calculated from a single image, and ejection fraction, from a pair of end-diastolic and end-systolic images. The validity of the rapid method was studied by comparison with summing the areas of the chamber in multiple contiguous slices in 25 normal persons and 20 patients with previous myocardial infarction. The single-slice method requires only 9 minutes of acquisition time for both volume and ejection fraction. In 25 other normal subjects the left ventricle was measured in vertical and horizontal long axis planes (Fig 1–11).

The 2 methods of measuring volume agreed well in normal individuals but less well in patients with previous infarction, where the mean difference was 4.5 ml. Discrepancy in ejection fraction estimates was most marked where wall motion was very abnormal and the ejection fraction was low. Agreement between single-plane volume measurements in the vertical and horizontal long axis planes was good.

Vertical long axis magnetic resonance images of the left ventricle are an efficient means of estimating ventricular volume. Combined with regional wall motion studies, both global and regional left ventricular function can be rapidly assessed. Ejection fraction estimates should be interpreted cautiously in patients with abnormal ventricles.

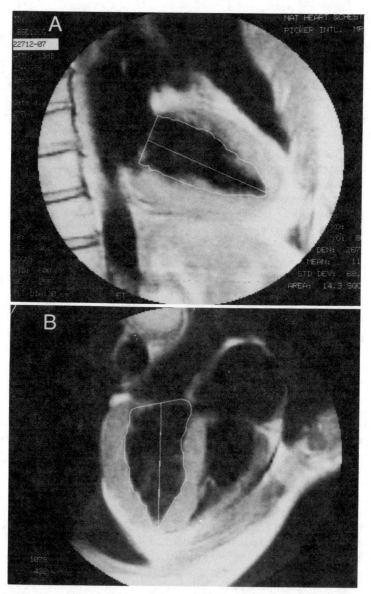

Fig 1–11.—Area and length of left ventricle in vertical (**A**) and horizontal long axis planes (**B**) were measured by tracing on computer screen. Images displayed are of normal subject with end diastolic volume of 125 ml. (Courtesy of Underwood SR, Gill CRW, Firmin DN, et al: *Br Heart J* 60:188–195, September 1988.)

▶ As indicated above, nuclear magnetic resonance imaging (NMRI) is being used with increased frequency to study patients with cardiac disease, but it has been primarily used as a research tool and its clinical indications are currently being assessed and defined. Other less expensive and more readily available noninvasive techniques frequently provide the necessary diagnostic information. However, for certain diagnoses (e.g., dissecting thoracic aortic aneurysm), NMRI is extremely valuable. The above study demonstrates the accuracy of left ventricular volumes obtained by single plane image analysis in normal subjects. However, as in other studies utilizing alternative techniques, biplane image analysis is more accurate when segmental wall motion abnormalities are present or when the left ventricle is markedly dilated.— R.A. O'Rourke, M.D.

Value and Limitation of Stress Thallium-201 Single Photon Emission Computed Tomography: Comparison With Nitrogen-13 Ammonia Positron Tomography

Tamaki N, Yonekura Y, Senda M, Yamashita K, Koide H, Saji H, Hashimoto T, Fudo T, Kambara H, Kawai C, Konishi J (Kyoto Univ, Kyoto, Japan)

J Nucl Med 29:1181–1188, July 1988   1–43

Thallium 201 single-photon emission computed tomography (SPECT) is useful for assessing myocardial perfusion in coronary artery disease; however, the technique might not be suitable for determining subtle changes in perfusion. A study was conducted to compare ^{210}TI SPECT with nitrogen 13 ammonia positron emission tomography (PET) in assessing coronary artery disease.

Fifty-one patients underwent both stress ^{201}TI SPECT and stress [^{13}N] ammonia PET; of these patients, 38 had histories of myocardial infarction. Coronary angiography was performed in multiple views.

Stress thallium SPECT showed abnormal perfusion in 46 of 48 patients with angiographically documented coronary artery disease; stress [^{13}N] ammonia PET showed abnormal perfusion in 47. The sensitivity for detecting disease in individual coronary arteries was 81% for SPECT and 88% for PET. The SPECT and PET findings concurred in 79% of 765 myocardial segments when interpretations were classified as normal, transient defect, and fixed defect. However, 66 segments showed a fixed defect by SPECT that was called a transient defect by PET, and 9 segments showed a transient defect by SPECT but a fixed defect by PET.

Both stress SPECT and PET showed high sensitivity for detecting coronary artery disease and specific stenosed vessels. However, stress-delayed SPECT with single tracer injection detects transient perfusion defects less often than stress-rest PET with 2 separate injections. The current SPECT protocol may underestimate the presence of myocardial ischemia.

▶ Fixed perfusion defects on thallium scan do not necessarily mean irreversible infarcted myocardium as reported previously by Brunken and associates (*J*

Am Coll Cardiol 10:557–567, 1987). One of the potential reasons for the detection of more transient defects by PET is the higher resolution and count density images of PET.—R.A. O'Rourke, M.D.

A list of additional references concerning the use of noninvasive cardiovascular methods of diagnosis is as follows:

1. Becker RC, Alpert JS: Electrocardiographic ST segment depression in coronary heart disease. *Am Heart J* 115:862–868, 1988.
2. Nath A, Alpert MA, Terry BE, et al: Sensitivity and specificity of electrocardiographic criteria for left and right ventricular hypertrophy in morbid obesity. *Am J Cardiol* 62:126–130, 1988.
3. Douglas PS, O'Toole ML, Hiller WDB, et al: Electrocardiographic diagnosis of exercise-induced left ventricular hypertrophy. *Am Heart J* 116:784–790, 1988.
4. Allen BJ, Casey TP, Brodsky MA, et al: Exercise testing in patients with life-threatening ventricular tachyarrhythmias: Results and correlation with clinical and arrhythmia factors. *Am Heart J* 116:997–1002, 1988.
5. David D, Lang RM, Borow KM: Clinical utility of exercise, pacing, and pharmacologic stress testing for the noninvasive determination of myocardial contractility and reserve. *Am Heart J* 116:235–247, 1988.
6. Allen BJ, Brodsky MA, Lazarus M, et al: Failure of ambulatory electrocardiographic monitoring to predict results of programmed electrical stimulation. Studies in patients with clinical ventricular tachyarrhythmias. *Chest* 93:699–704, 1988.
7. Machac J, Weiss A, Winters SL, et al: A comparative study of frequency domain and time domain analysis of signal-averaged electrocardiograms in patients with ventricular tachycardia. *J Am Coll Cardiol* 11:284–296, 1988.
8. Bolger AF, Eigler NL, Pfaff JM, et al: Computer analysis of Doppler color flow mapping images for quantitative assessment of in vitro fluid jets. *J Am Coll Cardiol* 12:450–457, 1988.
9. Delemarre BJ, Bot H, Visser CA, et al: Phasic flow in the left ventricular inflow tract: The importance of Doppler sample volume position. *J Clin Ultrasound* 16:227–232, 1988.
10. Eisner R, Churchwell A, Noever T, et al: Quantitative analysis of the tomographic thallium-201 myocardial bullseye display: Critical role of correcting for patient motion. *J Nucl Med* 29:91–97, 1988.

Newer Diagnostic and Therapeutic Techniques

Technetium-99m Methoxyisobutyl Isonitrile (RP30) for Quantification of Myocardial Ischemia and Reperfusion in Dogs
Li Q-S, Frank TL, Franceschi D, Wagner HN Jr, Becker LC (Johns Hopkins Med Institutions, Baltimore)
J Nucl Med 29:1539–1548, September 1988   1–44

Because of their flow-related distribution in the myocardium, a number of hexakis (isonitrile) technetium analogues can be used as substitutes for thallium 201 in assessing patients with suspected or proved coronary artery disease. The analogue ^{99m}Tc-methoxyisobutyl isonitrile (RP30) is rapidly cleared from the lungs and accumulates less in the liver than do other isonitrile compounds. A study was done using ^{99m}Tc-RP30 to assess myocardial blood flow during ischemic and reperfusion in dogs with temporary occlusion of the left anterior descending or left circumflex coronary artery. Studies also were done with ^{153}Gd-labeled microspheres and ^{125}I-labeled microspheres.

Image subtraction aided the quantification of flow during reperfusion. Tomographic studies in which RP30 was injected during ischemia clearly showed perfusion defects in the appropriate areas of myocardium wherever microsphere studies confirmed ischemia. Correlation between the normalized activity ratio for RP30 and the normalized microsphere ratio in the center of the ischemic zone was very high. Injection of RP30 after reperfusion demonstrated reperfusion in 7 of 8 animals with initial defects. The remaining animal had persistent ischemia on both RP30 and microsphere studies.

Repeated injections of the isonitrile RP30 can serve to quantify serial changes in regional myocardial blood flow. Clinical use of this approach will require precise image alignment so that subtraction can take place without creating artifact defects.

▶ This is one of many basic and clinical research studies utilizing the radionuclide technetium 99m methoxyisobutyl isonitrile and standard scintigraphic cameras. The results are quite promising. Because minimal myocardial redistribution occurs with the use of this compound, it is suitable for serial perfusion studies on the same day. However, the lack of redistribution limits its usefulness for separating areas of exercise-induced ischemia from areas of prior myocardial infarction (utilizing 1 injection of isotope) as compared with thallium 201.—R.A. O'Rourke, M.D.

Cardiac Imaging and Myocardial Kinetics of Technetium-Tertiary Butyl-Isonitrile During Dipyridamole-Induced Hyperemia

Okada RD, Williams SJ, Glover DK, Dragatokis D (Univ of Oklahoma, Tulsa; E I DuPont de Nemours & Co, Inc, Billerica, Mass)
Am Heart J 116:979–988, October 1988   1–45

Animal studies have shown excellent myocardial uptake of ^{99m}Tc-tertiary butyl-isonitrile (Tc-TBI). The properties of this nuclide may be better than those of ^{201}T1 for gamma camera imaging. The myocardial kinetics of Tc-TBI during dipyridamole-induced hyperemia were studied in dogs having partial occlusion of the circumflex coronary artery. Activity was monitored in the left anterior descending and circumflex vessels by gamma camera imaging for a period of 3 hours after infusion of dipyridamole. Regional myocardial flow was estimated by the microsphere technique.

The ratio of circumflex to left anterior descending blood flow was significantly reduced during dipyridamole infusion. Three-hour fractional Tc-TBI clearance rates were equal in the left anterior descending and cir-

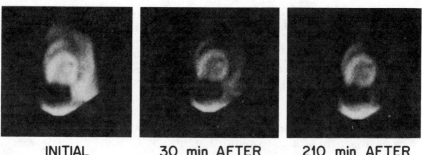

INITIAL   30 min AFTER   210 min AFTER
                    INJECTION   INJECTION

Fig 1–12.—Gamma camera images from control dog showing uniform tracer uptake throughout left ventricular myocardium. (Courtesy Okada RD, Williams SJ, Glover DK, et al: *Am Heart J* 116:979–988, October 1988.)

cumflex arteries. Excellent images were recorded in all dogs, showing the circumflex defect (Fig 1–12). The coefficient of correlation between regional myocardial flow and initial Tc-TBI distribution was 0.98.

Technetium 99m-tertiary butyl-isonitrile is a reliable tracer of regional myocardial blood flow. It is not ideal for clinical imaging because of early lung activity and accumulation in the liver, but it is an excellent tracer of regional myocardial flow because of marked extraction by the heart.

▶ This study utilized an isonitrile technetium analogue closely related to that used in the prior study (Abstract 1–44). Since intravenous dipyridamole has been used to accentuate differences in thallium 201 uptake between normal and ischemic myocardium (particularly in patients unable to exercise), Tc-TBI was injected after intravenous dipyridamole in dogs with a partial circumflex artery occlusion. Distribution of Tc-TBI was proportional to regional myocardial blood flow post dipyridamole, which unmasked coronary stenoses (microsphere data) in dogs with no flow disparities at rest. Isonitrile analogues will likely be used with intravenous dipyridamole, when both are clinically available, to detect myocardial ischemia in coronary disease in patients with no areas of reduced uptake at rest.—R.A. O'Rourke, M.D.

---

¹¹¹In-Labeled Platelet Scintigraphy and Two-Dimensional Echocardiography for Detection of Left Atrial Appendage Thrombi: Studies in a New Canine Model

Vandenberg BF, Seabold JE, Conrad GR, Kieso R, Johnson J, Fox-Eastham K, Ponto J, Bruch P, Kerber RE (Univ of Iowa)
Circulation 78:1040–1046, October 1988   1–46

Platelet scintigraphy with ¹¹¹In-labeled platelets is helpful in detecting left ventricular thrombi. Its usefulness in detecting left atrial thrombi was compared with that of 2-dimensional echocardiography in dogs with "acute" and "chronic" thrombosis. Platelets were injected 24 hours or 4 to 8 days after induction of thrombus. Thrombi were produced by clamping the atrial appendage and instilling thrombin and blood via a catheter.

With echocardiography, 3 of 17 acute thrombi and 3 of 10 chronic thrombi were detected. All the acute thrombi but only 2 chronic thrombi were detected with scintigraphy. The scintigraphic studies were blood pool-corrected.

Platelet scintigraphy consistently detected acute but not chronic thrombi in this model. It is probable that thrombus propagation and incorporation of labeled platelets decrease as the thrombus ages. Platelet scintigraphy may be a useful clinical means of detecting acute or fresh left atrial thrombi.

▶ Whereas noninvasive techniques, particularly 2-dimensional echocardiography, have been valuable for detecting ventricular thrombi, their accuracy and sensitivity for detecting left atrial thrombi has been disappointing. More patients with atrial fibrillation but no valvular heart disease would be followed without anticoagulation if a reliable noninvasive method for excluding left atrial thrombi was available. In the study by Vandenberg and associates, ^{111}In-labeled platelet scintigraphy and 2-dimensional echocardiography were relatively insensitive in detecting left atrial appendage thrombi in dogs. Studies by others utilizing transesophageal echocardiography and computed tomographic scanning suggest that they may be more sensitive, but confirmation in large numbers of patients is still needed.— R.A. O'Rourke, M.D.

Quantitative Assessment of Regional Left Ventricular Function by Densitometric Analysis of Digital-Subtraction Ventriculograms: Correlation with Myocardial Systolic Shortening in Dogs
Chappuis F, Widmann T, Guth B, Nicod P, Peterson KL (Univ of California, San Diego)
Circulation 77:457–467, February 1988   1–47

The usual form of wall motion analysis of contrast ventriculograms assesses only the part of the heart wall tangential to the x-ray beam. Left ventricular function may be evaluated in 3 dimensions using a computerized method based on densitrometric analysis of digital subtraction left ventriculograms. Time-volume curves are generated in individual wall segments to demonstrate regional volume changes throughout the cardiac cycle.

This method was validated in open-chest dogs, each having a circumflex artery occluder in place. Ventriculography was done at varying levels of inferior wall dysfunction produced by stenosing the circumflex coronary artery. Systolic shortening decreased in the ischemic myocardial wall. Regional ejection fraction decreased in the ischemic region, as did regional amplitude and peak ejection rate (Fig 1–13). Regional ejection fraction and amplitude were correlated well with myocardial systolic shortening. Regional peak ejection rate and phase were less closely related to systolic shortening.

Densitometric analysis of digital subtraction ventriculograms is a use-

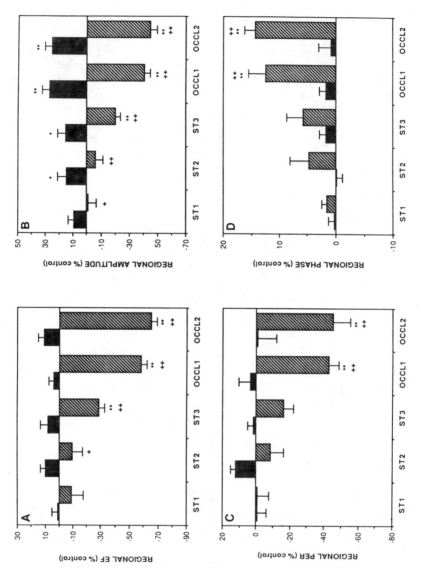

Fig 1–13.—Changes in regional left ventricular function (in % of control) as assessed by densitometric analysis of digital-subtraction ventriculograms in normal anterior *(black)* and ischemic inferior *(cross-hatched)* segments of left ventricle in 9 open-chest dogs. Ischemic dysfunction of inferior region was produced by mild, moderate, and severe stenoses *(ST1, ST2, ST3)*, and 15 and 30 sec occlusions *(OCCL1, OCCL2)* of circumflex coronary artery. Regional ejection fraction and amplitude (**A** and **B**) progressively decreased in ischemic region. Regional amplitude also demonstrated significant compensatory hyperkinesia in normal region. Regional peak ejection rate and phase (**C** and **D**) changed significantly in ischemic region only with complete coronary occlusion. (Courtesy of Chappuis F, Widmann T, Guth B, et al: *Circulation* 77:457–467, February 1988.)

ful means of evaluating left ventricular function in 3 dimensions. It is faster and more reproducible than conventional geometric methods of wall motion analysis. Subtle changes in contraction following treatment may be detected using this method, as may mild stress-induced abnormalities in patients with subclinical coronary heart disease.

▶ Many noninvasive and invasive imaging techniques have been used to assess regional ventricular systolic function in patients with coronary artery stenoses, but all are suboptimal because of limitations due to less than 3-dimensional assessment or inadequate spatial and temporal resolution or both.

In the above study densitometric analysis of digital-subtraction ventriculograms yielded measurements of regional ventricular function (e.g., ejection fraction) that correlated well in dogs during transient coronary artery occlusion with sonomicrometer measurements of regional left ventricular function. Although preliminary results in patients with coronary artery disease appear promising, additional clinical studies are necessary to define the usefulness of this technique for demonstrating subtle alterations in regional function during or after therapeutic interventions in patients with ischemic heart disease or for detecting mild stress-induced abnormalities in regional systolic function in patients without other clinical manifestations of their coronary artery stenoses.—R.A. O'Rourke, M.D.

Additional recent references of interest concerning noninvasive diagnostic methods for assessing ventricular performance, for measuring cardiac output, and for determining myocardial perfusion are listed below:

1. Monaghan MJ, Quigley PJ, Metcalfe JM, et al: Digital subtraction contrast echocardiography: A new method for evaluation of regional myocardial perfusion. *Br Heart J* 59:12–19, 1988.
2. Nicolosi GL, Pungercic E, Cervesato E, et al: Feasibility and variability of six methods for the echocardiographic and Doppler determination of cardiac output. *Br Heart J* 59:299–303, 1988.
3. McKelvie RS, Heigenhauser GJF, Jones NL: Measurement of cardiac output by CO_2 rebreathing in unsteady state exercise. *Chest* 92:777–782, 1987.
4. Feiring AJ, Rumberger JA, Reiter SJ, et al: Sectional and segmental variability of left ventricular function: Experimental and clinical studies using ultrafast computed tomography. *J Am Coll Cardiol* 12:415–425, 1988.
5. Sporn V, Balino NP, Holman BL, et al: Simultaneous measurement of ventricular function and myocardial perfusion using the technetium-99m isonitriles. *Clin Nucl Med* 13:77–81, 1988.
6. Zimmerman R, Tillmanns H, Knapp WH, et al: Regional myocardial nitrogen-13 glutamate uptake in patients with coronary artery disease: Inverse post-stress relation to thallium-201 uptake in ischemia. *J Am Coll Cardiol* 11:549–556, 1988.
7. Jackman WM, Friday KJ, Yeung-Lai-Wah JA, et al: New catheter technique for recording left free-wall accessory atrioventricular pathway activation: Identification of pathway fiber orientation. *Circulation* 78:598–610, 1988.

Sudden Death and CPR

Autonomic Mechanisms and Sudden Death: New Insights from Analysis of Baroreceptor Reflexes in Conscious Dogs With and Without a Myocardial Infarction
Schwartz PJ, Vanoli E, Stramba-Badiale M, De Ferrari GM, Billman GE, Foreman RD (Univ of Oklahoma, Oklahoma City; Università degli Studi di Milano, Milan, Italy)
Circulation 78:969–979, October 1988   1–48

In the conscious dog, depressed baroreflex sensitivity (BRS) is associated with an increased risk of ventricular fibrillation in the setting of healed anterior wall myocardial infarction. Fibrillation is induced by a brief ischemic episode during exercise stress. The goal of the present study in dogs was to determine whether myocardial infarction actually alters BRS and whether analysis of BRS before infarction can predict the outcome of acute myocardial ischemia after infarction.

Ventricular fibrillation occurred in 55% of dogs after a 2-minute circumflex coronary occlusion during exercise stress testing. Baroreflex sensitivity, assessed by the phenylephrine method, was significantly lower in susceptible than in resistant dogs. The risk of sudden death increased as the BRS declined. A control study demonstrated a decrease in BRS 4 weeks after myocardial infarction. However susceptible dogs had a lower BRS even before infarction.

Depressed BRS can identify dogs at high risk of ventricular fibrillation during acute myocardial ischemia. Preliminary data from infarction patients corroborate these findings. Because daily exercise improves depressed BRS, and vagal stimulation during acute ischemia is highly protective, means of preventing sudden cardiac deaths may be at hand.

▶ This animal study is consistent with 3 clinical studies (La Rovere et al: *Circulation* 78:816–824, 1988; Kleiger et al: *Am J Cardiol* 59:256–262, 1987; Martin et al: *Am J Cardiol* 60:86–89, 1987) indicating that the risk of a subsequent cardiac death of a postinfarction patient increases when either a depressed baroreflex sensitivity or a reduced heart rate variability is present. Both conditions suggest the presence of a derangement in the autonomic balance due to a reduced vagal activity probably associated with increased sympathetic activity.—R.A. O'Rourke, M.D.

Failure of Epinephrine to Improve the Balance Between Myocardial Oxygen Supply and Demand During Closed-Chest Resuscitation in Dogs
Ditchey RV, Lindenfeld J (Univ of Colorado, Denver)
Circulation 78:382–389, August 1988   1–49

Epinephrine often is given in high doses during cardiopulmonary resuscitation to increase arterial pressure and coronary blood flow. Coronary flow does increase, but myocardial oxygen requirements are augmented by epinephrine. The balance of oxygen supply and demand was studied in dogs by estimating myocardial adenosine 5'-triphosphate and lactate before and after 10 minutes of cardiopulmonary resuscitation. Study animals received a 1-mg bolus of epinephrine followed by an infusion of 0.2 mg/min.

Left ventricular myocardial blood flow during cardiopulmonary resuscitation, measured by the radioactive microsphere method, was significantly higher in epinephrine-treated animals. Myocardial lactate was increased significantly in both groups, more in the epinephrine group. Myocardial adenosine 5'-triphosphate declined significantly in both groups.

Large doses of epinephrine may not improve the balance between myocardial oxygen supply and demand during cardiopulmonary resuscitation, even if a substantial increase in coronary flow results. The increase in myocardial lactate tended to be greater in epinephrine-treated dogs. Benefit from epinephrine may reflect factors other than improved myocardial oxygenation. In addition to primary electrophysiologic effects, epinephrine may help by preventing coronary stasis and washing out metabolic products. It is not clear whether treatment aimed at improving myocardial oxygenation will make successful cardiopulmonary resuscitation more likely.

▶ The findings in this study suggest that the apparent benefit of epinephrine during attempted cardiopulmonary resuscitation may be due to factors other than improved myocardial oxygenation. The increment in coronary blood flow due to epinephrine likely prevents stasis in the coronary circulation and augments the washout of metabolic end products. Whether more pure α-adrenergic agents or alternative drugs that reduce the disparity between myocardial oxygen demand and supply are more effective than epinephrine in facilitating successful cardiopulmonary resuscitation remains to be established.—R.A. O'Rourke, M.D.

Expired Carbon Dioxide: A Noninvasive Monitor of Cardiopulmonary Resuscitation

Gudipati CV, Weil MH, Bisera J, Deshmukh HG, Rackow EC (University of Health Sciences, North Chicago, Ill)
Circulation 77:234–239, January 1988   1–50

The end-tidal CO_2 concentration ($ETCO_2$) could serve as a simple noninvasive measure of blood flow during precordial compression. The $ETCO_2$ was related to cardiac output in a mechanically ventilated porcine model of ventricular fibrillation, induced by a 5-mamp alternating current delivered to the right ventricular endocardium.

The onset of fibrillation was accompanied by a rapid decline in $ETCO_2$ from 4% to less than 0.7%. A rise to 1.9% occurred on precordial compression. Successfully defibrillated animals had an immediate increase in $ETCO_2$. Changes in $ETCO_2$ were correlated closely with changes in car-

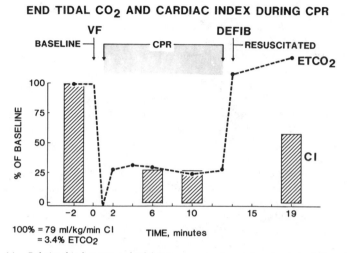

Fig 1–14.—Relationship between end-tidal CO_2 concentration and cardiac index before cardiac arrest, during cardiopulmonary resuscitation with external cardiac compression, and after restoration of spontaneous circulation. (Courtesy of Gudipati CV, Weil MH, Bisera J, et al: *Circulation* 77:234–239, January 1988.)

diac output (Fig 1–14). A similar correlation was observed during open-chest cardiac massage, when correlation coefficients averaged .95.

The $ETCO_2$ is predictive of the outcome during cardiopulmonary resuscitation. It can serve to immediately identify the restoration of spontaneous circulation in a noninvasive manner.

► This animal study and preliminary observations in patients suggest that the end-tidal CO_2 concentration during precordial compression is a useful clinical indicator of prognosis and identifies restoration of spontaneous circulation.— R.A. O'Rourke, M.D.

2 Cardiovascular Disease in Infants and Children

Introduction

This was another good year for expanding our knowledge about heart disease in people ranging from the fetus with heart defect or arrhythmia to the adult with congenital heart disease. While the year saw no newly described ailments, diagnostic techniques, or treatments, it nonetheless contributed short- and intermediate-term follow-ups on new techniques, especially those utilizing the balloon in treatment. In addition, it provided truly long-term follow-up on surgical treatment of large series of valvular aortic and also of pulmonic stenosis and of tetralogy of Fallot with pulmonary atresia. It added more data for comparison of balloon dilatation versus surgical valvotomy for congenital aortic stenosis.

We learned more about intermediate-term results in a large series of infants operated upon by open-heart surgery for tetralogy of Fallot and in several centers, for transposition of the great arteries by arterial switch.

As we think about long-term results, it is appropriate to pay our respects to Étienne-Louis Arthur Fallot. This was the centenary year of his clinical-pathologic correlates of "la maladie bleue." It was celebrated appropriately with a program in his honor in France.

In medical aspects of congenital heart disease, we had the opportunity to learn about its incidence and prevalence at high altitude in China and to note an increased incidence in Alberta, Canada, where ascertainment is high and medical care is free.

Those interested in unusual arrhythmias have an opportunity to review 2 reports on automatic atrial tachycardia. Cross-reference to the section entitled "Pharmacology" provides new information on amiodarone, flecainide, and even on the old drug digitalis.

Several forms of myocardial impairment are covered in the section on cardiomyopathy—myocarditis. Included is an analysis of cases of dilated cardiomyopathy that may help in decisions regarding cardiac transplantation.

Echocardiographic studies continue to impress us with their diagnostic accuracy. Fetal echocardiography was separated from the rest of echocardiography this year and called "Fetal Cardiology," to give status to that phase of an infant's prenatal life that involves not only diagnosis but also options for management.

Exercise testing was used in evaluation of aortic stenosis, in postoperative patients with residual pulmonary regurgitation, and in those undergoing the Fontan operation. To stress the situation by exercise often uncovers abnormalities in asymptomatic individuals.

Imaging other than echocardiography provided some interesting anatomical and physiologic information. Noteworthy and newsworthy was the study with cine magnetic resonance imaging.

Intermediate and long-term (up to 18 years) results of epicardial pacing were presented with respect to longevity and problems.

This year was both instructive and varied in publications of high quality in the field of pediatric cardiology. Many more were published than could be presented in the following abstracted articles. May these simply whet your appetites!

Mary Allen Engle, M.D.

Arrhythmias

Ectopic Automatic Atrial Tachycardia in Children: Clinical Characteristics, Management, and Follow-up
Mehta AV, Sanchez GR, Sacks EJ, Casta A, Dunn JM, Donner RM (St Christopher's Hosp for Children, Philadelphia; Temple Univ; Thomas Jefferson Univ; Univ of Texas Med Branch, Galveston)
J Am Coll Cardiol 11:379–385, February 1988   2–1

Ectopic automatic atrial tachycardia, an uncommon arrhythmia found primarily in infants and children, is difficult to treat. Its most common place of origin is the high right atrium. Family history, left ventricular dysfunction, and congenital heart defects have all been associated with the arrhythmia, but these were not found to be important risk factors in this study. Spontaneous resolution is known to occur, especially among young patients.

A series of drug therapies was tried with a group of 10 infants and children. Except for a girl aged 7.5 years, the patients were all aged younger than 3 years. Digoxin was given first, followed by 1 or more of the following if necessary: propranolol, administered orally, intravenously, or both; procainamide, administered orally, intravenously, or both; quinidine; and phenytoin. Digoxin continued to be given until 1 of the other drugs was found successful and improvement was noted in left ventricular dysfunction. Amiodarone, recently approved by the Food and Drug Administration for use in the United States, was used if all other therapies failed.

Digoxin slowed the tachycardia rate but did not control it. Propranolol proved successful for 5 patients, and amiodarone suppressed the arrhythmia in 4. Quinidine, procainamide, and phenytoin were not only ineffective, but worsened the rate in 3 patients. Four children were free from tachycardia and no longer needed medication on follow-up examination. Four others continued to do well with drug therapy. No serious side effects were observed with propranolol or amiodarone, making these medications preferable to surgery with its higher degree of risk.

▶ An arrhythmia that is fortunately uncommon at all ages, and rarely seen in adults, is automatic ectopic atrial tachycardia. The bad news is that it is very difficult to control. Digitalization merely slows the rate. Class I antiarrhythmics are ineffective. The good news is that in the 10 infants and children herein described, intravenous and oral propranolol and amiodarone suppressed the arrhythmia in two thirds to three fourths. The best news is that the arrhythmia tends spontaneously to abate.—M.A. Engle, M.D.

Atrial Automatic Tachycardia in Children
Koike K, Hesslein PS, Finlay CD, Williams WG, Izukawa T, Freedom RM (Hosp for Sick Children, Toronto)
Am J Cardiol 61:1127–1130, May 1, 1988   2–2

Atrial automatic tachycardia is a rare arrhythmia, usually occurring in children, which is characterized by abnormalities in atrial rate and distinct P waves with normal or slightly prolonged PR intervals. Nine children were seen with atrial automatic tachycardia. Age at onset of tachycardia ranged from prenatal to 14.3 years (median age, 6.6 years). In 8 patients, a tachycardia rate greater than 220 beats per minute ruled out sinus tachycardia. Normal P waves were seen intermittently, but long-term ambulatory monitoring was necessary to observe these pauses in tachycardia. Eight patients underwent electrophysiologic cardiac catheterization, during which there was spontaneous clinical tachycardia that could neither be initiated nor terminated by standard programmed atrial stimulation techniques.

A total of 33 drug trials was undertaken, beginning with digoxin; however, digoxin alone or in combination with other drugs achieved no better than partial control. Trials with newer drugs achieved somewhat better results. Full or good control with medical treatment was achieved in 5 of 9 patients. Cryoablation or resection or both were undertaken in 3 patients not helped by medical treatment. These patients remained in sinus rhythm and were arrhythmia-free at 1- to 3-year follow-up.

Based on these data, sotalol is recommended as the first-choice drug followed by a class 1C drug for this particular arrhythmia. Although more than half of the patients in this series had associated dilated cardiomyopathy, all patients showed improvement of left ventricular function with either medical or surgical treatment. Although there is no doubt that surgery is sometimes necessary, it is recommended that atrial automatic tachycardia in children initially be treated medically. Surgical intervention is mandated by drug failure, intolerable side effects, progressive cardiomyopathy, or failure to resolve with medical therapy.

▶ The experience over an 8-year period at The Hospital for Sick Children in Toronto is recounted for this rare but challenging arrhythmia. Based on careful studies of 9 children and their trials of therapy, they recommend medical therapy first as worth attempting. Because the usual drugs often failed to control the arrhythmia, they recommend sotalol, followed if needed by a class 1C drug.

If drug therapy fails or serious side effects or progressive cardiomyopathy ensue, they advise surgical ablation.

The bright sides of their experience are that, as in Mehta's report (Abstract 2–1), spontaneous remission occurred in one third of the patients, that dilated cardiomyopathy improved on restoration of sinus rhythm, and that surgery succeeded in the 3 children subjected to cryoablation or resection of the automatic focus or both.—M.A. Engle, M.D.

Cardiomyopathies

Arrhythmia and Prognosis in Infants, Children, and Adolescents With Hypertrophic Cardiomyopathy

McKenna WJ, Franklin RCG, Nihoyannopoulos P, Robinson KC, Deanfield JE, Dickie S, Krikler SJ (Hammersmith Hosp, Hosp for Sick Children, London)
J Am Coll Cardiol 11:147–153, January 1988   2–3

In adults with hypertrophic cardiomyopathy, the annual mortality associated with sudden death is 2% to 3%. Those at greatest risk can be singled out through ECG monitoring for episodes of ventricular tachycardia. Among children, for whom the annual mortality for this condition is 6%, the high-risk patient is harder to identify.

The significance of arrhythmia in children with hypertrophic cardiomyopathy and its relationship to sudden death was studied. Fifty-three children, aged 6 months to 21 years, underwent 2 days of ECG monitoring. Arrhythmias were rare in the group as a whole, but 4 adolescents had nonsustained supraventricular tachycardia and 5 others had nonsustained ventricular tachycardia. These 5 patients showed more symptoms as well as evidence of more severe left and right ventricular hypertrophy.

Five patients died suddenly and 2 survived ventricular fibrillation; none of the 5 who died showed signs of increased risk during the ECG monitoring. The 2 adolescents who were successfully resuscitated were considered to have a greater risk because of family history. Most children who die suddenly have no indications of increased risk. Unlike adults, the risk for children seems to be associated with a hemodynamic event brought on by exercise or emotion-related tachycardia, not a result of a primary arrhythmia.

The management of children with hypertrophic cardiomyopathy is not clear. Low-dose amiodarone is used successfully for adults and may benefit children as well. In this study, it was given to those with known risk factors. All of these patients survived the follow-up period, and none of the 5 who died had taken amiodarone.

▶ It is well known that in adults with hypertrophic cardiomyopathy there is a small but significant risk of sudden death, on exercise but also at rest. What is less well known is that, in infants and children, the rate of sudden death is even higher; 6% annual mortality versus 2% for adults.

The authors therefore performed Holter monitoring for at least 2 days in a series of 6 infants, 14 children, and 33 adolescents with this diagnosis in order to determine the incidence and types of arrhythmia and the prognosis for each. They found that arrhythmias were rare in infants and children, but in adolescents, paroxysmal supraventricular tachycardia was found in 4 and nonsustained ventricular tachycardia was recorded in 18%. Seven patients died suddently (15%) and 2 were resuscitated, but none of these had showed ventricular or supraventricular arrhythmia on monitoring.

Holter monitoring provides a marker for risk of sudden death in adults when nonsustained ventricular tachycardia is recorded. However, in young subjects, the absence of that arrhythmia does not indicate a low risk of sudden death.

What to do? The authors favor use of amiodarone in a low dose for those with recorded ventricular tachycardia.—M.A. Engle, M.D.

Effects of Verapamil on Left Ventricular Diastolic Filling in Children With Hypertrophic Cardiomyopathy
Shaffer EM, Rocchini AP, Spicer RL, Juni J, Snider R, Crowley DC, Rosenthal A
(Univ of Michigan)
Am J Cardiol 61:413–417, Feb 15, 1988   2–4

Symptomatic improvement from verapamil in patients with hypertrophic cardiomyopathy may reflect improved left ventricular (LV) diastolic filling. Ten children aged 7 to 18 years with clinical and angiographic findings of hypertrophic cardiomyopathy received long-term oral verapamil therapy. Half the patients initially had a resting or provoked LV outflow tract gradient of 30 mm Hg or greater. The mean LV end-diastolic pressure was 15 mm Hg. After intravenous verapamil in the catheterization laboratory, patients received 4 to 6 mg/kg daily, orally, for a mean time of 1.8 years.

On grated equilibrium blood pool scintigraphy, the LV ejection fraction was not changed significantly during long-term verapamil therapy. Both peak filling rate and time to peak filling improved significantly, indicating better diastolic filling. All the patients improved symptomatically. Dyspnea, chest pain, and dizziness all were less marked or absent during long-term treatment. Exercise endurance increased in 8 of 9 patients.

Diastolic abnormalities are more closely related to symptoms of hypertrophic cardiomyopathy than are systolic changes, and affected patients have markedly abnormal diastolic function. It is not yet clear how verapamil improves diastolic function, and it remains to be learned whether long-term treatment will improve the prognosis for children with hypertrophic cardiomyopathy.

▶ Hypertrophic cardiomyopathy continues to be an intriguing and poorly understood condition, difficult to improve with treatment and well nigh impossible to cure. This study of the effects of oral verapamil provides an explanation for the symptomatic improvement reported by some children and adults on this calcium antagonist because of hypertrophic cardiomyopathy. The mechanism of the improvement in diastolic function is not yet clear.—M.A. Engle, M.D.

Pathological Features of Coronary Arteries in Children With Kawasaki Disease in Which Coronary Arterial Aneurysm Was Absent at Autopsy: Quantitative Analysis

Fujiwara T, Fujiwara H, Nakano H (Kyoto Women's Univ, Kyoto Univ, Kyoto, Japan; Shizuoka Children's Hosp, Shizuoka, Japan)
Circulation 78:345–350, August 1988
2–5

In available published autopsy studies of Kawasaki disease, most children had coronary aneurysms at autopsy. Because there are no reports on whether a coronary arterial (CA) lesion can also develop in patients with Kawasaki disease but no CA aneurysm, the coronary arteries in 6 patients who had died of Kawasaki disease, but who had no CA aneurysms at autopsy, were studied.

The 5 boys and 1 girl, who ranged in age from 3 months to 4 years 7 months at the time of death, were Japanese. All children had typical clinical signs and symptoms of Kawasaki disease when they were in the acute stage. Twenty-one autopsied children without Kawasaki disease, 12 boys and 9 girls aged 2 months to 4 years, were studied as controls. Four children died of myocarditis at the acute stage of the disease, and the other 2 children died when the disease was in the healed stage. One of the latter 2 children died of *Staphylococcus aureus* sepsis, and the other child died 2 days after experiencing acute myocardial infarction that occurred during follow-up cineangiography.

At autopsy, the 6 children with Kawasaki disease had no thrombi, recanalization, or stenosis greater than 50% in the major coronary arteries. Three patients who died during the acute stage had dilatation of the major coronary arteries at autopsy. Two of these 3 patients showed slight dilatation of coronary arteries and abnormal thickening of the intima caused by panvasculitis. In 1 child who died at the healed stage, dilatation of the coronary arteries had disappeared, and no dilatation of any of the major coronary arteries was seen at autopsy. However, this child showed abnormal fibrous intimal thickening of the major coronary arteries but no inflammatory changes.

The other 3 children had no dilatation of the major coronary arteries at the acute stage. Two children had slight inflammation, but no signs of abnormal intimal thickening. The third child showed no dilatation during the clinical course, and no inflammatory changes or abnormal intimal thickening were found at autopsy.

Patients with Kawasaki disease have angiitis of the major coronary arteries, even if coronary dilatation is not present at the acute stage. Abnormal thickening of the intima may or may not remain at the healed stage in such patients.

▶ We continue to learn more about the puzzling disease that Dr. Kawasaki of Japan described more than 2 decades ago. Extensive vasculitis and pancarditis characterize this illness of as yet unknown etiology. Coronary aneurysms, which sometimes spontaneously regress, are a common and dreaded complication in 20% to 25% of the children. These doctors from Japan described the pathologic features in the coronary arteries of patients dying from the disease but not affected by coronary aneurysms. They reported that coronary vasculitis of major coronary arteries was present even without detected coronary aneurysms and that abnormal intimal thickening can persist even in the healed stage. Certainly it is important to terminate this illness promptly and to prevent coronary aneurysms. Intravenous gamma globulin in the acute phase of the first 2 weeks offers this possibility and hope.— M.A. Engle, M.D.

Prevention of Giant Coronary Artery Aneurysms in Kawasaki Disease by Intravenous Gamma Globulin Therapy
Rowley AH, Duffy CE, Shulman ST (Children's Mem Hosp, Chicago; Northwestern Univ)
J Pediatr 113:290–294, August 1988   2–6

When intravenous gamma globulin (IVGG) is administered within the first 10 days of Kawasaki disease, it reportedly decreases the prevalence of coronary artery abnormalities in these patients. However, there is still controversy over the efficacy or advisability of its widespread use in this illness. The experience of a single institution was retrospectively reviewed in the use of IVGG as early treatment in patients with Kawasaki disease.

During an 8-year study period, 113 boys and 74 girls, with a mean age of 31 months, were treated for Kawasaki disease. The patients were divided into 3 temporal groups based on the time of their admission. The first 75 patients were admitted before IVGG was used to treat Kawasaki disease. The next 49 patients were admitted just about when IVGG was used in a phase 1 trial; 11 children were thus treated with IVGG. Fifty-seven of the most recently admitted 63 children had diagnoses during the first 10 days of illness and were treated with IVGG plus aspirin. The other 6 children did not have diagnoses within the first 10 days of illness and were not treated with IVGG.

Coronary artery abnormalities developed in only 3 (4%) of the 68 children treated with IVGG, 1 of whom already had echocardiographic abnormalities before IVGG therapy was initiated. In contrast, coronary artery abnormalities developed in 39 (33%) of the 119 untreated patients. None of the 68 IVGG-treated patients had giant coronary artery aneurysms, compared with 7 (6%) of the 119 children who were not treated with IVGG.

The IVGG appears to be effective not only in reducing the overall incidence of coronary artery abnormalities of Kawasaki disease, but also in preventing the formation of giant CA aneurysms which are the most serious consequence of this disorder.

► These investigators with considerable experience in management of children with Kawasaki disease continue to report their results with early use of intravenous gamma globulin (IVGG). The emphasis in this study is giant aneurysms of coronary arteries, the most severe manifestation of the process in coronary arteries. Giant aneurysms developed in none of the 68 patients treated with IVGG but in 7 (6%) of 119 patients not so treated.—M.A. Engle, M.D.

A Genetic Marker for Rheumatic Heart Disease
Rajapakse CNA, Halim K, Al-Orainey I, Al-Nozha M, Al-Aska AK (King Khalid Univ Hosp, King Saud Univ, Riyadh, Saudi Arabia)
Br Heart J 58:659–662, December 1987   2–7

Genetic factors are thought to predispose to rheumatic heart disease, but studies of human leukocyte antigen (HLA) types have not conclusively shown a marker for this predisposition. The possible role of HLA, and in particular the DR antigens, in predisposing a person to rheumatic fever was investigated.

Twenty-five patients with chronic rheumatic heart disease and 15 patients with acute rheumatic fever were evaluated for the frequency of antigen types A, B, C, and DR and were compared with 100 control persons. All persons were Arabs of Saudi origin.

The only antigen type that varied significantly between subjects and controls was HLA-DR4. The incidence of HLA-DR4 was 72% in patients with chronic rheumatic heart disease and 53% in patients with acute rheumatic fever, for an overall incidence of 65%. However, only 12% of controls had HLA-DR4. The incidence of HLA-DR4 antigen was 83% in 12 patients with mitral stenosis and 70% in 7 patients with aortic incompetence. In 17 non-Saudi Arab patients, the frequency of HLA-DR4 was 65%, which was identical to that in Saudi patients.

These results may have implications for the pathogenesis of rheumatic fever and rheumatic heart disease. Studies of families of patients with these diseases may confirm these findings.

▶ About 50 years ago, the late Dr. Maye Wilson of the New York Hospital CUMC became convinced that there was genetic susceptibility to rheumatic fever. She and her associates conducted studies then in those New York City families, using the genetic methodology of the time, chiefly pedigree analysis. Then the incidence of rheumatic fever in the United States declined so dramatically that little further work was done. Recently Dr. John Zabriskie of Rockefeller University, in studying children from the Caribbean where rheumatic fever had not disappeared, applied modern metholodogy and found a genetic marker.

This report comes from Saudi Arabia, where these workers found in 25 patients with chronic and 15 with acute rheumatic fever a frequency of HLA-DR4 significantly higher than in a control group of 100 healthy volunteers. In 17 non-Saudi subjects with acute rheumatic fever, they found an identically high frequency (65%) of HLA-DR4. They consider this HLA type to be a genetic marker for rheumatic fever.

Now that there is in several regions of the United States a resurgence of cases of rheumatic fever in children, it will be interesting to study them and a control group for HLA types.—M.A. Engle, M.D.

Dilated Cardiomyopathy in Infants and Children

Griffin ML, Hernandez A, Martin TC, Goldring D, Bolman RM, Spray TL, Strauss AW (Washington Univ)
J Am Coll Cardiol 11:139–144, January 1988   2–8

Cardiac transplantation offers hope of increased survival in patients with dilated cardiomyopathy who do not respond to conventional treatment. An index to predict which patients might respond to medical management and which might be suitable candidates for cardiac transplantation was developed.

Records of infants and children in whom dilated cardiomyopathy was diagnosed from 1975 to 1985 were reviewed. Group 1 included 20 patients aged younger than 2 years of age; group 2 included 12 patients aged older than 2 years. Follow-up data were obtained from clinical records and parent interviews. Two patients in group 1 were unavailable for follow-up.

Group 1 had a significantly better survival rate than group 2 at all stages of follow-up (Fig 2–1). The mean patient age at presentation in group 1 was 9 months. Average follow-up was 4 years. Seventy percent of patients had congestive heart failure; 40% had mitral regurgitation. Five patients died. Autopsies showed endocardial fibroelastosis in 4 patients; this finding was also indicated on angiocardiography in 93% of survivors. Ten surviving patients showed improved cardiac status, and 5 remained unchanged.

Group 2 had a mean age of 10 years. Average follow-up was 2 years. Eighty-three percent of patients had congestive heart failure. Unlike the younger group, there was a family history of death caused by dilated cardiomyopathy in 25% of patients. All patients in this group died. These patients had more significant rhythm disturbances and a more rapid course to death than the younger patients.

Risk factors for poor outcome in both groups included persistent cardiomegaly and the development of significant arrhythmias. Cardiac transplantation is recommended for children with onset of dilated cardiomyopathy after age 2 years who survive 1 month. Patients aged younger than 2 years who remain unimproved after 1 year and who have persistent

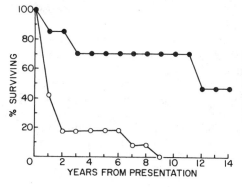

Fig 2–1.—Life-table analysis of 32 patients with dilated cardiomyopathy, 12 (group 1, *shaded circles*) presenting at younger than age 2 years and 12 (group 2, *open circles*) presenting at older than age 2 years. (Courtesy of Griffin ML, Hernandez A, Martin TC, et al: *J Am Coll Cardiol* 11:139–144, January 1988.)

cardiomegaly or complex ventricular arrhythmias might also benefit from transplantation.

▶ Outcome from medical treatment of congestive cardiomyopathy in patients of all ages is poor. This study from St. Louis looks at the question in the pediatric age group. It compromises 20 infants aged younger than 2 years at presentation and 12 patients aged older than 2 years. All 12 older children died, but only 5 of the infants died and 10 improved. The authors identified some significant differences between the 2 age groups that affected outcome and that could be used in prognosis. Group II had a higher incidence of similarly affected family members and had more arrhythmias and a shorter course to death. Group I patients had a diagnosis of endocardial fibroelastosis at autopsy in 4 and on angiocardiography in 93% of survivors. In both groups, risk factors for fatal termination were persistent cardiomegaly and arrhythmias.

With cardiac transplantation currently enjoying greater early success and 5-year survival even in children, this kind of analysis can be useful in deciding about that option.—M.A. Engle, M.D.

Congenital Heart Disease, Medical Aspects

Atrial Septal Defect in Older Adults: Atypical Radiographic Appearances
Sanders C, Bittner V, Nath PH, Breatnach ES, Soto BS (Univ of Alabama in Birmingham; Mater Misericordiae Hosp, Dublin)
Radiology 167:123–127, April 1988   2–9

Patients aged younger than 30 years with atrial septal defect (ASD) generally have typical clinical and radiographic findings, but this is less often the case for older patients. Seventy patients aged older than 50 years with ASD who were seen from 1978 to 1985 were compared with 50 patients aged younger than 50 years. The respective mean ages were 61 and 31 years. All but 2 of the older group were symptomatic at diagnosis. Fifty-three patients had ostium secundum defects.

Nearly one third of the older patients had atypical radiographic findings, such as apparently normal vascularity, left atrial enlargement, pulmonary venous hypertension, and pulmonary edema. Only 6% of the younger patients with ASD had atypical findings. In older patients, pulmonary venous hypertension and pulmonary edema were correlated with smaller defects and higher rates of mitral valve disease, left ventricular dysfunction, and pulmonary arterial hypertension. Older patients with normal vascularity had smaller defects and smaller shunts than those with typical radiographic features of ASD.

Older patients with ASD frequently have atypical radiographic findings. Pulmonary venous hypertension and pulmonary edema in ASD likely are related to the decreased right atrial and ventricular compliance that characterizes aging. An absence of the usual radiographic findings does not rule out ASD in an older patient, especially if mitral valve disease is present.

▶ The most common congenital cardiac anomaly in adults is atrial septal defect. Auscultatory clues may be subtle: the soft systolic murmur in the pulmonary area, the widely and fixedly split second heart sound. Although radiographic features of right-sided and pulmonary arterial volume overload tend to be seen in younger adults, this paper says that, of patients older than 50 years, 30% had atypical and even misleading radiologic findings.—M.A. Engle, M.D.

Progressive Vascular Lesions in Williams-Beuren Syndrome

Ino T, Nishimoto K, Iwahara M, Akimoto K, Boku H, Kaneko K, Tokita A, Yabuta K, Tanaka J (Juntendo Univ, Tokyo)
Pediatr Cardiol 9:55–58, 1988   2–10

Most reported patients with Williams-Beuren syndrome, supravalvular aortic stenosis, and mental retardation have had a variety of cardiovascular anomalies, including peripheral pulmonary stenosis, aortic coarctation, and intracardiac defects. Two patients recently were seen, 1 with progressively severe hypertension due to coarctation of the aorta and the other with progressive renovascular hypertension.

The first patient presented at 1 year of age with poor growth, diffuse ascending aortic hypoplasia, and multiple peripheral pulmonary stenoses. Hypertension appeared at age 10 years, and persisted after a subclavian flap repair of coarctation of the aorta. The patient has been without symptoms on daily calcium antagonist therapy. The second patient presented at age 5 years with diffuse aortic hypoplasia, supravalvular narrowing, and multiple peripheral pulmonary stenoses. The left renal artery was absent and the right one was mildly stenotic. A calcium antagonist and angiotensin-converting enzyme inhibitor were given after renovascular hypertension was diagnosed at age 11 years.

Progressive vascular lesions in Williams-Beuren syndrome may be related to latent abnormalities of calcium metabolism.

▶ Pediatric cardiologists have learned that many congenital cardiac anomalies can change over time and have come to respect the importance of long-term follow-up. For example, ventricular septal defects can close and subaortic and subpulmonic stenosis can develop. This article teaches that long-term follow-up of arterial lesions in Williams-Beuren supravalvular syndrome is important, too.—M.A. Engle, M.D.

Tetralogy of Fallot: A Centennial Review

Anderson RH, Tynan M (Brompton Hosp, London; Guy's Hosp, London)
Int J Cardiol 21:219–232, December 1988   2–11

In tetralogy of Fallot, abnormal anterocephalad location of the outlet septum may unite the various morphologic features (Fig 2–2). The outlet septum is malaligned relative to the rest of the ventricular septum and is attached only within the morphologically right ventricle. This feature

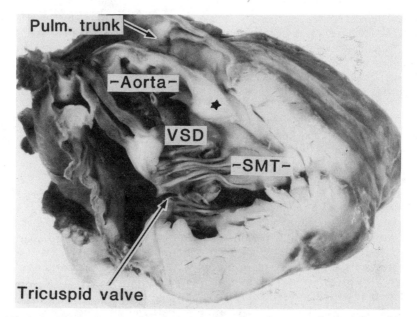

Fig 2–2.—This heart, sectioned in plane to simulate subcostal paracoronal echocardiographic cut, shows salient features of tetralogy of Fallot. *VSD,* ventricular septal defect; *SMT,* septomarginal trabeculation; *Star,* outlet septum. (Courtesy of Anderson RH, Tynan M: *Int J Cardiol* 21:219–232, December 1988.)

highlights the large subaortic ventricular septal defect, the narrowed subpulmonary infundibulum, and the biventricular connection of the overriding aortic valve. Right ventricular hypertrophy is a result of the various anatomical derangements.

The ventricular septal defect in tetralogy is a malalignment defect and is definitely subaortic in location. When the posterior limb of the septomarginal trabeculation is fused with the ventriculoinfundibular fold, discontinuity between the aortic and tricuspid leaflets results. The proximal extent of the subpulmonary infundibulum usually is marked by a prominent muscular orifice. There is considerable variation in the degree of overriding of the aortic valve leaflets.

Associated malformations can affect all parts of the heart. They include interatrial communication, pulmonary artery stenoses, right-sided aortic arch, atrioventricular septal defect, and coronary artery anomalies. Cases of tetralogy with pulmonary atresia are among the many cases in which pulmonary atresia coexists with a ventricular septal defect.

▶ One hundred years ago, Fallot described in cyanotic patients the 4 components of a malformation that bears his name. Fifty years ago Helen Taussig made it meaningful through her diagnostic acumen. Forty-five years ago, Blalock and Taussig made it come to life with the first "blue baby" operation. Now Anderson and Tynan bring the story up to date with their clinical and pathologic insights.—M.A. Engle, M.D.

Congenital Heart Disease: Incidence in the First Year of Life: The Alberta Heritage Pediatric Cardiology Program

Grabitz RG, Joffres MR, Collins-Nakai RL (Univ of Alberta)
Am J Epidemiol 128:381–388, August 1988   2–12

The advent of echocardiography has changed the methods of investigation and follow-up in patients with congenital heart disease. However, recently published studies from Europe and the United States show major variations in the rate of congenital heart disease during the first year of life. These differences may be ascribed to different entry criteria and the use of invasive vs. noninvasive diagnostic methods.

Data on congenital heart disease in northern and central Alberta, Canada, were compared with data from the recently published studies. In Alberta, all cardiac diagnostic procedures, operations, and therapy are provided without direct cost to the patients and their parents. Furthermore, the Heritage Pediatric Cardiology Program offers pediatric cardiology services in 25 outreach clinics in northern and central Alberta.

During a 4-year study period, there were 103,411 live births in the study region, 573 of which were diagnosed with congenital heart disease. All cases were confirmed by a pediatric cardiologist plus echocardiography, with or without 1 or more invasive diagnostic methods. Thus, the prevalence of congenital heart disease for this study was 5.54/1,000 live births.

This prevalence was significantly higher than that reported for the Baltimore–Washington Infant Study, which was 3.69/1,000 live births for noninvasive methods and 2.38/1,000 live births for invasive methods. Although the rates of some lesions were similar to those found in other studies, the number of double outlet right ventricles was 4.4 times higher and the number of atrial septal defects was 2.9 times higher than those reported for the New England Regional Infant Cardiac Program.

During the 4-year study period, the overall congenital heart disease rate in northern and central Alberta increased 47%, and the rate of ventricular septal defects doubled. Analytic studies are presently underway to find out why the incidence of congenital heart disease has increased so much in northern and central Alberta during recent years.

▶ If one includes the usually silent congenital anomaly of bicuspid aortic valve, the incidence of congenital heart disease is probably 1 in 100. It seems to be pretty constant around the world, although certain differences do exist: for instance, the frequency of subpulmonic ventricular septal defects and the paucity of coarctation of the aorta among Oriental persons. Several prospective studies of incidence have been reported in this modern era of accurate noninvasive as well as invasive confirmation of diagnosis.

This study is noteworthy because it was conducted in a well-defined area in Canada with expert pediatric cardiologic capabilities in hospitals and in outreach clinics in a health care setup with full access to free care. The study was prospective, and ascertainment of incidence of congenital heart disease extended from birth through the first birthday. A startling finding was the 47% increase in overall incidence of congenital heart disease and the doubling of incidence of ventricular septal defect.—M.A. Engle, M.D.

Prevalence of Congenital Cardiac Anomalies at High Altitude
Miao C-Y, Zuberbuhler JS, Zuberbuhler JR (High Altitude Research Inst, Xining, China; Children's Hosp of Pittsburgh)
J Am Coll Cardiol 12:224–228, July 1988   2–13

Birth at high altitude reportedly is associated with an increased incidence of patent ductus arteriosus. The effects of altitude on the prevalence of congenital lesions were studied in 1,116 schoolchildren at 4 study sites in China, ranging in altitude from sea level to 4,500 m above sea level. Children suspected of having anomalies underwent echocardiography and ECG study.

Altitude was progressively correlated with an increasing rate of patent ductus arteriosus and atrial septal defect. Both of these anomalies may be related to the lower atmospheric oxygen tension present at high altitude. Patent ductus arteriosus was diagnosed in 9 children, and atrial septal defect, in 18. Fourteen of the latter children had echocardiographic evidence of right ventricular enlargement.

Failure of a lower oxygen tension to constrict the ductus arteriosus explains patent ductus arteriosus at high altitude. It is reasonable to think that persistent high pulmonary vascular resistance and high right heart pressures inhibit early closure of the foramen ovale, and subsequent growth may lead to an atrial septal defect. In the setting of birth at high altitude, atrial septal defect and patent ductus arteriosus probably are not actually congenital cardiac malformations but may reflect hypoxemia-induced failure of normal neonatal processes.

▶ After examining 1,116 schoolchildren at 4 different altitudes from sea level to 4,500 m above sea level, this Chinese-American team confirmed what we have known about greater prevalence of patent ductus arteriosus in children at higher altitudes, but they also found a greater prevalence of atrial septal defect.—M.A. Engle, M.D.

Cardiac Malformations in Relatives of Children With Truncus Arteriosus or Interruption of the Aortic Arch
Pierpont MEM, Gobel JW, Moller JH, Edwards JE (Univ of Minnesota; United Hosp, St Paul)
Am J Cardiol 61:423–427, Feb 15, 1988   2–14

The risk of recurring uncommon congenital cardiac malformations is uncertain. The occurrence of such malformations was examined in relatives of patients seen from 1955 to 1985 with either truncus arteriosus or interruption of the aortic arch (IAA). Fifty-three families with truncus arteriosus and 38 with IAA in an index case were identified.

Two (2.1%) of 98 siblings of patients with IAA had congenital cardiac malformations. All recurrences were in families of patients with type B IAA. Of 106 siblings of patients with truncus arteriosus, 7 (6.6%) had congenital cardiac malformations. Two of them had truncus arteriosus, and 3 had other conotruncal anomalies. Two parents had congenital malformations, including 1 with truncus arteriosus. Five of 7 malformations in second- and third-degree relatives were conotruncal.

Both IAA type B and complex truncus arteriosus are frequently associated with familial recurrence. Families with a child having these anomalies should know of the increased risk in subsequent children. Fetal echocardiography may help in the diagnosis of malformations in subsequent pregnancies.

▶ Now that there are many long-term survivors of congenital heart disease into adulthood, the question of risk of familial clustering of congenital cardiac anomalies is beginning to be answered. The group from the University of Minnesota focused attention on 2 relatively rare anomalies and found that, for interrupted aortic arch, the recurrence rate in siblings was 2.1%; for truncus arteriosus, it was 6.6%; and for complex forms of truncus, it was 13.6%, suggesting single gene inheritance.—M.A. Engle, M.D.

Congenital Heart Disease, Surgical Aspects

Surgical Spectrum of Aortic Stenosis in Children: A Thirty-Year Experience With 257 Children

Brown JW, Stevens LS, Holly S, Robison R, Rodefeld M, Grayson T, Marts B, Caldwell RA, Hurwitz RA, Girod DA, King H (Indiana Univ, Indianapolis)
Ann Thorac Surg 45:393–403, April 1988   2–15

Between 5% and 6% of all children treated for congenital heart disease present with aortic stenosis. The operative results and follow-up for 257

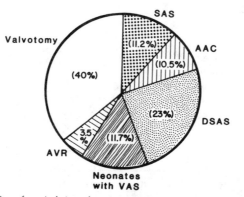

Fig 2–3.—Distribution of surgical sites of aortic stenosis in 257 children. *SAS,* supravalvular aortic stenosis; *AAC,* apicoaortic conduit; *DSAS,* discrete subvalvular aortic stenosis; *VAS,* valvular aortic stenosis; *AVR,* aortic valve replacement. (Courtesy of Brown JW, Stevens LS, Holly S, et al: *Ann Thorac Surg* 45:393—403, April 1988.)

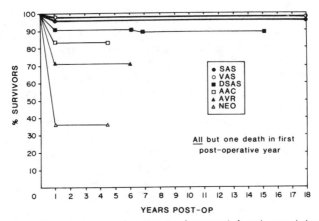

Fig 2–4.—Actuarial survival curves after operation for congenital aortic stenosis in children. *SAS,* supravalvular aortic stenosis; *VAS,* valvular aortic stenosis; *DSAS,* discrete subvalvular aortic stenosis; *AAL,* apicoaortic conduit; *AVR,* aortic valve replacement; *NEO,* aortic valvotomy in neonates. (Courtesy of Brown JW, Stevens LS, Holly S, et al: *Ann Thorac Surg* 45:393–403, April 1988.)

patients who underwent 379 operations in the treatment of congenital aortic stenosis and associated cardiac anomalies during the past 30 years are reviewed.

The patient population consisted of 77 girls and 180 boys aged 1 day to 19 years, with a mean age of 9.6 years. For this analysis the patients were divided into 6 categories by surgical site (Fig 2–3). Twenty-nine (11.2%) had supravalvular aortic stenosis, 104 (40%) had valvular aortic stenosis, 58 (23%) had discrete subvalvular aortic stenosis, 27 (10.5%) had apicoaortic conduit, 9 (3.5%) had aortic valve replacement, and 30 (11.7%) were neonates who had aortic valvotomy.

Angina, syncope, dyspnea, and cardiogenic shock were present in 60% of these patients. Cardiac catheterization was performed in 99% of patients. Mean preoperative gradient for the entire series was 88 mm Hg.

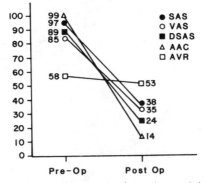

Fig 2–5.—Mean gradient reduction after operation for aortic stenosis in children. *SAS,* supravalvular aortic stenosis; *VAS,* valvular aortic stenosis; *DSAS,* discrete subvalvular aortic stenosis; *AAC,* apicoaortic conduit; *AVR,* aortic valve replacement. (Courtesy of Brown JW, Stevens LS, Holly S, et al: *Ann Thorac Surg* 45:393–403, April 1988.)

There were 28 (11%) early deaths after operation. Excluding the 18 early deaths in the neonatal aortic valvotomy group reduced the operative mortality to 4%. Mean follow-up for the 229 surviving patients was 4.8 years. There were 6 (2%) late deaths (Fig 2–4). Fourteen patients had nonfatal complications, including 2 cases of complete heart block.

Twenty-nine patients (13%) underwent reoperation for residual or recurrent left ventricular outflow tract disease. Postoperative cardiac catheterization was performed in 80% of the surviving patients. Mean postoperative gradient for the entire group was 31 mm Hg, representing an overall gradient reduction of 57 mm Hg (Fig 2–5).

Operative mortality among children older than neonates with single-level aortic stenosis is low, and the patients attain good hemodynamic benefits from operation. The mortality among neonates and those with complex anatomy remains high, but survivors have acceptable hemodynamic benefits.

▶ Congenital aortic stenosis is usually valvar but sometimes supravalvar or subvalvar or both. It is one of the 8 or 10 most common congenital anomalies, and in the extensive experience of the pediatric cardiologists and surgeons at Indianapolis, it constituted 5% to 6% of infants and children operated on for congenital heart disease. This review covers 30 years' experience and includes a follow-up as long as 19 years.

Overall, 89% of those operated upon survived surgery and 84% of survivors had symptomatic relief. The least favorable outcome, not unexpectedly, was in the newborns with critically severe aortic stenosis. Often moribund on admission, these babies required emergency treatment. Excluding them reduced operative mortality to 4%. Aortic insufficiency developed in 42%. Reoperation was needed by 13%. Endocarditis occurred in 5%.

The detailed tables and analyses are very helpful to all of us with the responsibility of caring for these patients in their infancy, childhood, and adult life.—M.A. Engle, M.D.

Long-term Outcome of Patients Undergoing Surgical Repair of Isolated Pulmonary Valve Stenosis: Follow-up at 20–30 Years

Kopecky SL, Gersh BJ, McGoon MD, Mair DD, Porter CJ, Ilstrup DM, McGoon DC, Kirklin JW, Danielson GK (Mayo Clinic, Mayo Found, Rochester, Minn)
Circulation 78:1150–1156, November 1988   2–16

A total of 191 patients had surgery for isolated pulmonary valvular stenosis at the Mayo Clinic during 1956–1967 and were followed for 20 years or longer. Ischemic cardiac arrest was the rule. The mean cardiopulmonary bypass time was 41 minutes, and the mean aortic cross-clamp time was 17 minutes. Eighteen patients received a transvalvular pulmonary outflow patch, most often of prosthetic material. After repair the mean peak systolic right ventricular pressure fell 76 mm Hg.

Eight patients died within 30 days of surgery. The 183 surviving patients, followed for a mean of 24 years, had a mortality of 9.2%, significantly but not markedly greater than expected in a normal population. There were 11 deaths caused by cardiovascular disease, 3 of them sudden. Nine other patients had cardiovascular events during follow-up. Five of them were reoperated on for pulmonary stenosis, and 2 had a permanent pacemaker implanted. Functional disability in late-surviving patients was minimal. No patient reported symptoms at last follow-up.

Excellent survival and cardiac function are possible 20 to 30 years after the repair of isolated pulmonary valve stenosis. Late survival is good, though somewhat less than in an age- and sex-matched control group.

▶ If one could choose which anomaly the patient with congenital heart disease has, the choices would be one of these: patent ductus arteriosus, atrial septal defect, or valvar pulmonic stenosis. All can be easily diagnosed and successfully treated surgically. This long-term follow-up study shows that life expectancy is normal for patients undergoing valvotomy before the age of 21 years.— M.A. Engle, M.D.

Late Results in Patients With Tetralogy of Fallot Repaired During Infancy

Walsh EP, Rockenmacher S, Keane JF, Hougen TJ, Lock JE, Castaneda AR (Harvard Med School)
Circulation 77:1062–1067, May 1988   2–17

The early results of primary repair of tetralogy of Fallot in infancy are encouraging. The late results in 220 infants repaired at age 18 months or younger were analyzed. The mean age at operation was 7 months. Seventeen infants died within a month of surgery, and 184 of the surviving infants were followed up for a mean time of 5 years. Of the original infants, 69% had uncomplicated tetralogy of Fallot and 11% had tetralogy of Fallot with pulmonary atresia. A patch was placed across a hypoplastic or atretic pulmonary anulus in 85% of cases.

On postoperative hemodynamic assessment 15 months after repair, 24 patients had right ventricular peak systolic gradients exceeding 40 mm Hg, usually associated with residual infundibular or pulmonary artery narrowing. Reoperation was required by 24 patients during follow-up, but only 10% of surviving infants with uncomplicated tetralogy of Fallot had further surgery. Only 1 patient has had symptomatic arrhythmia, and no patient currently is on antiarrhythmic drug treatment. One of 3 late deaths was ascribed to pulmonary vascular disease in a patient with large aortopulmonary collaterals.

The infrequent occurrence of significant arrhythmias after primary repair of tetralogy of Fallot in infancy is encouraging. Arrhythmias may be less likely after early relief of right ventricular hypertension, normalization of left ventricular volume, and correction of systemic desaturation.

▶ A trend of the past decade and a half has been that of open repair of tetralogy of Fallot in infancy instead of initial palliation followed later by open heart surgery. Boston's Children's Hospital has led the way, and now its cardiologic and surgical teams report their results in 91% of long-term survivors. Early mortality was 7.7%; late mortality was 2%. Reoperation or interventional catheterization took place in 17%. Incidence of ventricular ectopy or sudden death was low, and hemodynamic outcome was generally acceptable.—M.A. Engle, M.D.

Survival, Functional Status, and Reoperation After Repair of Tetralogy of Fallot With Pulmonary Atresia
Kirklin JW, Blackstone EH, Shimazaki Y, Maehara T, Pacifico AD, Kirklin JK, Bargeron LM Jr (Univ of Alabama in Birmingham; Alabama Congenital Heart Disease Diagnosis and Treatment Ctr, Birmingham)
J Thorac Cardiovasc Surg 96:102–116, July 1988   2–18

Survival was analyzed for up to 20 years in 139 patients who underwent repair of tetralogy of Fallot with pulmonary atresia in 1967–1986. Twenty-nine percent of patients had not undergone surgery before repair. One hundred patients were alive at the end of follow-up. Twenty-two patients died in hospital, and 17 died after discharge.

Survival 1 month after operation was 85%. Survival rates after 1, 5, 10, and 20 years were 82%, 76%, 69%, and 58%, respectively. The hazard function declined from immediately after operation, but a low level of hazard persisted for the duration of follow-up. The factor most predictive of death after repair was the postrepair ratio of peak right and left ventricular pressures, followed by the time on cardiopulmonary bypass. Among morphologic abnormalities, the size of the pulmonary arteries was most informative, followed by the number of large aortopulmonary collateral arteries. Three percent of hospital survivors required reoperation for recurrent or residual ventricular septal defect. Most survivors were in New York Heart Association class I at follow-up.

Survival is poorer after repair of tetralogy with pulmonary atresia than after that of tetralogy with pulmonary stenosis. The postrepair peak right ventricular/left ventricular pressure ratio and the risk of death both are related inversely to the size of the pulmonary arteries and directly to the number of large aortopulmonary collateral arteries. Current data indicate that reoperation will be necessary less often with the use of allograft valved conduits than with xenograft valved conduits.

▶ This excellent analysis of a large and carefully followed series of patients with that form of tetralogy of Fallot in which pulmonary atresia occurs offers indicators of outcome up to 20 years after surgical repair. It is comforting to know that nearly 70% can be expected to survive for 10 years and almost 60% for 20 years in New York Heart Association class I, a real turnaround from what would be expected from the natural history of this condition.—M.A. Engle, M.D.

Anatomic Repair of Anomalies of Ventriculoarterial Connection Associated With Ventricular Septal Defect: I. Criteria of Surgical Decision

Sakata R, Lecompte Y, Batisse A, Borromée L, Durandy Y (Centre Médico-Chirurgical de la Porte de Choisy, Paris)

J Thorac Cardiovasc Surg 95:90–95, January 1988   2–19

Congenital malformations of the heart appear in many forms, and the choice of surgical repair is not always clear. An attempt has been made to classify malformations according to a simplified and practical method.

All ventriculoarterial connections that are not normal are called anomalous. In this context anatomical repair is any procedure that seeks to connect, without an external conduit, the left ventricle to the aorta and the right ventricle to the pulmonary artery.

Three types of repair are currently used: intraventricular, in which a patch is used to achieve a normal ventriculoarterial connection; the arterial switch operation; and réparation à l'étage ventriculaire (REV) in which the right ventricle is connected to the pulmonary artery. The first type is the simplest and often best choice, but REV should be used when pulmonary outflow tract obstruction occurs, and arterial switch is suitable for cases of pulmonary regurgitation.

In 2 studies, 1 retrospective and 1 prospective, the records of 104 patients who were undergoing surgery for ventriculoarterial anomalies were analyzed. The distance between the tricuspid anulus and pulmonary anulus was crucial and determined the means of connecting the left ventricle to the aorta. Echocardiography was judged to be more accurate than angiography at estimating distances. Only 1 case required a prosthetic conduit for surgical repair. Experience with these patients showed that preoperative pulmonary blood flow should be low to avoid pulmonary regurgitation.

Anatomic Repair of Anomalies of Ventriculoarterial Connection Associated With Ventricular Septal Defect: II. Clinical Results in 50 Patients With Pulmonary Outflow Tract Obstruction

Borromée L, Lecompte Y, Batisse A, Lemoine G, Vouhé P, Sakata R, Leca F, Zannini L, Neveux J-Y (Centre Médico-Chirurgical de la Porte de Choisy, Paris; Hôpital Laennec, Paris)

J Thorac Cardiovasc Surg 95:96–102, January 1988   2–20

During a 5-year period 50 patients aged 4 months to 13 years underwent réparation à l'étage ventriculaire (REV). Twenty-four of the children had a variety of anomalies, which made it impossible to connect the right ventricle to the pulmonary artery by using the pulmonary orifice, the method used in "classic" transposition of the great arteries.

The surgical technique was similar in the 50 patients: resection of the infundibular septum; connection of the aorta to the left ventricle with a patch; and translocation of the pulmonary artery, with pulmonary bifurcation placed anterior or posterior to the ascending aorta, according to the initial position of the great arteries.

Nine patients died in the hospital. Fewer deaths were reported as the surgeons became more experienced with the REV procedure. One late death occurred and 6 patients had complications. Twenty-six of the 29 patients who were followed up for longer than 1 year enjoyed excellent clinical status and required no further treatment.

When septal resection is used, no external conduit is required. A prosthetic device is not desirable in small children because of its lack of growth potential. Results from this group of 50 children suggest that REV is a valuable technique for treating children with ventriculoarterial anomalies.

▶ These 2 companion articles (Abstracts 2–19 and 2–20) from the team in Paris first reported their simplified nomenclature for a variety of complex malformations of ventriculoarterial connection and their analysis of surgical approaches based on anatomical and physiologic concepts and then presented the results of their reconstructive surgery for patients who had ventricular septal defect and pulmonic stenosis together with abnormal ventriculoatrial connection.

The simplified nomenclature has merit, for there are so many variations and degrees of abnormalities in this large group that encompasses double outlet right ventricle (including Taussig-Bing anomaly) and double outlet left ventricle as well as transposition of the great arteries with ventricular septal defect. Their goals at operation are commendable: to connect the left ventricle to the aorta and right ventricle to the pulmonary artery and to avoid an external conduit. They accomplished these goals in 82% of 50 children with ventricular septal defect and pulmonary stenosis as part of the malformation.—M.A. Engle, M.D.

Doppler Echocardiographic Comparison of Haemodynamic Results of One- and Two-Stage Anatomic Correction of Complete Transposition
Gibbs JL, Qureshi SA, Wilson N, Radley Smith R, Yacoub MH (Killingbeck Hosp, Leeds; Harefield Hosp, Middlesex, England)
Int J Cardiol 18:85–92, 1987   2–21

A recent study reported that Doppler echocardiography provides extensive hemodynamic data after anatomical correction of transposition of the great arteries using the arterial switch operation. Whether Doppler ultrasound can also detect hemodynamic changes after 1-stage and 2-stage anatomical correction of complete transposition was examined.

Cross-sectional echocardiography and pulsed and continuous wave Doppler ultrasound were used to study 36 children with complete transposition, 18 of whom had undergone 1-stage anatomical correction and 18 who had undergone 2-stage operations. All children were operated on when they were between 1 week and 3 years old.

After single-stage operation, peak mitral flow velocities showed no significant difference from normal, but peak mitral flow velocities were significantly higher than normal after 2-stage correction. Peak tricuspid flow velocities were significantly higher than normal in both groups. The significance of increased peak flow velocities across the tricuspid valve after both types of repair and across the mitral valve after 2-stage repair is not yet known. There was no significant difference in pulmonary artery flow velocities between the 2 groups. Peak velocities in the ascending aorta were within normal limits after single-stage correction but were lower than normal in 2-stage patients. Twenty-two percent of the single-stage patients and 55% of the 2-stage patients had mild aortic regurgitation.

Doppler ultrasound is useful in the postoperative investigation of hemodynamic patterns in children who have undergone either single-stage or 2-stage anatomical correction of complete transposition of the great arteries, as it allows accurate assessment of ventricular filling patterns and ventricular diastolic behavior.

▶ In mid- and long-term evaluation that is so crucial for a relatively new surgical procedure such as the arterial switch repair of transposition of the great arteries, noninvasive procedures offer a great advantage in serial studies. This team from the United Kingdom has regularly reported their results and has shared with us what they have learned. This Doppler echo study provided a new approach to assessing ventricular filling patterns and diastolic behavior. It compared the flow velocities after 1-stage or 2-stage repair. In both, tricuspid peak flow velocities were higher than normal and there was mild supravalvular pulmonic stenosis, but mild aortic regurgitation was more common in 2-stage than after 1-stage repair (55% versus 22%).—M.A. Engle, M.D.

Arterial Switch in Simple and Complex Transposition of the Great Arteries

Idriss FS, Ilbawi MN, DeLeon SY, Duffy CE, Muster AJ, Berry TE, Paul MH (Children's Mem Hosp, Chicago; Northwestern Univ, Chicago)
J Thorac Cardiovasc Surg 95:29–36, January 1988   2–22

Arterial switch is an alternative to intra-atrial venous rerouting in the operative treatment of transposition of the great arteries. The results of arterial switching (Fig 2–6) in 53 infants and children since October 1983 at Children's Memorial Hospital are reported. The patients were divided into group I, 25 infants with intact ventricular septums who had primary repair within their first month of life; group II, 13 patients with an intact ventricular septum who had anatomical repair after a preliminary procedure; and group III, 15 infants with a ventricular septal defect.

Six patients in group III had a Taussig-Bing abnormality, 9 had pulmonary artery banding, and 3 had previous coarctation of the aorta. Four infants in group III were aged younger than 2 weeks at operation.

Overall early operative mortality was 9.4%. Mortality in group I was 8%, in group II it was 7.6%, and in group III it was 13.3%. Three late deaths occurred in group II.

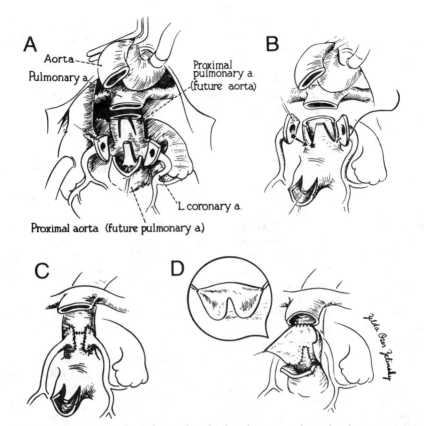

Fig 2–6.—Steps in arterial switch procedure detailing dissection and transfer of coronary arteries and implantation of coronary artery cuffs in off-axis location (**B**). Reconstruction of pulmonary artery (**D**) with pantaloon *(inset)* pericardial patch. Incision in pulmonary artery and final location of coronary artery cuffs are fairly distal (**A, B, C**) so as not to interfere with new aortic valve function and at same time to minimize kinking of coronary arteries. *a,* artery. *L,* left. (Courtesy of Idriss FS, Ilbawi MN, De-Leon SY, et al: *J Thorac Cardiovasc Surg* 95:29–36, January 1988.)

The surviving patients generally continue to do well and nearly all have normal sinus rhythm. Ventricular function was within normal range in all but 2 patients. Right ventricular pressure was 27 to 42 mm Hg in 12 patients and was 55 mm Hg in 2. There was no aortic stenosis.

The arterial switch is effective in treating transposition of the great arteries with or without ventricular septal defect in neonates and children.

▶ The cardiologists and cardiac surgeons from Chicago have had a long and extensive experience with children who have transposed great arteries, from the early days of cardiac surgery with the Baffee's partial venous rerouting procedure to the present report of the results of the arterial switch operation of Jatene. They analyzed 53 patients who could be divided into 3 groups: intact ventricular septum and primary repair in the first month, intact septum repaired after pulmonary artery banding, and ventricular septal defect. Five died early (mortality, 9.4%), and 3 died later. Early results were good, with moderate pulmonic stenosis in 2 and aortic insufficiency in 4 survivors. Results such as these have now been reported from several centers.—M.A. Engle, M.D.

Surgical Risk Factors in Total Anomalous Pulmonary Venous Connection
Lincoln CR, Rigby ML, Mercanti C, Al-Fagih M, Joseph MC, Miller GA, Shinebourne EA (Brompton Hosp, London)
Am J Cardiol 61:608–611, March 1, 1988   2–23

Some infants with total anomalous pulmonary venous connection may die if surgery is postponed. But surgery at an early age has been considered risky because of factors that include preoperative condition and anatomical types. A retrospective review of 83 patients treated by 1 surgeon in a 13-year period was conducted to determine the importance of risk factors in treatment for total anomalous pulmonary venous connection.

The infants were divided into 4 groups: 32 had supracardiac drainage; 16 had infracardiac drainage; in 27, the connection was to the coronary sinus; 8 had connection to the right atrium or mixed anomalous drainage. Median age at the time of operation was 60 days. Fifteen patients underwent conventional cardiopulmonary bypass with profound to moderate hypothermia. In 68, surgical correction was achieved using profound hypothermia and circulatory arrest.

Twelve patients died within 30 days of the operation, and 6 died at later times after surgery. Seven infants required a second operation. A review of 30-day survival rates found that significant risk factors for early death were infracardiac anomalous connection, postoperative pulmonary hypertensive crises, and preoperative heart and renal failure. Girls had a higher death rate than boys, and mortality decreased over the years of the operation.

Because improvement of survival occurred when the infants underwent echocardiography but not cardiac catheterization and angiography, echocardiography is now recommended by the authors as the definitive diagnostic test. Their recent experience reveals only 1 mistaken anatomical diagnosis, and the patient survived.

▶ The points of entry of anomalously draining pulmonary veins as well as the presence or absence of obstruction to flow determine the severity of symptoms and thus the time of presentation of those born with this unusual anomaly. It is still easier to diagnose than it is successfully to treat this fortunately uncommon anomaly. In the first 30 days postoperatively, 8.5% of the patients died, whereas 10% died later and 10% required late reoperation. Actuarial survival for the whole group was 75% at 7 years, but outlook was less favorable for those with infradiaphragmatic than with supradiaphragmatic drainage.

On an optimistic note, it is encouraging to know that use of echocardiographic definitive diagnosis and avoidance of preoperative cardiac catheterization in these newborns who are critically ill has had a favorable effect on their postoperative course and survival.—M.A. Engle, M.D.

Fate of the Pulmonic Valve After Proximal Pulmonary Artery-to-Ascending Aorta Anastomosis for Aortic Outflow Obstruction
Chin AJ, Barber G, Helton JG, Alboliras ET, Aglira BA, Pigott JD, Norwood WI
(Children's Hosp of Philadelphia; Univ of Pennsylvania)
Am J Cardiol 62:435–438, Sept 1, 1988   2–24

Transection of the main pulmonary artery and end-to-side anastomosis of the proximal pulmonary artery to the ascending aorta are increasingly being selected for the palliative treatment of cardiac malformations, such as hypoplastic left heart syndrome and single ventricle with small outlet foramen. Pulmonary valve competence after this procedure was evaluated, using color Doppler ultrasound flow mapping.

The study was done with 45 survivors of anastomosis of the pulmonary artery to ascending aorta who underwent their first color Doppler examination at a median of 202 days after operation. At the time of anastomosis, the 37 infants with hypoplastic left heart syndrome ranged in age from 1 to 63 days, and the 8 infants with other lesions, from 5 to 377 days. The patients' ages at the time of Doppler examination ranged from 4 days to 2.8 years.

Although none of the 37 patients with hypoplastic left heart syndrome had pulmonary regurgitation or abnormal pulmonary valve morphology before operation, mild regurgitation was detected in 9 (24%) patients, and moderate regurgitation, in 1 (3%), postoperatively. Among the 8 patients with other lesions, mild regurgitation was detected in 2 patients and moderate regurgitation, in 1 patient. The latter patient expired on the third postoperative day before cardiac catheterization and angiography could be performed. Regurgitation was detected in 7 of the 11 patients who were imaged more than 12 months postoperatively.

Pulmonary regurgitation appeared at some time after palliative surgery in approximately one fourth of patients who survived pulmonary artery-to-ascending aorta anastomosis. However, it was usually mild, and pulmonary regurgitation of this degree should not be considered a contraindication to this procedure.

▶ The modern era of surgery for congenital heart disease has created 2 situations in which the pulmonic valve is required to function as the aortic valve during systole and diastole. The 2 procedures that cause this anomaly of function are (1) the arterial switch operation devised by Jatene for complete transposition of the great arteries (TGA) and (2) the palliative Norwood operation for hypoplastic left heart (HLH) syndromes. Is the pulmonic valve up to the task? Early follow-up reports from several centers describe the occurrence of "aortic" regurgitation in some children after the arterial switch operation for TGA, and this report from Norwood's group describes mild regurgitation in 24% and moderate regurgitation in 3% of 37 survivors with HLH followed up for as long as 202 days. It seems that we cannot take for granted that the semilunar valve designed for a low-pressure system will function adequately in a high-pressure circuit.—M.A. Engle, M.D.

Echocardiography

Impact of Two-Dimensional and Doppler Echocardiography on Care of Children Aged Two Years and Younger

Alboliras ET, Seward JB, Hagler DJ, Danielson GK, Puga FJ, Tajik AJ (Mayo Clinic, Mayo Found, Rochester, Minn)
Am J Cardiol 61:166–169, Jan 1, 1988   2–25

The influence of 2-dimensional and Doppler echocardiography on young children with suspected heart disease was assessed by comparing management of and outcome for 161 patients seen in 1975 with those related to 206 patients seen in 1985, when these techniques were available. Only children aged 2 years and younger participated in the study. M-mode echocardiography was not widely used in 1975. In subsequent years, 77% of patients underwent 2-D echocardiography. Most patients had pulsed-wave or continuous-wave Doppler studies as well.

The rate of catheterization declined from 48% to 21%, and recatheterization also was less prevalent when echocardiography was routinely practiced. More of the later patients underwent surgery without first having catheterization. In infants with several common anomalies, preoperative catheterization was omitted. Operative mortality was similar in the 2 periods. In 1985, mortality was similar whether or not preoperative catheterization was carried out. The primary diagnosis did not change after catheterization in 1985, but echocardiography altered the diagnosis in 18% of cases.

Catheterization is required less often in young infants as echocardiography becomes widely available. Today cardiac catheterization is goal-directed and is used to delineate specific hemodynamic features. In addition, catheterization is used for therapeutic purposes such as balloon angioplasty.

▶ All pediatric cardiologists attest to the tremendous impact that development of 2-dimensional echocardiographic imaging has had. In older children it has often rendered unnecessary the performance of preoperative and postoperative cardiac catheterization. This analysis by Mayo Clinic physicians of the change in their practice as it affects children aged younger than 2 years established that, in infants as well, 2-D and Doppler echocardiography often substitute satisfactorily for cardiac catheterization.—M.A. Engle, M.D.

Accuracy of Doppler Echocardiography in Quantification of Left to Right Shunts in Adult Patients With Atrial Septal Defect

Dittman H, Jacksch R, Voelker W, Karsch K-R, Seipel L (Univ of Tübingen, West Germany)
J Am Coll Cardiol 11:338–342, February 1988   2–26

The ratio of pulmonary to systemic flow in various cardiac shunt lesions was accurately estimated with Doppler echocardiography in experimental and pediatric studies. The accuracy of pulsed Doppler echocardiography in determining the volume of shunt flow in adult patients with ostium secundum type atrial septal defects was investigated.

The pulmonary and systemic flows were measured with Doppler echocardiography in the right and left ventricular outflow tracts in 32 patients evenly divided between those who had heart disease and those who did not. The ratio of pulmonary to systemic flow by oximetry was compared with the Doppler findings.

There was a significant correlation between the 2 methods in the 16 patients with an ostium secundum type atrial defect. When the group was taken as a whole, the correlation was even higher. There were no systemic differences between the invasive and noninvasive shunt calculations.

With high-quality echocardiograms, the magnitude of left to right shunt can be accurately assessed with pulsed Doppler echocardiography in adult patients with atrial septal defects of the secundum type. In the absence of pulmonary hypertension, this method provides precise information affecting the decision for conservative or operative treatment.

▶ In pediatric cardiology we have come to rely heavily on 2-dimensional echocardiography with Doppler studies to confirm the diagnosis of atrial septal defect (ASD) and to identify its site, size, and shape and the drainage of the pulmonary veins. The study has replaced preoperative cardiac catheterization in typical cases. This study is an evaluation of the utility of this methodology in adults with ASD, with a finding that, in the absence of pulmonary hypertension, pulsed Doppler echocardiography provides precise assessment of the left-to-right shunt across secundum-type ASDs.—M.A. Engle, M.D.

Accuracy of Two-Dimensional Echocardiography in the Diagnosis of Aortic Arch Obstruction
Nihoyannopoulos P, Karas S, Sapsford RN, Hallidie-Smith K, Foale R (Royal Postgraduate Med School, Hammersmith Hosp, London)
J Am Coll Cardiol 10:1072–1077, November 1987   2–27

Obstruction at the level of the aortic arch has traditionally been diagnosed with cardiac catheterization. Recent studies have shown that aortic arch obstruction can be accurately diagnosed with the use of 2-dimensional echocardiography aided by conventional or color flow-imaging techniques. Doppler and color flow-imaging techniques and the expertise to use these techniques are less widely available than 2-dimensional echocardiography.

In a 2-year study, the predictive accuracy of 2-dimensional echocardiography in diagnosing aortic arch obstruction was evaluated in 540 consecutive patients, aged 2 days to 15 years, who subsequently underwent cardiac catheterization and angiography for verification of the echocardiographic findings.

At angiography, 51 patients were found to have aortic arch obstruc-

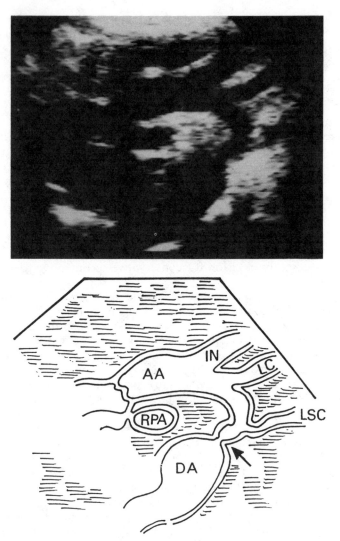

Fig 2–7.—Suprasternal echocardiographic view of aortic arch from patient with juxtaductal coarctation. Note localized infolding of posterior descending aorta *(DA, arrow)* followed by poststenotic dilation. *AA,* ascending aorta; *IN,* right innominate artery; *LC,* left carotid artery; *LSC,* left subclavian artery; and *RPA,* right pulmonary artery. (Courtesy of Nihoyannopoulos P, Karas S, Sapsford RN, et al: *J Am Coll Cardiol* 10:1072–1077, November 1987.)

tion, including 35 with juxtaductal coarctation, 15 with isthmic hypoplasia, and 1 with a type B interrupted aortic arch. Three of the 51 patients died before cardiac catheterization could be performed, and 5 other patients died after cardiac catheterization while awaiting surgical correction. All 43 remaining patients underwent surgical repair of the narrowed segment of the aortic arch. Two more patients died during the immediate postoperative period.

Two-dimensional echocardiography was used to correctly identify aortic arch obstruction in 45 of 51 patients, for an overall sensitivity of 88%; correctly define juxtaductal coarctation in 33 of 35 patients (Fig 2–7), for a sensitivity of 94%; and correctly identify isthmic hypoplasia in 13 of 15 patients, for a sensitivity of 73%. However, 2-dimensional echocardiography was used to incorrectly identify the presence of aortic arch obstruction in 9 of the 489 patients who did not have such an obstruction, for an overall specificity of 98%.

These results show that 2-dimensional echocardiography is highly specific for diagnosing aortic arch obstruction and is reliable for distinguishing juxtaductal coarctation from isthmic hypoplasia. However, the technique is less sensitive for predicting isthmic hypoplasia during the neonatal period.

▶ These authors from London report remarkable diagnostic accuracy with 2-dimensional echocardiography (2-D-E) in identifying abnormalities of the obstructed aortic arch and in recognizing associated intracardiac defects. This is especially significant information for pediatric cardiologists dealing with critically sick newborns with suspected coarctation of the aorta and frequently with accompanying intracardiac malformations. If one can make the correct diagnosis noninvasively, then immediate medical management of cardiac failure and metabolic or respiratory acidosis can be followed by surgical repair without intervening cardiac catheterization.

In this study with echocardiographic diagnosis before catheterization, 51 of 540 infants and children had aortic arch obstruction. Overall sensitivity was 88%. Sensitivity was 94% for juxtaductal coarctation (33 of 35 patients) but 73% (13 of 15 patients) for isthmic hypoplasia. Overall specificity was 98%; 2-D-E was used to wrongly diagnose aortic arch obstruction in 9 of 489 patients who did not have it.

The authors are right when they say that Doppler studies should provide even greater diagnostic accuracy.— M.A. Engle, M.D.

Color Doppler Flow Mapping in Patients With Coarctation of the Aorta: New Observations and Improved Evaluation With Color Flow Diameter and Proximal Acceleration as Predictors of Severity
Simpson IA, Sahn DJ, Valdes-Cruz LM, Chung KJ, Sherman FS, Swensson RE
(Univ of California, San Diego, La Jolla)
Circulation 77:736–744, April 1988   2–28

Color Doppler flow mapping was performed in 15 patients with coarctation of the aorta that was later confirmed with angiography or surgery. The goal was to accurately delineate the extent of narrowing of flow at the site of coarctation. The patients (aged 1 week to 17 years) had native coarctation or, in 3 instances, mild recoarctation after surgical repair. A digital analysis package served to analyze the color Doppler flow maps.

Satisfactory echographic images and color flow maps were obtained in all patients but 1. The diameter in the area of coarctation was correlated well with the measured diameter at angiography. However, 2-dimensional echographic estimates of coarctation diameter were not predictive of the angiographic severity of coarctation. Narrowing of the area of acceleration in the proximal descending aorta also was correlated with angiographic severity. Highly turbulent flow was evident distal to the coarctation and continued into diastole in patients with increased diastolic flow velocity on continuous-wave Doppler imaging.

Color Doppler flow mapping improves the noninvasive evaluation of patients with coarctation of the aorta. Flow velocity is depicted spatially in relation to structural detail. In conjunction with digital video computer analysis, this method will provide insight into circulatory events in the descending aorta in patients with coarctation.

▶ Diagnosis of coarctation of the aorta is made at the bedside. One palpates simultaneously the radial pulses and then radial and femoral pulses. Stronger radial than femoral pulse, together with lower pressure in the legs than arms, makes the diagnosis. One often hears a systolic murmur in the left interscapular area over the site of narrowing. Ribnotching on x-ray films is the effect of collateral circulation. Doppler echocardiography confirms the diagnosis. Now this study with color flow mapping enhances the accuracy of that study and provides interesting information about turbulence and the mechanism of poststenotic dilatation.— M.A. Engle, M.D.

Doppler Ultrasound Evaluation of Valvar Pulmonary Stenosis From Multiple Transducer Positions in Children Requiring Pulmonary Valvuloplasty
Frantz EG, Silverman NH (Univ of California, San Francisco)
Am J Cardiol 61:844–849, April 1, 1988   2–29

The peak pressure differences across stenotic pulmonary valves can be determined using the modified Bernoulli equation. If the direction of the poststenotic jet is eccentric in relation to the axis of the pulmonary artery, the maximal velocity determined from the parasternal transducer position may inaccurately estimate peak pressure difference. A study was conducted to determine whether the use of multiple transducer positions would improve the accuracy of pressure-difference estimates in children undergoing balloon pulmonary valvuloplasty.

Doppler-derived estimates of pressure difference from the subcostal, parasternal, apical, and suprasternal notch transducer positions were compared with peak-to-peak pulmonary artery to right ventricle catheter withdrawal pressure differences in 24 patients. Studies were performed both before and after valvuloplasty.

Before cardiac catheterization, suprasternal, subcostal, or apical transducer positions produced higher maximal velocities than did the parasternal transducer position in 12 of 24 patients. This was also true in 8 of 12 patients studied during catheterization. The transducer position yielding the highest maximum velocity in a given patient was the same before and after valvuloplasty. The correlation with pressure at cardiac catheterization improved when the highest maximal velocity, rather than the parasternal maximal velocity, was used.

Multiple transducer positions improve the accuracy of estimates of pressure difference. The highest correlation with pressure at catheterization is achieved by using the highest maximal velocity.

▶ Noninvasive modalities in cardiac diagnosis begin with the stethoscope and careful attention to heart sounds and murmurs, then to interpretation of the ECG for hypertrophy or "strain" and the x-ray film for volume load. In no instance of congenital heart disease is this bedside evaluation more accurate in making the diagnosis and assessing its severity than in valvular pulmonic stenosis. Echocardiography with Doppler sampling is the single most useful diagnostic study that is next employed in patients with congenital heart disease. In the case of pulmonary stenosis, the correlation of Doppler estimates of pressure gradient with cardiac catheterization has been less good than with the aforementioned simple methods. The reason for this is that the jet through the stenotic valve may be eccentric. Doctors Frantz and Silverman found that the correlation is improved by seeking the highest maximal velocity rather than using a standard parasternal view to judge the gradient.—M.A. Engle, M.D.

An Echocardiographic Study of the Association of Ventricular Septal Defect and Right Ventricular Muscle Bundles With a Fixed Subaortic Abnormality
Vogel M, Smallhorn JF, Freedom RM, Coles J, Williams WG, Trusler GA (Univ of Toronto; Hosp for Sick Children, Toronto)
Am J Cardiol 61:857–860, April 1, 1988   2–30

The incidence of subaortic abnormality in patients with anomalous right ventricular muscle bundles and ventricular septal defect (VSD) has not been established. Thirty-six patients with combined right ventricular muscle bundles and perimembranous VSD were studied to determine the frequency of associated subaortic abnormality.

Patients were assessed with Doppler echocardiography. To determine the frequency of the association of right ventricular muscle bundles and VSD with a subaortic abnormality, the incidence of each abnormality alone was determined for the same time period.

There was echocardiographic evidence of a subaortic abnormality in 88% of patients with combined VSD and right ventricular muscle bundles. All but 3 patients had a typical subaortic ridge protruding from the crest of the interventricular septum. The others had an echodense area in this location. Surgical confirmation was available for 26 patients; surgical and echocardiographic findings were correlated in all patients. Only 10 patients had resting Doppler gradients greater than or equal to 10 mm Hg. Six patients had evidence of progression of their gradient.

The incidence of subaortic abnormality in association with right ventricular muscle bundles and VSD appears to be far more frequent than previously believed. The exact significance of this finding in the absence of a measurable pressure gradient remains to be discovered, although data suggest progression in some patients. Resection of the subaortic ab-normality at the time of surgical correction of the associated lesions is recommended.

▶ The natural history of ventricular septal defect (VSD) continues to evolve. In the really early days of our knowledge of congenital heart disease, VSD was regarded as a benign condition with no cardiopulmonary burden. Eisenmenger syndrome was recognized at autopsy, then during life with studies at cardiac catheterization that measured the pulmonary hypertension and elevated pulmonary vascular resistance that led to right-to-left shunting. It was not until the mid-1950s that we appreciated that large VSDs were common and that they caused cardiac failure and often death or, in survivors, an Eisenmenger reaction. About that time we also learned that large and small defects could spontaneously decrease in size or close and also that infundibular pulmonic stenosis could be acquired, especially in Orientals.

This manuscript describes what we are now recognizing with increasing frequency because of 2-dimensional echocardiography: the development of fixed subaortic stenosis that may itself call for surgery.—M.A. Engle, M.D.

The Cross Sectional Anatomy of Ventricular Septal Defects: A Reappraisal
Baker EJ, Leung MP, Anderson RH, Fischer DR, Zuberbuhler JR (Children's Hosp of Pittsburgh)
Br Heart J 59:339–351, March 1988   2–31

An attempt was made to learn which morphological features of ventricular septal defects (VSDs) are more important in interpreting cross-sectional echocardiographic images. Analysis of 100 specimens of VSD revealed 3 groups of defects: those abutting the central fibrous body, those with a margin formed partly by an area of fibrous continuity between the aortic and pulmonary valve leaflets, and those with solely muscular margins. These groups had distinctive features in cross section. Defects opening between the 2 ventricular inlets and those opening between the 2 subarterial outlets were evident in cross-sectional images, as were defects that extended solely into the trabecular septum.

This classification is equally applicable to hearts having discordant atrioventricular connection, discordant ventriculoarterial connection, common arterial trunk, or double outlet from the morphological right ventricle. Cross-sectional imaging is the most informative approach to studying ventricular septal defects, because it defines morphological detail at the defect margins very clearly.

▶ Ventricular septal defect is probably the single most common and most interesting congenital cardiac malformation. It comes in various sizes and locations in the septum, and these aspects affect that patient's health and prognosis. Echocardiographic imaging and Doppler sampling of flows and pressures have been enormously valuable. This study combines a clinical-pathologic approach to standardization of nomenclature that should be applicable to all situations involving a ventricular septal defect.—M.A. Engle, M.D.

Electrophysiology

Conduction Disturbances After Correction of Tetralogy of Fallot: Are Electrophysiologic Studies of Prognostic Value?

Friedli B, Bolens M, Taktak M (Hôpital Cantonal Universitaire, Geneva; Hôpital La Rabta, Tunis, Tunisia)
J Am Coll Cardiol 11:162–165, January 1988   2–32

Late sudden death and syncopal episodes occasionally occur after successful correction of tetralogy of Fallot. This type of late complication usually results from either ventricular arrhythmia or advanced conduction disturbances. To determine whether electrophysiologic study (EPS) could identify patients at risk of having late conduction disturbances, 57 persons aged 1.5 to 20 years underwent EPS 2 months to 7 years after undergoing correction of tetralogy of Fallot or of double outlet right ventricle. These patients were followed up for 1–13 years after the first postoperative investigation.

Electrophysiologic study was used to identify 13 children with conduction intervals that were abnormal for age. Pacing-induced atrioventricular block at the supra-His bundle level occurred in 48 studies. Seven patients had Wenckebach block during atrial pacing at rates lower than expected for age, suggesting atrioventricular node dysfunction. Five patients were unavailable for follow-up. There was 1 sudden death 7 years after EPS, 11 years after correction of double outlet right ventricle. Death was caused by ventricular arrhythmia and not by a conduction disturbance. Late complete heart block occurred 2 years after EPS in 1 patient and 5 years after EPS in another patient. Both patients had a prolonged HV interval. Progressive lengthening of the HV interval was demonstrated at 2 subsequent EPS studies performed 1 year apart. Another 5 patients with a prolonged HV interval had normally conducted sinus rhythm up to 11 years after EPS. Atrial pacing at increasing rates during EPS was the best predictor for late heart block, as 2 of the 3 children with block below the bundle of His occurring at pacing rates of less than 180 per minute experienced late complete heart block.

Electrophysiologic study of the conduction system is useful in predicting late complete heart block in children who have undergone correction of tetralogy of Fallot and who have a history of transient postoperative heart block or of a prolonged PR interval.

▶ When cardiac surgery for open repair of tetralogy of Fallot was begun in the mid-1950s by the pioneering work of Dr. C. Walton Lillehei, surgeons knew little about the anatomy of the conduction system of the human heart. Complete heart block occurred too often. This led to the development of artificial pacemakers to save lives and also to studies by Dr. Maurice Lev that enabled surgeons to know critical areas to avoid in their suturing and intracardiac manipulation. Postsurgical heart block in the operating room became a rarity.

Freidli and colleagues address what I believe to be the rare occurrence of late complete heart block several years after repair. They reported one late death due to ventricular arrhythmia and 2 cases of late complete heart block 2 and 5 years postoperatively. They studied 57 postoperative children, whom they followed up for a mean of 6.5 years and as long as 13 years after the electrophysiologic studies. They noted lengthening of the HV interval before the block developed in these 2, whereas another 5 with this same finding still had normally conducted rhythm up to 11 years later.

Alertness to the possibility of the unusual late development of complete heart block is important, but the significant aspect of postoperative follow-up and management is that consistent long-term overall cardiac observation by well-informed cardiologists is important for all patients surviving surgical repair of tetralogy.—M.A. Engle, M.D.

Electrophysiologic Consequences of the Mustard Repair of d-Transposition of the Great Arteries
Vetter VL, Tanner CS, Horowitz LN (Children's Hosp of Philadelphia, Univ of Pennsylvania)
J Am Coll Cardiol 10:1265–1273, December 1987   2–33

The Mustard repair of d-transposition of the great arteries is commonly associated with postoperative arrhythmias, including supraventricular tachyarrhythmias, sinus node dysfunction, ectopic atrial rhythms, slow junctional rhythms, and complete heart block. The postoperative incidence of sudden death has been reported at 2% to 8%.

The electrophysiologic effects of the Mustard operation on sinus node, conduction, and refractoriness in the atrium, atrioventricular node, and ventricle were evaluated in 64 patients who underwent surgery for d-transposition of the great arteries. Patients included 48 boys and 16 girls aged 2 months to 10 years, 3 months. A total of 72 electrophysiologic studies were carried out in these patients. Of these 64 patients, 43 had an intact ventricular septum, 2 had significant patent ductus arteriosus, 14 had a ventricular septal defect, 4 had pulmonary stenosis, and 1 had coarctation of the aorta.

Catheter endocardial atrial mapping, available for 67 of 72 studies, showed that 33 patients had sinus rhythm in the atria, 26 had ectopic atrial rhythm, and 8 had junctional rhythm. Three other patients had junctional rhythm that alternated with sinus rhythm or ectopic atrial rhythm. Only 9 of the 64 study patients had normal sinus node function.

Electrophysiologic study revealed significant abnormalities of sinus node function, atrial conduction, and refractoriness in patients with transposition of the great arteries after undergoing the Mustard operation. Most of these abnormalities were significant enough to predispose the patient to sudden death.

▶ Physiologic repair for transposition of the great arteries by switching the venous return to match the transposed arteries (venous switch operation) has saved lives and provided a good quality of life to hundreds of children with this common form of cyanotic congenital heart disease. The price paid for this excellent salvage at low risk is the occurrence of arrhythmias in increasing proportions with passage of time.

Dr. Vetter and colleagues addressed this issue by performing electrophysiologic studies on 64 patients from 1 month to 15 years after the surgery, which had been performed at the ages of 2 months to 10 years. They found that only 9 had normal sinus node function and 33 had sinus rhythm in the atria. Approximately half had abnormal atrial refractoriness, and half developed sustained atrial reentry on pacing. Episodes of atrial flutter spontaneously developed in half of the latter.

These children were operated upon during all stages of the learning curve for that kind of intra-atrial surgery. Whether continued analysis of results such as these will lead to success in future minimizing of arrhythmic tendencies remains to be seen. It is not yet clear whether long-term results of arterial switch or venous switch will be better. Each has sequelae of different kinds, the importance of which needs to be continually assessed.— M.A. Engle, M.D.

Electrophysiologic Consequences of the Arterial Switch Repair of d-Transposition of the Great Arteries
Vetter VL, Tanner CS (Children's Hosp of Philadelphia; Univ of Pennsylvania)
J Am Coll Cardiol 12:229–237, July 1988   2–34

The intra-atrial repair of d-transposition of the great arteries is commonly associated with postoperative cardiac arrhythmias caused by electrophysiologic abnormalities after this type of surgical repair. It has been suggested that the arterial switch repair will prevent the cardiac arrhythmias associated with intra-atrial repair. The electrophysiologic consequences occurring 1 year after successful arterial switch repair for d-transposition of the great arteries are reported.

During a 2-year study period, 6 girls and 14 boys, aged 1 to 120 days, underwent the arterial switch repair of d-transposition of the great arteries, including 9 who had simple transposition of the great arteries and 11 who had transposition with ventricular defect. One patient also had an interrupted aortic arch. All atrial septal defects were closed primarily with sutures, whereas ventricular septal defects were closed through the atrium in 8 patients and through a ventriculotomy in 1 patient. Two smaller ventricular septal defects were not closed. Electrophysiologic studies were performed 7 to 25 months after operation.

One patient had an ectopic atrial rhythm on the preoperative rest ECG, and the other 19 patients had normal sinus rhythm on their preoperative ECGs. Postoperative rest ECGs showed transient postoperative ectopic atrial or junctional rhythms in 2 patients, intermittent ectopic atrial rhythms in 2 patients, and right bundle branch block in 9 patients.

Ambulatory monitor ECG recordings showed infrequent premature ventricular complexes in 5 patients.

Postoperative electrophysiologic abnormalities were mild and infrequent and included mild abnormalities of sinus node function in 6 patients, slightly increased sinoatrial conduction time in 4 patients, and distal right bundle branch block in 9 patients. All 20 patients had a normal ratio of sinus node recovery time to sinus cycle length, and all had normal atrial effective and functional refractory periods. Programmed stimulation did not induce atrial arrhythmias in any patients.

Few arrhythmias and few electrophysiologic abnormalities seem to occur after the arterial switch repair of d-transposition of the great arteries. However, longer follow-up will be required to determine whether any late arrhythmias will occur.

▶ Dr. Vetter continued her exploration of electrophysiologic events in children born with transposed great arteries who survive, thanks to pediatric cardiologic and surgical treatment. In this sequel to her other reports, she studied survivors of the arterial switch operation. Not surprisingly, because that operation involves little insult to the atria other than for caval cannulation, 18 children had normal sinus rhythm and 1 had junctional rhythm and atrial activation was normal.

A well-known axiom is that everything is a trade-off. The venous switch operation tends to produce more supraventricular arrhythmias and obstruction to venous return, whereas the arterial switch produces more supravalvular pulmonic stenosis and aortic regurgitation.—M.A. Engle, M.D.

Exercise Testing

Comparison of the Cardiac Output and Stroke Volume Response to Upright Exercise in Children With Valvular and Subvalvular Aortic Stenosis

Cyran SE, James FW, Daniels S, Mays W, Shukla R, Kaplan S (Children's Hosp Med Ctr, Cincinnati; Univ of Cincinnati)
J Am Coll Cardiol 11:651–658, March 1988   2–35

Measures of cardiac performance during upright maximal exercise in children with mild or moderate aortic valve obstruction have not been extensively evaluated. Cardiac output and stroke volume were assessed in 17 children with discrete subvalvular and valvular aortic stenosis during submaximal and maximal cycle ergometry.

Patients were subgrouped according to the type of left ventricular outflow obstruction. Group I had discrete membranous subvalvular aortic stenosis; group II had valvular aortic stenosis. Patients were matched with 17 controls. Cardiac and stroke indexes were calculated by the acetylene rebreathing method at each exercise level.

The stroke-volume index in group I was significantly greater at rest than indexes in controls or group II. Patients in group I were unable to increase their stroke volume indexes from rest to submaximal exercise. At maximal exercise levels, stroke volume index decreased in these patients. The cardiovascular response was similar to that of patients with hypertrophic cardiomyopathy. The response is characterized by maintenance of supernormal stroke volume from rest to submaximal exercise levels, followed by a significant decrease at maximal exercise.

Patients with mild valvular aortic stenosis (group IIA) had a normal exercise response. In group IIB, patients with severe valvular aortic stenosis, the stroke volume response was blunted at rest and at each level of exercise. These patients also had signs of myocardial ischemia during maximal exercise.

Measurement of cardiac output during exercise permits analysis of stroke volume patterns that differ by anatomical type and severity of left ventricular outflow tract obstruction. These findings should be considered when planning exercise prescriptions for children with aortic stenosis. Children with subvalvular aortic stenosis are probably capable of tolerating various degrees of submaximal exercise, but maximal exercise could have adverse clinical effects. Children with mild valvular disease probably require no restrictions, but those with severe disease should be considered for relief of obstruction and should avoid significant physical exercise.

▶ Because most children tend to be asymptomatic whether their congenital heart disease is mild, moderate, or severe and because the ECG often underestimates left ventricular hypertrophy accompanying aortic stenosis, it is good that we have other noninvasive ways to assess the situation. One of these is exercise stress testing on the treadmill or bicycle.

The group from Cincinnati reports a sophisticated modification of upright exercise testing in which they assess cardiac output and stroke volume in a control group of 17 patients, in 7 with mild to moderate discrete subaortic stenosis (mean outflow tract gradient, 21 ± 12 mm Hg), 5 with mild valvular aortic stenosis (mean gradient, 23 ± 4 mm Hg), and 5 with valvular aortic stenosis and a mean gradient of 54 ± 18 mm Hg.

Not unexpectedly, those with mild valvular aortic stenosis performed very well and those with severe cases did not. They had blunted stroke volumes and ischemic changes in ST segments. The interesting new finding was that those with mild, discrete subaortic stenosis had a response to upright exercise that was similar to that of patients with hypertrophic cardiomyopathy. They had a supernormal stroke volume through submaximal exercise and a significant decrease at maximal exercise.—M.A. Engle, M.D.

Noninvasive Assessment of Hemodynamic Responses to Exercise in Pulmonary Regurgitation After Operations to Correct Pulmonary Outflow Obstruction

Marx GR, Hicks RW, Allen HD, Goldberg SJ (Univ of Arizona)
Am J Cardiol 61:595–601, March 1, 1988   2–36

Pulmonary regurgitation (PR) is frequent after surgery for placement of a nonvalved conduit from the right ventricle to pulmonary arteries. The effect of regurgitation on exercise capacity was studied, using the Doppler-measured regurgitant fraction, in 31 patients with postoperative PR. Patients less than 6 years of age and those with a right ventricular outflow tract gradient more than 20 mm Hg were excluded. Doppler echocardiography was carried out in conjunction with supine cycle exercise at half maximal and maximal oxygen consumption.

Nine patients with mild, 10 with moderate, and 8 with severe PR were compared with control subjects matched with the patients for age, size, and sex. The patients with PR had larger right ventricles and a lower heart rate response to exercise than the controls. Their maximal oxygen consumption was lower and the patients worked at a lower load than the controls. The exercise factor was the same in both groups. The exercise response was normal only in patients with mild PR. Patients with severe PR had lower cardiac output responses than the others.

For hemodynamically significant PR to occur there should be no functional valve in the pulmonary position and the distal pulmonary pressure should be elevated. In these patients, elevated distal pulmonary pressure was secondary to peripheral pulmonary stenosis. Significant PR is associated with right ventricular hypertension. Although exercise capacity is lowered in patients with moderate or severe PR, many patients are able to attend school and lead active lives.

▶ Pulmonary regurgitation is a condition well known to pediatric cardiologists but rarely seen by medical cardiologists except in patients who are intravenous drug abusers. We see it commonly in patients with congenital heart disease who have had relief of pulmonary valvular stenosis and also in those with severe Eisenmenger syndrome. We have learned that the condition is benign unless there is resistance to flow in the distal pulmonary tree (branch stenosis, pulmonary vascular obstructive disease, for example, or unless there is a sizable proximal shunt (residual ventricular septal defect). This study quantitates the effects of PR in mild to severe degree with the challenge of exercise and shows that the condition is not always well tolerated.—M.A. Engle, M.D.

Cardiorespiratory Response to Exercise After the Fontan Procedure for Tricuspid Atresia

Grant GP, Mansell AL, Garofano RP, Hayes CJ, Bowman FO Jr, Gersony WM (Columbia Univ)

Pediatr Res 24:1–5, July 1988   2–37

A maldistribution of pulmonary perfusion is expected after the Fontan operation for tricuspid atresia. Noninvasive exercise testing of 13 such patients aged 6–25 years was done in order to assess gas exchange. Twelve of the patients were in New York Heart Association class I. Five of the patients had a preexisting Glenn shunt. Control data were collected from 28 age- and sex-matched subjects.

The patients had higher heart rates and ventilation, based on oxygen consumption, than did the controls. The mean oxygen saturation was 92% at rest and 87% after exercise. Similar results were observed in patients having had the Glenn operation and those who had not. Low expired CO_2 also was characteristic of the operated patients.

Patients with tricuspid atresia who undergo the Fontan repair have a high heart rate for oxygen consumption, a low expired CO_2, and oxygen desaturation on exercise. An elevated physiologic dead space and ventilation-perfusion mismatching are consistent with maldistribution of pulmonary blood flow in patients with connections either from right atrium to pulmonary artery or right atrium to right ventricle, with or without a previous Glenn shunt. The clinical implications require further study. All of the present patients were clinically well and active at the time of study.

▶ Clinical well-being can sometimes exceed physiologic measurements after cardiac surgery. Twelve of 13 patients were in New York Heart Association class I but all showed high heart rates for oxygen consumption and other evidence of elevated physiologic dead space and ventilation perfusion mismatch 2 years or more after the Fontan procedure. Whether this will affect activity and good health in longer follow-up is unknown.—M.A. Engle, M.D.

Fetal Cardiology

Prenatal Detection of Congenital Heart Disease: Factors Affecting Obstetric Management and Survival
Crawford DC, Chita SK, Allan LD (Guy's Hosp, London)
Am J Obstet Gynecol 159:352–356, August 1988   2–38

A total of 989 antenatal patients had 1,757 fetal echocardiographic studies during an 18-month period because of increased risk of congenital heart disease. Maternal risk factors included a family history of such disease, diabetes, and exposure to a potential teratogen. Fetal risk factors included extracardiac fetal anomalies, growth retardation, and fetal cardiac dysrhythmia.

Cardiac defects were accurately predicted in 74 cases. Associated extracardiac or chromosomal anomalies were present in 34 of these cases. Twenty-three pregnancies underwent elective termination. The survival rate for ongoing pregnancies was 17%. The most frequent specific anomalies diagnosed were atrioventricular septal defect, ventricular septal defect, and left-sided anomalies such as coarctation and mitral atresia. There were 16 false-negative diagnoses, a majority involving minor anomalies having good prognoses. The survival rate in these cases was 81%.

Congenital heart defects in fetuses means that they are at high risk of chromosomal and extracardiac anomalies. Cardiac defects that are detectable in pregnancy usually are severe and carry a poor long-term outlook. If a severe anomaly is found early in pregnancy, termination may be a reasonable consideration. However, a multidisciplinary approach to decision making is preferred in this setting.

▶ Now that fetal diagnosis of congenital heart disease (CHD) has become accepted practice in the hands of experts, questions logically arise concerning the chance of error in diagnosis and the options for management. This expert team reported its most recent experience with 1,747 fetal echocardiograms with accurate prediction of congenital heart disease in 74 cases. Remarkable is the fact that 34 of these had extracardiac or chromosomal anomalies.—M.A. Engle, M.D.

Obstetric Importance, Diagnosis, and Management of Fetal Tachycardias
Maxwell DJ, Crawford DC, Curry PVM, Tynan MJ, Allan LD (Guy's Hosp, London)
Br Med J 297:107–110, July 9, 1988   2–39

Fetal tachycardias exceeding 200 beats per minute require investigation because uncontrolled atrial tachycardia may lead to cardiac failure in utero. Twenty-three pregnancies of 22 to 38 weeks' gestation, encountered during a 7-year period, underwent study for fetal atrial tachycardia.

Twelve patients had supraventricular tachycardia, and 8 had atrial flutter. In 3 cases the rhythm varied between supraventricular tachycardia and atrial flutter. Nonimmune fetal hydrops had developed in 11 fetuses previously, and another became hydropic during treatment. Antiarrhythmic therapy was given to 22 mothers; 1 infant was delivered prematurely. Digoxin alone was effective in 5 cases, and digoxin combined with verapamil was effective in 9 instances. Arrhythmia was controlled in 7 nonhydropic fetuses, and all were delivered at term. Seven of 12 hydropic fetuses gained control, but only 3 were delivered close to term. The 2 deaths were in the hydropic group. Five neonates in this series had severe complications of prematurity.

Atrial tachycardia, which may be intermittent, can cause nonimmune hydrops and should be considered in all cases of fetal hydrops. Transplacental treatment is worth trying in all cases; it may avert preterm delivery with its attendant morbidity.

▶ Now that it is known to be possible to recognize and to terminate some fetal tachyarrhythmias, it is good to learn about the 7-year experience in 23 babies with this problem who were treated by a team experienced in fetal cardiology. They achieved the goal of converting the arrhythmia and prolonging gestation of only 3 of 11 high-risk hydropic babies, but they controlled the arrhythmia in 7 of 10 nonhydropic infants, all delivered at term.—M.A. Engle, M.D.

Pediatric Thoracic Aorta: Normal Measurements Determined With CT
Fitzgerald SW, Donaldson JS, Poznanski AK (Northwestern Univ; Children's Mem Hosp, Chicago)
Radiology 165:667–669, December 1987   2–40

Computed tomography (CT) of the chest has many applications in children. Normal thoracic aortic dimensions in adults have been determined with CT, but no similar pediatric standards have been established. A study was undertaken to provide a range of normal thoracic aortic dimensions in a pediatric population.

Contrast-enhanced CT scans of 97 patients ranging in age from 2 weeks to 19 years were reviewed. The ascending and descending thoracic aortas were measured perpendicularly to the long axis of the arch at 3 levels, and the measurements were adjusted for interobserver and intraobserver variances. Aortic diameters were analyzed with respect to age, sex, and vertebral body size.

Thoracic vertebral body width had a linear relationship to age at all levels; however, there was no significant correlation between aortic size and thoracic body width independent of age. There were no significant differences when patients were separated by sex. In all patients, the diameter of the ascending aorta was larger than or equal to the diameter of the descending aorta at the same level. The descending aortic diameter never increased from level A to level C. Variances within and among observers showed good reproducibility.

These data demonstrate the linear relationship of aortic diameter to age in the pediatric population. The derived standards can be used to distinguish normal from abnormal thoracic aortas on axial CT scans of the chest.

▶ Computed tomography (CT) is one of those magical tests that have found many applications. It is not by any means used as a routine cardiac diagnostic procedure, nor should it be. But when questions arise concerning aneurysmal dilatation of the ascending aorta, or hypoplasia of the transverse arch, or pre-stenotic and poststenotic segments of the descending aorta with coarctation, the normal standards offered by this CT study of 97 children without cardiovascular abnormality should be useful.—M.A. Engle, M.D.

The Structure of the Pulmonary Circulation in Tetralogy of Fallot With Pulmonary Atresia: A Quantitative Cineangiographic Study
Shimazaki Y, Maehara T, Blackstone EH, Kirklin JW, Bargeron LM Jr (Univ of Alabama in Birmingham; Alabama Congenital Heart Disease Diagnosis and Treatment Ctr, Birmingham)
J Thorac Cardiovasc Surg 95:1048–1058, June 1988   2–41

The variability and interrelations of the gross structure of the pulmonary circulation in tetralogy of Fallot and pulmonary atresia were studied and compared with those in tetralogy of Fallot and pulmonary stenosis.

The 172 patients with tetralogy of Fallot and pulmonary atresia had 6 different types of operations: 85 had repair and 46 had classic aortopulmonary shunt. Investigators studied cineangiograms to classify the size and distribution of pulmonary arteries. The status of the central portion of pulmonary arteries was considered in relation to the age of the patient.

In 132 patients there was confluence of the right and left pulmonary arteries, and 70 had incomplete arborization (distribution) of 1 or both arteries. Twenty-eight patients lacked a central portion of 1 or both arteries, with 23 showing incomplete arborization. Twelve patients had an ineffective central portion of 1 pulmonary artery. Completeness of arborization had an inverse relationship to the number of large aortopulmonary collateral arteries.

The range of morphological anomalies (in ascending order) occurs in tetralogy of Fallot with pulmonary stenosis, tetralogy with pulmonary atresia, and tetralogy with pulmonary atresia and congenitally nonconfluent left and right pulmonary arteries.

Surgical intervention in tetralogy of Fallot with pulmonary atresia seeks to effect an enlargement of the pulmonary arteries; an increase in arborization, when necessary; and the connection of pulmonary vascular segments, whenever possible, to the central portion of the pulmonary arteries.

▶ Dr. Bargeron is noted for the high quality of his angiocardiographic studies and interpretations. This report analyzed the complexity of malformations of the pulmonary arterial tree when there is absolute atresia of the outflow tract of the right ventricle in tetralogy of Fallot. In the individual patient being evaluated for palliation or repair, it is important to know whether there is a central pulmonary artery (PA) and whether there is continuity with right and left PA branches. In this large series of 172 patients, 77% had confluence, but half of these had abnormalities of arborization distally. Incomplete arborization was present in 58%. Stenosis of the left PA was more common (23%) than obstruction at the origin of the right branch. Stenoses of lobar or segmental PAs were less common (5%). Large aorticopulmonary collaterals were found in 65% of patients, and in 100% of those with nonconfluent pulmonary arteries.—M.A. Engle, M.D.

Cine Magnetic Resonance Imaging for Evaluation of Anatomy and Flow Relations in Infants and Children With Coarctation of the Aorta
Simpson IA, Chung KJ, Glass RF, Sahn DJ, Sherman FS, Hesselink J (Univ of California, San Diego)
Circulation 78:142–148, July 1988   2–42

It may be difficult to adequately image the site of aortic coarctation in older patients and in patients after surgery. Sixteen cine magnetic resonance imaging (MRI) studies were carried out in 14 patients aged 1 week to 17 years who had coarctation confirmed angiographically or surgically. Initially, conventional echocardiographic-gated MRI served to identify slice locations for the cine study. Cine imaging utilized gradient-recalled acquisition in steady state with a 30-degree flip angle, a 12-msec echo time, and a 22-msec pulse repetition time.

The anatomy was very well defined in all patients except 1 who had vascular clips at the repair site. The smallest descending aortic flow diameter, estimated using cine MRI, agreed very well with angiography. The length of a lucent jet of high-velocity flow, where present, was correlated well with the severity of coarctation on angiography. Both patients who underwent repeat study after repair showed normal flow patterns.

Cine MRI is an effective means of visualizing flow and the vascular anatomy in cases of coarctation of the aorta. The finding of a lucent jet at the coarctation site indicates significant obstruction, but its absence does not rule out significant coarctation. Oblique plane imaging is helpful. The study is noninvasive, making it useful for serially assessing patients after coarctation repair or balloon angioplasty.

▶ Simpson and colleagues report a new, noninvasive imaging technique that compared favorably with angiography in depicting the anatomy and flow patterns in coarctation of the aorta in 16 studies in 14 children. Oblique plane imaging was essential. A drawback is that the richness of collateral circulation was not depicted. An advantage is that it can be used in noninvasive serial assessment.—M.A. Engle, M.D.

Invasive Cardiology

Percutaneous Balloon Angioplasty for Native Coarctation of the Aorta
Beekman RH, Rocchini AP, Dick M II, Snider AR, Crowley DC, Serwer GA, Spicer RL, Rosenthal A (Univ of Michigan)
J Am Coll Cardiol 10:1078–1084, November 1987   2–43

Percutaneous balloon angioplasty is well accepted for the treatment of children with recurrent postoperative coarctation of the aorta, but its use in children with a native coarctation is more controversial. Although balloon angioplasty has been shown to acutely reduce the gradient of a native coarctation, results of a small series suggest that such relief may be short-lived or that late aneurysm formation may occur.

Fifteen boys and 11 girls aged 5 weeks to 14.7 years, with a native coarctation of the aorta, underwent percutaneous balloon angioplasty. All patients had discrete thoracic coarctation with a resting systolic gradient of 30 mm Hg or higher and systolic hypertension in the arms. Two infants had congestive heart failure. Patients with a long-segment coarctation or severe isthmic hypoplasia were excluded from the study. Fifteen patients were followed for at least 12 months, and 14 have undergone repeated cardiac catheterization and angiography to evaluate long-term outcome.

At follow-up, the average residual gradient was 11.7 mm Hg, unchanged from that measured immediately after angioplasty, but the average systolic pressure in the ascending aorta had improved substantially from 143.9 to 116.0 mm Hg. Nine (64%) children who had a preangioplasty gradient of less than 50 mm Hg had good results, defined as a residual gradient of less than 20 mm Hg, and no aneurysm formation (Fig 2–8). Five children with preangioplasty gradients of 50 mm Hg or higher had poor results, defined as a residual gradient of 20 mm Hg or higher, or aneurysm formation. Two of 4 children with residual gradients greater than 20 mm Hg were the youngest in the study, whereas in the other 2,

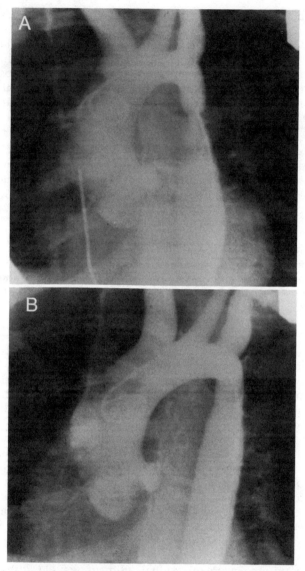

Fig 2–8.—A, preangioplasty aortogram of girl aged 4 years with discrete membranous coarctation and rest gradient of 32 mm Hg. **B,** aortogram obtained 18 months after angioplasty demonstrating virtually normal aorta. No residual gradient was present. (Courtesy of Beekman RH, Rocchini AP, Dick M II, et al: *J Am Coll Cardiol* 10:1078–1084, November 1987.)

the aorta had been inadvertently dilated with a balloon 4–5 mm smaller than the isthmus diameter. An aneurysm was found at the dilatation site in 1 child (Fig 2–9).

These results show that children with a native coarctation who have a preangioplasty gradient of less than 50 mm Hg are good candidates for percutaneous balloon angioplasty.

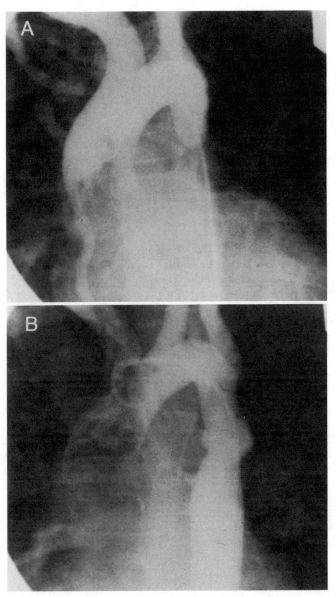

Fig 2–9.—**A,** preangioplasty aortogram of boy aged 8 years who had 52-mm Hg coarctation gradient. **B,** follow-up aortogram 26 months later demonstrates small saccular aneurysm at angioplasty site. A 1-mm Hg residual gradient was present. (Courtesy of Beekman RH, Rocchini AP, Dick M II, et al: *J Am Coll Cardiol* 10:1078–1084, November 1987.)

▶ Because we are still in the learning curve for risks and rewards of balloon dilatation of native coarctation of the aorta, it behooves us to consider the experience of those investigators who are cautiously, carefully evaluating this method of relief of obstruction. In 26 infants and children at Ann Arbor, the gradient was reduced acutely in all, and at 12–26 months' follow-up in 14 children, that improvement persisted. Overall, that reduction of gradient plus the absence of mortality are the rewards, but this good news is modified by the fact that, whereas 9 of 14 could be classed as having a good result with gradients less than 20 mm Hg and no aneurysm, 4 patients had a higher residual gradient. Now for the risk: 1 child had an aneurysm at the dilation site. The fate of such an aneurysm is unknown, but at the least, it is of great concern.—M.A. Engle, M.D.

Balloon Angioplasty for Coarctation of the Aorta: Immediate and Long-Term Results
Rao PS, Najjar HN, Mardini MK, Solymar L, Thapar MK (King Faisal Hosp, Riyadh, Saudi Arabia; Univ of Wisconsin–Madison)
Am Heart J 115:657–665, March 1988   2–44

Twenty-five infants and children had balloon dilation of coarctation of the aorta during a 28-month period. The procedure utilized a no. 4 F and no. 5 F Grüntzig or Medi-Tech balloon dilation catheter. In 2 cases, the catheter was placed antegrade from the pulmonary artery via the ductus arteriosus. The balloon was at least twice the size of the coarcted segment but no larger than the size of the descending aorta at the level of the diaphragm. Three or more dilations were done at least 5 minutes apart. No catheter or guide wire was manipulated over the freshly dilated area.

Two balloons ruptured during angioplasty without adverse effects. Five infants had significant blood loss and required transfusions. One child required thrombectomy for femoral artery occlusion. The systolic pressure gradient across the coarctation decreased from 48 to 10 mm Hg after angioplasty. The coarcted segment increased in diameter from 3.2 to 7.8 mm. Femoral pulses became palpable and had increased volume after the procedure. Infants who were in heart failure improved, and systemic hypertension also lessened after the procedure. One of 14 patients who had recatheterization a mean of 11 months after angioplasty had a significant gradient with recoarctation and responded to repeat balloon dilation. Another had surgical resection of coarctation elsewhere. No aneurysms were found in the area of dilated coarctation. All patients were clinically well at late follow-up.

Apparently coarctation is relieved when balloon dilation produces an intimal and medial tear. Inadvertent manipulation in the area of dilation may lead to aortic perforation and death. Aneurysm formation may not occur if the size of the balloon is limited to that of the descending aorta at the level of the diaphragm. Balloon dilation is a safe and effective alternative to surgical resection of coarctation in neonates and young infants.

▶ The controlled intimal damage by balloon dilatation has been generally well tolerated and has been of lasting benefit in adults with obstructions in proximal coronary arteries that can be reached by the balloon-tipped catheter. In an artery as large as the aorta, it is also possible to relieve the obstruction and often to maintain reduction of the pressure gradient, but aneurysm of the aorta at the site has also been reported. In the dilemma of the learning curve of this new procedure, this paper by Rao and collaborators should prove helpful. They describe meticulously their procedure that has yielded effective relief of the coarctation and has produced no evidence of aneurysm formation in a follow-up period up to 22 months postangioplasty.—M.A. Engle, M.D.

Percutaneous Balloon Dilatation of Aortic Valve Stenosis in Neonates and Infants
Wren C, Sullivan I, Bull C, Deanfield J (Freeman Hosp, Newcastle upon Tyne, England; Hosp for Sick Children, London)
Br Heart J 58:608–612, December 1987   2–45

Management of critical aortic valvular stenosis in infants is difficult, and surgical mortality is high. Surgical palliation by valvotomy is possible, but repeat procedures are often necessary. Isolated reports of effective balloon dilatation in infancy led to a trial of this management technique in 13 consecutive patients younger than 1 year of age, 7 of them neonates. The median age was 4 weeks. Three patients had undergone surgical valvotomy, and all except 3 patients had signs of heart failure at the time of balloon dilatation. The procedure involved a balloon at least 1–2 mm smaller than the cineaortographic valve diameter.

In 2 patients the valve was not crossed, and both died during subsequent operations. Two other infants died during manipulation of the balloon catheter. In 1 patient who later died during surgery, there was no significant benefit. In 8 patients the aortic valve pressure gradient declined from a mean of 63 mm Hg to 23 mm Hg. Two of these patients later died of heart failure related to other cardiac lesions, but the 6 survivors have done well clinically, despite evidence of an increasing valve gradient on follow-up after 2–23 months. None of these infants had signs of heart failure and none required diuretics.

Improved balloon dilatation of aortic valve stenosis may be expected as experience is gained and balloon catheter design and patient selection improve. However, patients weighing less than 3 kg are likely to continue to have significant mortality, whether treated operatively or by balloon catheter.

▶ These cardiologists in the United Kingdom attempted balloon dilatation under the most difficult but also very usual circumstance: the critically severe congenital stenosis in 7 neonates and 6 infants. Their keen analysis presents a sobering statement for balloon watchers.—M.A. Engle, M.D.

Balloon Dilation of Congenital Aortic Valve Stenosis: Results and Influence of Technical and Morphological Features on Outcome
Sholler GF, Keane JF, Perry SB, Sanders SP, Lock JE (Harvard Med School)
Circulation 78:351–360, August 1988   2–46

Seventy-five patients aged 1 day to 39 years underwent 80 balloon dilations for congenital aortic valve stenosis during 1984–1987. Fifteen patients had undergone previous surgical valvotomy. In 74 instances retrograde dilation was performed via a percutaneous femoral approach. The initial catheter was chosen to provide a ratio of balloon to anulus diameter of 90% to 100%.

Neither a history of survival after valvotomy nor the use of 1 or 2 dilating balloons influenced the reduction in valvular gradient. However, aortic regurgitation was induced more often when the balloon-anulus ratio exceeded 100%. Relief of obstruction determined on postdilation echocardiography was related to apparent commissural division. Substantial increases in regurgitation occurred in 3 of 8 unicommissural valves and in 1 of 50 bicommissural valves.

Patients with unicommissural aortic valves may be at increased risk of significant regurgitation after balloon dilation. In patients with thick valves, the reduction in valve gradient may be less satisfactory. The risk of a major increase in regurgitation can be minimized by avoiding a balloon-anulus ratio diameter greater than 100%.

▶ This invasive cardiologic technique is much more controversial than pulmonary balloon valvuloplasty for several reasons that this expert team at Boston Children's Hospital analyzes for us. The bottom line is that severe congenital aortic stenosis, which often presents in a critically ill newborn, by its morphology often defies surgical or invasive cardiologic or medical management.— M.A. Engle, M.D.

Balloon Dilatation in Infants and Children With Dysplastic Pulmonary Valves: Short-Term and Intermediate-Term Results
Rao PS (King Faisal Specialist Hosp and Research Ctr, Riyadh, Saudi Arabia)
Am Heart J 116:1168–1173, November 1988   2–47

Fairly good results have been reported with balloon pulmonary valvuloplasty, but as many as one third of patients have had recurrent valve obstruction. Results have been considered less favorable for dysplastic valves. In a series of 56 patients aged 1 week to 20 years who underwent balloon dilation of the pulmonic valve for isolated valvular stenosis during a 50-month period through 1987, follow-up catheterization was possible in 36 cases, a mean of 11 months after valvuloplasty. Thirteen had dysplastic valves.

Overall, the right ventricular peak systolic pressure and pulmonary valve gradient remained improved 6–34 months after valvuloplasty and were similar in both groups with and without dysplasia. Two of 13 patients with dysplastic valves and 3 of the 23 other patients required repeated valvuloplasty. Residual gradients greater than 30 mm Hg were found in 3 of 13 with dysplastic valves and in 4 of 23 without.

Balloon valvuloplasty can be effective even for patients with dysplastic pulmonary valves. Valve dysplasia did not dispose to poor results in the present series. The use of larger balloons may be helpful in these cases.

▶ During the period of the learning curve for balloon dilatation to relieve valvular and vascular obstructions the procedure has come into wide acceptance for patients with nondysplastic pulmonary valvular stenosis. It has generally been thought to be less helpful or even contraindicated for dysplastic valves. Not so, says Dr. Rao in this comparative analysis, and he tells us why.—M.A. Engle, M.D.

Pacemakers

Epicardial Ventricular Pacemaker Electrode Longevity in Children
Serwer GA, Mericle JM, Armstrong BE (Duke Univ)
Am J Cardiol 61:104–106, Jan 1, 1988   2–48

The increased life expectancy of children with pacemakers compared with adults makes system longevity very important. The longevity of a pacing system is dependent on the longevity of the pulse generator and pacing electrode. Epicardially implanted electrodes are widely used in children for ventricular pacing, but their expected longevity is unknown. The useful life of 126 such electrodes implanted between 1970 and 1985 was evaluated in 81 children.

Age at implant ranged from 1 day to 18 years; the median age was 7 years. One to 5 electrodes were implanted in each child. Seventy-six of the 81 children had structural heart disease, and all had undergone previous cardiac surgery. Forty-one electrodes were suture fixated; 85 were of the sutureless helical type. All electrodes were connected to a pulse generator implanted in an abdominal pocket. Electrode failure was defined as either loss of capture with a high pacing threshold discovered at surgery or sensing failure.

Thirty-eight electrodes failed 1–157 months after implant (median time of failure, 37 months). The mode of failure was high threshold with high impedance in 15 patients, low impedance in 6, inability to pace in 8, high threshold without measured impedance in 7, and sensing failure in 2. Actuarial survival was 88% at 6 months and remained constant until 53 months, when survival steadily decreased to 49% at 101 months. From 101 months to 157 months, there was no significant decrease. The failure rate within the first 6 months was 12%. Electrodes surviving 6 months were highly likely to survive 53 months; of these, 74% were likely to survive 120 months.

Long-term pacemaker follow-up requires evaluation of both battery reserves and electrode characteristics, including determination of pulse width necessary to pace at a minimum of 2 amplitudes; electrode impedance; and intrinsic QRS amplitude seen by the pulse generator in the non-pacemaker-dependent patient.

▶ Pacemaker therapy in the few infants and children who need it has advanced remarkably over the almost 3 decades that it has been in use. Yet the life expectancy of pacemakers implanted epicardially (the most frequent way) has not been clearly defined. The authors report on 126 pacemakers implanted between 1970 and 1985, with follow-up as long as 16 years on 81 children. Electrode failure occurred in 38 units. The first 6-month period was the time of greatest risk of failure: 12%. Beyond that, the chances of electrode survival up to 4.5 years (53 months) were excellent. Of pacemakers lasting that long, 74% would be expected to last 10 years.

While this is reassuring information overall, nonetheless it behooves the cardiologist to maintain long-term follow-up on individual patients with pacemakers to evaluate electrode and battery characteristics with aging.— M.A. Engle, M.D.

Pharmacology

Comparison of the Digitalis Receptor in Erythrocytes from Preterm Infants and Adults

Koren G, Long D, Klein J, Beatie D, Bologa-Campeanu M, Livne A, Kirpalani H (Univ of Toronto; Ben Gurion Univ, Beer Sheva, Israel)
Pediatr Res 23:414–417, April 1988   2–49

Infants and children require more digoxin per unit body weight than do adults to achieve similar serum concentrations because of more rapid clearance. It has not been proved that less mature individuals are less sensitive to digoxin. The digitalis receptor in 31 newborn infants with a mean postnatal age of 12 days was compared with that in 12 healthy adults. Measurements of rubidium 86 uptake served to reflect the function of the $Na^+,K^+,ATPase$ enzyme system in terms of binding capacity and affinity.

Total uptake was significantly higher in neonates than in adults, as was specific uptake. The percentage of specific uptake from total uptake also was higher in infants. Affinity constants were comparable in the 2 groups of subjects. Serum potassium levels greater than 5.4 mEq/L in infants were related to greater specific uptake, even after excluding infants given adult packed cells. Creatinine clearance did not explain differing potassium concentrations.

Uptake of red cell rubidium is greater in preterm infants than in adults. Both total binding and specific binding are higher in neonates. Greater binding capacity may mean that more glycoside is needed for a given pharmacologic or toxic effect. Because most infants with congestive failure do not receive digitalis only, it remains difficult to directly assess the effects of digitalis.

▶ It has long been known that infants in cardiac failure usually require more digitalis per kilogram than do older children and adults. This study focuses not on elimination of the drug but on receptors in red blood cells. They found that in neonates the uptake was significantly higher than in adults and found a difference between hyperkalemic and normokalemic preterm infants.— M.A. Engle, M.D.

Effect on Growth of Children With Cardiac Dysrhythmias Treated With Amiodarone

Ardura J, Hermoso F, Bermejo J (Univ Hosp, Valladolid, Spain)

Pediatr Cardiol 9:33–36, 1988   2–50

The problem of dysrhythmia in children has recently sparked much interest. In contrast with diagnostic techniques for identifying dysrhythmias, which have been considerably refined during recent years, treatment has evolved only marginally, as the ideal drug to treat these disorders has not yet been developed. Amiodarone is an almost ideal antiarrhythmic drug for adult patients, but experience with its use in children has thus far been limited. An accidental finding of a remarkable acceleration of bone aging in a child treated with amiodarone prompted this study.

Amiodarone was prescribed for 2 girls and 7 boys aged 15 days to 13 years because of dysrhythmia that had been resistant to treatment with conventional antiarrhythmic agents. Three patients had reciprocal rhythm tachycardia, 2 had atrial tachycardia, 1 had junctional tachycardia, 1 had ventricular tachycardia, and 2 had episodes of Wolff-Parkinson-White syndrome. The initial dose of amiodarone was 800 mg/1.73 m^2, administered for 2 weeks, followed by 400 mg/1.73 m^2 for 5 days a week. Duration of treatment ranged from 9 months to 19 months, for a mean duration of 13 months. After establishing baseline values, age, period of treatment, weight, height, growth velocity, and bone age were recorded every 4 months. In addition, each child had a chest radiograph, electrocardiogram, Holter monitoring, and eye examination and underwent laboratory studies of transaminase, triiodothyronine, thyroxine, and thyrotropin levels every 4 months.

Treatment with amiodarone resulted in complete remission in 5 (56%) children, whereas treatment of the other 4 was partially successful. Side effects were observed from 2 to 9 months after the start of treatment and included photosensitization in 2 patients and headaches in 1 patient. Three children showed excessive weight gain, 7 had a negative deviation of the height curve, and 6 had abnormal growth velocity curves. Concurrently, triiodothyronine values were increased in 2 children, and thyroxine values were increased in 5 children. Side effects persisted for 5 to 18 months after treatment had been discontinued.

Children with cardiac dysrhythmias should be treated with amiodarone only if they have critical dysrhythmias that are resistant to other therapies, and then only for no longer than 2 years.

▶ When recurrent arrhythmias resistant to conventional drugs develop in children, it is important to decide why this should be and what else should be done. These investigators selected amiodarone as an alternative therapy and quite wisely monitored these 9 children for untoward effects. They looked and found several undesirable and important side effects that began from 2 to 9 months after instituting therapy and that persisted for 5 to 18 months after stopping it. Initial hypothyroidism was followed by hyperthyroid reaction and growth was sufficiently affected that the authors advise limiting use of this drug in children to 2 years.—M.A. Engle, M.D.

Electrophysiologic Effects and Clinical Efficacy of Flecainide in Children with Recurrent Paroxysmal Supraventricular Tachycardia

Musto B, D'Onofrio A, Cavallaro C, Musto A, Greco R (Vincenzo Monaldi Hosp, Naples)
Am J Cardiol 62:229–233, August 1988   2–51

Reentrant paroxysmal supraventricular tachycardia (SVT), with or without Wolff-Parkinson-White syndrome, is the most common form of SVT in children. Because flecainide is effective in treating many arrhythmias in adults, its electrophysiologic effects were examined in 15 children with recurrent paroxysmal SVT and 1 with overt accessory pathway and a history of syncope. Eleven patients in all had an accessory pathway. Five of the other patients had an atrioventricular nodal reentrant tachycardia. The dose of intravenous flecainide was 1.5 mg/kg.

The effective refractory periods of the atrium and ventricle increased significantly after intravenous flecainide was administered, whereas the atrioventricular node refractory period did not change. Treatment blocked retrograde conduction in the accessory pathway in 4 patients and anterograde conduction in 8 of 9 cases. Tachycardia was noninducible in 7 patients after flecainide administration. In 4 others it was inducible but nonsustained.

Fifteen patients continued to use flecainide orally for a mean of 19 months. The dosage was 4–6 mg/kg. Tachycardia recurred in 4 patients.

Flecainide holds promise for both the short-term and long-term treatment of SVT in children. It could be a useful alternative when more conventional agents are ineffective.

▶ So few cardioactive drugs have been studied in children that it is a pleasure to see this study of effects and efficacy of flecainide in children with a common form of arrhythmia: recurrent supraventricular tachycardia. The rapid rhythm in the 16 children was due to accessory pathway in 11 (2 concealed) and to atrioventricular nodal reentrant tachycardia in 5. Intravenous flecainide lengthened the effective refractory period of atria and ventricles. The drug was effective in short- and long-term (19 ± 11 months) follow-up when given orally 2 or 3 times daily.—M.A. Engle, M.D.

3 Heart Disease in Adults

Introduction

The 15 articles dealing with valvular heart disease include papers on balloon valvuloplasty of the aortic and mitral valves; combined aortic balloon valvuloplasty and coronary angioplasty; the association of mitral valve disease and rheumatic heart disease; mechanisms of flow augmentation at the mitral and aortic valve; the accuracy of Doppler echocardiography in predicting the severity of aortic stenosis; the frequency of angina pectoris and coronary artery disease in aortic stenosis and aortic regurgitation; the therapy of aortic regurgitation with hydralazine; the coronary reserve in chronic aortic regurgitation; echocardiographic evaluation of prosthetic heart valves; valvular dysfunction in patients with lupus erythematosus; and color Doppler evaluation of valvular regurgitation in normal subjects.

The 7 articles on myocardial diseases deal with the demonstration of restrictive ventricular physiology by Doppler echocardiography; the Doppler echocardiographic estimation of the pressure difference in hypertrophic cardiomyopathy; myocarditis mimicking acute myocardial infarction; myocarditis in AIDS; the prospective detection of myocarditis in dilated cardiomyopathy; prevention of myocarditis with interferon; and the possible production of cardiomyopathy by a different interferon.

A fine article from Spain reviews 10 years of experience with a prospective protocol for the management of tuberculous pericarditis.

The 11 articles on disturbances of cardiac rhythm and conduction include studies on the prognosis of early ventricular fibrillation after myocardial infarction; the production of ST-segment depression by mental stress in patients with angina pectoris; reentry as a cause of ventricular tachycardia; the exercise response of patients with chronic atrial fibrillation; clinical experience with the automatic implantable cardioverter-defibrillator (AICD); criteria for the diagnosis of ventricular tachycardia in wide complex left bundle branch block morphology tachycardia; experience with the automatic external defibrillator in the management of out-of-hospital cardiac arrest; catheter ablation of accessory pathways; and the prognostic significance of signal-averaged ECGs during acute myocardial infarction.

Sixteen articles on miscellaneous topics describe the prevalence of patent foramen ovale in patients with stroke; the prognostic significance of the left ventricular ejection fraction after acute myocardial infarction; the potential value of captopril in preventing ventricular dilatation after myocardial infarction; antithrombotic therapy in patients with cardiac disease; the value of echocardiography in blunt chest trauma; the pharmacology and use of digitalis; the effects of cocaine upon the cardiovascular system; the clinical and echocardiographic studies of infective endocarditis in drug addicts; carotid sinus hypersensitivity in patients with syncope; the usefulness of high-dose dipyridamole echocardiography in women; skeletal muscle metabolism in heart failure; hemodynamics during cardiopulmonary resuscitation; and the prevalence and significance of left ventricular false tendons (bands).

Robert C. Schlant, M.D.

Valvular Heart Disease

Balloon Aortic Valvuloplasty in 170 Consecutive Patients

Safian RD, Berman AD, Diver DJ, McKay LL, Come PC, Riley MF, Warren SE, Cunningham MJ, Wyman RM, Weinstein JS, Grossman W, McKay RG (Beth Israel Hosp, Boston; Harvard Univ)
N Engl J Med 319:125–130, July 21, 1988   3–1

Percutaneous balloon aortic valvuloplasty (PBV) has recently been used successfully in elderly patients with aortic stenosis. Although long-term results are not yet available, short-term follow-up studies suggest that restenosis of the aortic valve may occur. The authors report their experience to date with PBV.

During a 2.5-year period, PBV was attempted in 170 patients with aortic valvular stenosis, 53% men and 47% women aged 35–94 years, with a mean age of 77 years, 115 (68%) of whom were considered poor candidates for cardiac surgery. Fifty-five (32%) patients had refused opera-

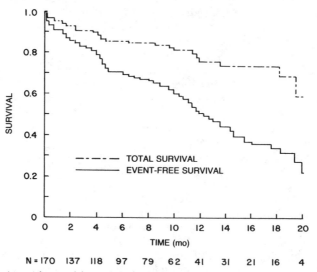

Fig 3–1.—Actuarial survival for patients treated by balloon aortic valvuloplasty. *Broken line* shows survival when only death is considered as end point. *Solid line* shows survival when death, aortic-valve replacement, and repeat valvuloplasty are considered as end points. N denotes number of patients alive at end of each follow-up interval. (Courtesy of Safian RD, Berman AD, Diver DJ, et al: *N Engl J Med* 319:125–130, July 21, 1988.)

tion as the initial therapy, 26 of whom were older than 80 years. Follow-up ranged from 1 to 23 months; the average was 9.1 months.

Percutaneous balloon aortic valvuloplasty was successfully completed in 168 patients and was aborted in 2 patients. However, 6 of the patients with successful PBVs, including 4 who were moribund before dilation, died in the hospital. Five other patients subsequently required aortic valve replacement. The PBVs resulted in significant increases in mean area of the aortic valve and cardiac output and yielded significant decreases in the peak aortic valve pressure gradient.

In 44 patients (28%), recurrent symptoms developed at a mean of 7.5 months after PBV: 16 underwent repeat PBV, 17 underwent aortic valve replacement, and 11 were treated conservatively. One of 2 patients who experienced a second restenosis underwent aortic valve replacement; the other had a third PBV procedure. There were 25 late deaths, including 5 from noncardiac causes. Life-table analysis indicated that the probability of survival for the entire study population at 1 year after PBV was 74% (Fig 3—1).

It is concluded that PBV is effective as palliative treatment for some elderly patients with symptomatic aortic stenosis, as symptoms improve in the majority of patients.

▶ This palliative procedure is best reserved for patients older than 80 years of age, patients with poor left ventricular function, and patients with serious additional problems (especially coronary, renal, or pulmonary). It is not appropriate for younger patients without other problems because of the high rate of restenosis, which occurred in nearly 50% of the patients by 1 year after valvuloplasty.

Letac et al. (1) report their experience in Rouen with 218 adult patients with valvular aortic stenosis. They recommend balloon aortic valvuloplasty as a bridge to surgery in some patients who are surgical candidates and as the treatment of choice in patients older than 75–80 years. Balloon aortic valvuloplasty may also be useful in the treatment of cardiogenic shock secondary to calcific aortic stenosis (2). Other reports have summarized the experience with 24 patients in Heidelberg (3); the experience of 90 patients at Massachusetts General Hospital (4); the short-term results in 55 patients at the Mayo Clinic (5), and the experience in 32 patients at Kings College Hospital in London (6). The mechanism of benefit appears to be predominantly by the production of fractures of cuspid calcium within the valves rather than commissural splitting (7).—R.C. Schlant, M.D.

References

1. Letac B, Cribier A, Koning R, et al: Results of percutaneous transluminal valvuloplasty in 218 patients with valvular aortic stenosis. *Am J Cardiol* 62:598–605, 1988.
2. Desnoyers MR, Salem DN, Rosenfield K, et al: Treatment of cardiogenic shock by emergency aortic balloon valvuloplasty. *Ann Intern Med* 108:833–835, 1988.
3. Kucherer H, Katus H, Dietz B, et al: Perkutane transfemorale valvulo-

plastie bei Patienten mit kalzifizierter Aortenstenose und deutlich er-
hohtem Operationsrisiko: Klinischer Verlauf und Wertigkeit der Dop-
plersonographic zur Beurteilung Therapieerfolges. *Klin Wochenschr*
66:571–578, 1988.

4. Block PC, Palacios IF: Clinical and hemodynamic follow-up after percutaneous aortic valvuloplasty in the elderly. *Am J Cardiol* 62:760–763,
   1988.
5. Nishimura RA, Holmes DR Jr, Reeder GS, et al: Doppler evaluation of
   the results of percutaneous aortic balloon valvuloplasty in calcific aortic
   stenosis. *Circulation* 78:791–799, 1988.
6. Sprigings DC, Jackson G, Chambers JB, et al: Balloon dilatation of the
   aortic valve for inoperable aortic stenosis. *Br Med J* 297:1007–1011,
   1988.
7. Kennedy KD, Hauck AJ, Edwards WD, et al: Mechanism of reduction
   of aortic valvular stenosis by percutaneous transluminal balloon valvuloplasty: Report of five cases and review of literature. *Mayo Clin Proc*
   63:769–776, 1988.

Combined Percutaneous Aortic Valvuloplasty and Transluminal Coronary Angioplasty in Adult Patients With Calcific Aortic Stenosis and Coronary Artery Disease

McKay RG, Safian RD, Berman AD, Diver DJ, Weinstein JS, Wyman RM, Cunningham MJ, McKay LL, Baim DS, Grossman W (Beth Israel Hosp, Boston; Harvard Univ)

Circulation 76:1298–1306, December 1987   3–2

The surgical risk is increased during aortic valve replacement in patients with coexisting coronary artery disease who subsequently require
coronary artery bypass grafting; the risk can be significant in elderly patients. The potential value of balloon aortic valvuloplasty and transluminal coronary angioplasty were evaluated in 9 adults with combined valvular and coronary artery disease. All had critical calcific aortic stenosis.
The mean age was 76 years. All patients were symptomatic; 7 had histories of pulmonary edema, 4 had previous subendocardial myocardial infarction, and 2 had undergone coronary artery bypass grafting.

Aortic valvuloplasty improved the peak aortic valve gradient and calculated aortic valve area. Single-vessel coronary angioplasty resulted in a
mean reduction of 29% to 91% in critical coronary stenosis. Complications included groin hematomas in 2 patients, transient left bundle
branch block in 1, and transient atrial fibrillation in another. Eight patients had significant improvement in symptoms of angina and congestive
heart failure. The ninth patient, who had persistent chest pain, was
treated successfully with aortic valve replacement and coronary artery
bypass grafting. Improvement persisted at 6-month follow-up in 7 patients. Valvular and coronary restenosis occurred in 1 patient.

Combined percutaneous aortic valvuloplasty and coronary angioplasty
is safe in older patients with calcific aortic stenosis and single-vessel coronary artery disease. The procedure may be useful with patients in whom
surgical intervention is contraindicated because of high surgical risk.

▶ The authors quite properly emphasize that combined aortic valvuloplasty and coronary angioplasty is still experimental but that it holds promise as a palliative treatment for selected elderly patients with angina and severe stenosis and single-vessel coronary artery disease who are not candidates for surgery. In the next article, the same group reports their experience when aortic balloon valvuloplasty is combined with mitral balloon valvuloplasty.— R.C. Schlant, M.D.

Combined Aortic and Mitral Balloon Valvuloplasty in Patients With Critical Aortic and Mitral Valve Stenosis: Results in Six Cases
Berman AD, Weinstein JS, Safian RD, Diver DJ, Grossman W, McKay RG (Beth Israel Hosp, Boston; Harvard Univ)
J Am Coll Cardiol 11:1213–1218, June 1988   3–3

Percutaneous balloon valvuloplasty may be a valuable nonsurgical alternative to valve replacement. Some patients with both aortic and mitral valve stenosis are at high risk for complications from surgery, and others may refuse an operation. In these patients, balloon valvuloplasty can be an effective treatment.

Six patients with severe combined aortic and mitral valve stenosis underwent double-valve balloon dilation as an alternative to valve replacement. All patients had severe stenosis, and 4 had a depressed cardiac index; only 1 patient was considered to be a good candidate for surgery. In each patient, a 20-mm balloon dilation catheter was passed retrograde through the aortic valve. Mitral valvuloplasty, with either a single- or double-balloon technique, was performed transseptally.

Cardiac output increased significantly in 3 patients, and left atrial pressure decreased markedly in 2 of these patients and in an additional patient. The only significant complication was a femoral artery thrombus, which was treated with catheter thrombectomy. Recovery from the procedure and hospital discharge were faster with valvuloplasty than with surgery.

Follow-up showed a decreased gradient across the aortic and mitral valves in 5 patients. Four patients continued to do well and were able to exercise. One patient sustained a hip fracture, and 1 died of metastatic lung cancer. At 6 months, 2 patients had probable restenosis. Combined valve valvuloplasty offers a well-tolerated procedure with at least temporary resolution of symptoms in patients who refuse or are not candidates for surgical valve replacement.

▶ The ages of the 6 patients in this report ranged from 60 to 83 years of age, and half of the patients had significant coronary artery disease. Five had contraindications to surgery, and 1 refused surgery. Most patients experienced a clinical improvement in symptoms, although the follow-up period was short and evidence of restenosis, particularly of the aortic valve, has developed in some. This combined procedure may be indicated for a few, highly select patients with conditions that prohibit surgery. A long-term follow-up of such patients will be very important.— R.C. Schlant, M.D.

Improvement in Exercise Capacity and Exercise Hemodynamics 3 Months After Double-Balloon, Catheter Balloon Valvuloplasty Treatment of Patients With Symptomatic Mitral Stenosis

McKay CR, Kawanishi DT, Kotlewski A, Parise K, Odom-Maryon T, Gonzalez A, Reid CL, Rahimtoola SH (Univ of Southern California)
Circulation 77:1013–1021, May 1988   3–4

Twenty-four of 27 patients having isolated mitral double-balloon catheter balloon valvuloplasty (CBV) survived and underwent clinical and hemodynamic evaluation after 3 months. The patients, treated for symptomatic mitral stenosis, had a mean age of 41 years. All but 3 patients were in New York Heart Association functional class III or IV preoperatively, and 7 patients were in atrial fibrillation.

Twenty-two of the 24 patients improved functionally after CBV and, after 3 months, were in functional class I or II. Treadmill time increased substantially after the operation. The mitral valve gradient fell from 17 mm Hg to 6 mm Hg immediately after CBV, and cardiac output rose from 4.3 L/minute to 5.0 L/minute. These changes persisted at 3 months. Exercise cardiac output also increased after operation. At maximum symptom-limited exercise, exercise time, maximum work load, and cardiac output all improved. No patient developed marked mitral regurgitation after valvuloplasty.

Mitral CBV with the double-balloon method effectively increases the mitral valve area and significantly improves resting and exercise hemodynamics. Symptoms have consistently resolved after the procedure. The hemodynamic changes provide a physiologic explanation of improved exercise performance after CBV in patients with mitral stenosis.

▶ This study documents that the majority of selected patients with mitral stenosis treated by double-balloon catheter balloon valvuloplasty (CBV) experienced an improvement in both New York Heart Association functional class and hemodynamics when studied 3 months later. The mitral valve area was significantly increased, whereas the mitral valve diastolic gradient and the left atrial and pulmonary artery pressures decreased. Six of the 24 surviving patients, however, had residual artery septal defects (Qp/Qs ranged from 1.2 to 1.6). Mitral regurgitation increased in 3 patients and decreased in 2. These results from a major center for CBV are encouraging for highly selected patients. It will be most important to learn whether or not the rate of restenosis over the next 5 to 7 years is similar to that following surgical commissurotomy. See the next article for more on mitral balloon valvuloplasty.— R.C. Schlant, M.D.

Percutaneous Balloon Mitral Valvotomy for Patients With Mitral Stenosis: Analysis of Factor Influencing Early Results

Herrmann HC, Wilkins GT, Abascal VM, Weyman AE, Block PC, Palacios IF (Massachusetts Gen Hosp, Boston)
J Thorac Cardiovasc Surg 96:33–38, July 1988   3–5

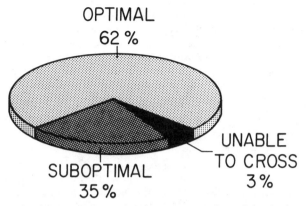

OPTIMAL
62 %

UNABLE
TO CROSS
3%

SUBOPTIMAL
35%

Fig 3–2.—Results of PMV in 49 patients (60 consecutive procedures). Suboptimal result was defined by (1) final mitral valve area ≤ 1.0 cm²; (2) final mean diastolic mitral valve gradient ≥ 10 mm Hg; or (3) increase in mitral valve area of ≤ 25%. (Courtesy of Herrmann HC, Wilkins GT, Abascal VM, et al: *J Thorac Cardiovasc Surg* 96:33–38, July 1988.)

Surgical mitral commissurotomy is effective treatment for many patients with mitral stenosis. Percutaneous mitral balloon valvotomy (PMV) is a recently developed, less invasive alternative to surgery. However, the immediate results of PMV have been inconsistent, and optimal hemodynamic improvement is not always attained. The authors analyzed their initial experience with PMV to identify factors that may influence the outcome of this procedure.

During an 18-month study period, 49 patients, 8 men and 41 women, aged 13 to 87 years with a mean of 50 years had a total of 60 consecutive PMV procedures; 11 patients each had 2 procedures. Based on hemodynamic results, the outcomes of PMV were retrospectively rated as optimal for 37 (62%) procedures and suboptimal for 21 (35%) procedures. Suboptimal results were defined as a final mitral valve area of 1.0 cm² or less, a final mean diastolic mitral valve gradient of 10 mm Hg or more, or an increase in mitral valve area of 25% or less. In the remaining 2 (3%) procedures, the catheter could not be passed across the mitral valve (Fig 3–2).

Following PMV, the mean mitral valve area for the total patient population increased from 0.8 to 1.6 cm². The mean diastolic mitral gradient fell from 18 to 7 mm Hg, and mean cardiac output increased from 3.8 to 4.5 L/minute. The results of univariate and multivariate analysis of 16 variables indicated that severe valve leaflet thickening or immobility and an extreme degree of subvalvular thickening and calcification on the echocardiogram were predictive of suboptimal results. A smaller effective balloon dilating area and the presence of atrial fibrillation were 2 other factors predictive of suboptimal outcome. Definite contraindications to PMV include left atrial thrombus, severe mitral regurgitation (>214 +), and inability to perform transseptal catheterization.

One patient died after emergency mitral valve replacement following an unsuccessful PMV. Other complications included conduction system abnormalities in 2 patients, transient loss of consciousness in 2 patients, and hepatic embolism in 1 patient.

The findings of this analysis suggest that most (62%) patients undergoing PMV may expect immediate hemodynamic benefit.

▶ This study, in which only 62% of the patients achieved a satisfactory result, was performed at one of the centers with the greatest experience in this procedure. All other centers attempting this palliative procedure should heed the definite and relative contraindications the authors have identified. In the meantime, the authors properly note that "optimism concerning PMV must be guarded."

In a separate article the same authors (1) reported that mitral balloon valvuloplasty is frequently associated with an increase in mitral regurgitation or the development of new regurgitation. The regurgitation was usually mild or moderate and could not be predicted. Three more articles from the same group are Palacios et al. (2); Wilkins et al. (3); and Block PC, Palacios IF (4). Come et al. (5) reported their experience in 37 patients undergoing balloon dilatation of the mitral valve.—R.C. Schlant, M.D.

References

1. Abascal VM, Wilkins GT, Choong CY, et al: Mitral regurgitation after percutaneous balloon mitral valvuloplasty in adults: Evaluation by pulsed doppler echocardiography. *J Am Coll Cardiol* 11:257–264, 1988.
2. Palacios I, Block PC, Brandi S, et al: Percutaneous balloon valvotomy for patients with severe mitral stenosis. *Circulation* 75:778–784, 1987.
3. Wilkins GT, Weyman A, Abascal VM, et al: Percutaneous balloon dilatation of the mitral valve: An analysis of echocardiographic variables related to outcome and the mechanism of dilatation. *Br Heart J* 60:299–308, 1988.
4. Block PC, Palacios IF: Pulmonary vascular dynamics after percutaneous mitral valvotomy. *J Thorac Cardiovasc Surg* 96:39–43, 1988.
5. Come PC, Riley MF, Diver DJ, et al: Noninvasive assessment of mitral stenosis before and after percutaneous balloon mitral valvuloplasty. *Am J Cardiol* 61:817–825, 1988.

Mitral Valve Prolapse in Patients With Prior Rheumatic Fever
Lembo NJ, Dell'Italia LJ, Crawford MH, Miller JF, Richards KL, O'Rourke RA
(Univ of Texas, VA Hospital, San Antonio)
Circulation 77:830–836, April 1988
3–6

Rheumatic heart disease often leads to isolated mitral regurgitation, and recent surgical studies suggest a high rate of mitral valve prolapse. The prevalence of valve prolapse was determined in a stable clinic population of 30 patients with a documented history of rheumatic fever and an apical systolic murmur. The 23 women and 7 men had a mean age of 31 years. Twenty-one patients had an early, mid, or late systolic murmur, whereas 9 had a pansystolic murmur.

Twenty patients had a murmur consistent with mitral regurgitation, whereas in 9 cases it was ascribed to aortic outflow turbulence. Only 1 patient had a right-sided murmur that increased on inspiration. Twenty-four (80%) patients had echographic evidence of mitral valve prolapse without mitral stenosis or other valve disease. Pulsed Doppler studies showed mild to moderate mitral regurgitation in 25 patients.

A systolic murmur in a patient with a history of rheumatic fever often represents isolated mitral regurgitation. However, mitral regurgitation in these patients often is secondary to mitral valve prolapse. The findings support an inflammatory cause of mitral prolapse in patients with a history of rheumatic fever. Whether long-term prophylaxis will prevent further valve inflammation remains to be learned.

▶ This study lends strong support to the proposal that rheumatic fever can produce inflammatory changes in the mitral valve that produce an acquired form of mitral valve prolapse (MVP). Larger and long-term studies both of patients with rheumatic fever and of patients with mitral valve prolapse are necessary to determine more accurately the frequency of this association. The finding of thickened mitral leaflets with prolapse of the anterior leaflet provides a clue to this form of acquired MVP.

Duren et al. (1) found that 100 of their 300 patients had a serious complication (ventricular tachycardia, infective endocarditis, severe mitral regurgitation, or cerebrovascular accidents) during an average follow-up of 6.1 years. The patients in this series were all symptomatic at the time of referral to the University of Amsterdam Medical Center. Two more recent articles dealt with the echocardiographic criteria for the diagnosis of mitral valve prolapse: Krivokapich et al. (2) and Levine et al. (3).—R.C. Schlant, M.D.

References

1. Duren DR, Becker AE, Dunning AJ: Long-term follow-up of idiopathic mitral valve prolapse in 300 patients: A prospective study. *J Am Coll Cardiol* 11:42–47, 1988.
2. Krivokapich J, Child JS, Dadourian BJ, et al: Reassessment of echocardiographic criteria for diagnosis of mitral valve prolapse. *Am J Cardiol* 61:131–135, 1988.
3. Levine RA, Stathogiannis E, Newell JB, et al: Reconsideration of echocardiographic standards for mitral valve prolapse: Lack of association between leaflet displacement isolated to the apical four chamber view and independent echocardiographic evidence of abnormality. *J Am Coll Cardiol* 11:1010–1019, 1988.

Differing Mechanisms of Exercise Flow Augmentation at the Mitral and Aortic Valves
Rassi A Jr, Crawford MH, Richards KL, Miller JF (Univ of Texas, VA Hosp, San Antonio)
Circulation 77:543–551, March 1988   3–7

During isotonic exercise, increases in both stroke volume and heart rate are responsible for the increase in cardiac output. The stroke volume is increased at both the mitral and the aortic valves. To determine the mechanism by which blood flow increases across the mitral and aortic valves during exercise, Doppler echocardiography was used to monitor 18 normal men during graded supine and upright bicycle exercise at matched workloads.

Heart rate increased by 124% during maximum supine exercise and by 104% during maximum upright exercise. Stroke volume increased by 20% during supine exercise and by 46% during upright exercise. These increases were statistically significant. At the ascending aorta, the increase in stroke volume was accomplished by an increase in the velocity-time integral of 15% during supine exercise and 48% during upright exercise. There was little change in the aortic cross section. However, at the mitral valve, the increase in stroke volume was accomplished by a 29% increase in mean diastolic cross-sectional area during supine exercise and a 34% increase during upright exercise. The velocity-time integral did not increase significantly.

It appears that the aorta and the mitral valve increase flow in response to exercise by different mechanisms. At the mitral valve, increased cross-sectional area is important, whereas increased velocity-time interval is important at the aortic valve. The heart rate times velocity integral can be used as an indicator of changes in cardiac output at the aortic valve, but is not appropriate for the mitral valve, where serial cross-sectional area measurements should be used. The effect of disease states that alter mitral valve mobility on exercise capacity is under investigation.

▶ The observation that the normal mitral valve orifice can increase significantly during exercise has important implications both for the normal mitral valve response to exercise and for a more complete undertaking of the factors responsible for the obstruction in rheumatic mitral stenosis and other conditions affecting the mitral valve.— R.C. Schlant, M.D.

Prediction of the Severity of Aortic Stenosis by Doppler Aortic Valve Area Determination: Prospective Doppler-Catheterization Correlation in 100 Patients

Oh JK, Taliercio CP, Holmes DR Jr, Reeder GS, Bailey KR, Seward JB, Tajik AJ (Mayo Clinic, Mayo Found, Rochester, Minn)
J Am Coll Cardiol 11:1227–1234, June 1988   3–8

Several studies have demonstrated an excellent correlation between pressure gradients determined by Doppler echocardiography and cardiac catheterization in the evaluation of aortic stenosis. However, the severity of aortic stenosis cannot always be determined on the basis of peak Doppler flow velocity or pressure gradient alone, because these parameters vary with cardiac output for a given aortic valve area. Recent studies have shown that aortic valve area could be reliably estimated from 2-dimensional and Doppler echocardiography using the continuity equation. The purpose of this study was to determine various Doppler variables predictive of the severity of aortic stenosis, and to compare Doppler- and catheterization-derived aortic valve areas.

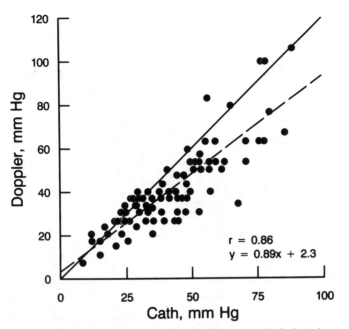

Fig 3–3.—Correlation between Doppler-derived and catheterization *(Cath)*-derived mean gradients across stenotic aortic valve in 100 patients. Mean standard error of estimation (estimation of catheterization mean gradient from Doppler mean gradient) was 10 mm Hg. (Courtesy of Oh JK, Taliercio CP, Holmes DR Jr, et al: *J Am Coll Cardiol* 11:1227–1234, June 1988.)

Two-dimensional and Doppler echocardiography were performed prospectively in 55 men and 45 women aged 53 to 95 years, with a mean age of 71 years, who had aortic stenosis and were undergoing cardiac catheterization for clinically valid reasons.

Doppler-derived mean gradient was correlated well with corresponding gradient measured by cardiac catheterization (Fig 3–3), but the peak Doppler aortic flow velocity or pressure gradient alone did not establish the severity of aortic stenosis in many patients. Peak Doppler aortic flow velocity and Doppler-derived mean aortic gradient were specific only for severe aortic stenosis but were not sensitive. Doppler-derived aortic valve area calculated by the continuity equation was correlated well with catheterization-derived aortic valve area calculated by the Gorlin equation (Fig 3–4).

The clinical implications of this study are, that in most patients, various Doppler variables and aortic valve area can be used to reliably estimate the severity of aortic stenosis by noninvasive techniques. Echocardiography provides additional data with regard to left ventricular function and other valvular lesions. Therefore, 2-dimensional and Doppler echocardiography should be the initial diagnostic procedure of choice for determining the severity of aortic stenosis.

▶ This study defines the value of 2-dimensional and Doppler echocardiography in evaluating patients with aortic stenosis, in whom it provides estimates of

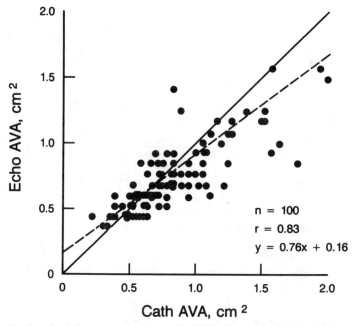

Fig 3–4.—Correlation between catheterization *(Cath)*-derived aortic valve area *(AVA)* and Doppler echocardiography *(Echo)*-derived aortic valve area with use of left ventricular outflow tract and aortic valve time velocity integral ratio in 100 patients. Mean standard error of estimation was 0.19 cm². (Courtesy of Oh JK, Taliercio CP, Holmes DR Jr, et al: *J Am Coll Cardiol* 11:1227–1234, June 1988.)

aortic valve area that usually agree well with valve areas calculated from cardiac catheterization. Catheterization is still advisable for many patients preoperatively, however, both to resolve conflicting clinical and Doppler data regarding the severity of stenosis and to study the coronary circulation in patients with symptoms of myocardial ischemia, men older than 40 years of age, women older than 50 years of age, or other patients at high risk of coronary artery disease (see Abstract 3–9).

Several other recent reports confirmed the value of Doppler echocardiography in the assessment of aortic stenosis: Harrison et al. (1), Jaffe et al. (2), Otto et al. (3), and Fan et al. (4).—R.C. Schlant, M.D.P

References

1. Harrison MR, Gurley JC, Smith MD, et al: A practical application of Doppler echocardiography for the assessment of severity of aortic stenosis. *Am Heart J* 115:622–628, 1988.
2. Jaffe WM, Roche AHG, Coverdale HA, et al: Clinical evaluation versus Doppler echocardiography in the quantitative assessment of valvular heart disease. *Circulation* 78:267–275, 1988.
3. Otto CM, Pearlman AS: Doppler echocardiography in adults with symptomatic aortic stenosis: Diagnostic utility and cost-effectiveness. *Arch Intern Med* 148:2553–2560, 1980.
4. Fan P-H, Kapur KK, Nanda NC: Color-guided Doppler echocardio-

graphic assessment of the aortic valve stenosis. *J Am Coll Cardiol* 12:441–449, 1988.

Frequency of Angina Pectoris and Coronary Artery Disease in Severe Isolated Valvular Aortic Stenosis
Vandeplas A, Willems JL, Piessens J, De Geest H (Univ Hosp Gasthuisberg, Leuven, Belgium)
Am J Cardiol 62:117–120, July 1, 1988   3–9

There is still much controversy over whether patients with severe aortic valve stenosis should routinely undergo coronary arteriography at cardiac catheterization before undergoing aortic valve replacement, even if they have no symptoms of coronary artery disease (CAD). Because previous recommendations to either omit or routinely perform coronary arteriography were based on studies with different sample sizes, mostly of less than 100 patients, the clinical and cardiac catheterization data from 192 patients who were treated during a 10-year period were reviewed.

The 121 men and 71 women aged 28–82 years, (mean, 59 years) underwent right-sided and left-sided cardiac catheterization, left ventriculography, aortography, and selective coronary angiography. Significant CAD was defined as a reduction of 50% or greater in the diameter of a major coronary artery or a major side branch.

Forty-seven (24%) of the 192 patients had significant CAD, and 145 did not. Thirty-nine (83%) of the 47 CAD patients and 88 (61%) of the 145 non-CAD patients had angina pectoris, for a total of 127 (66%) patients with angina and 65 (34%) patients without angina. However, 8 (12%) of the latter 65 patients had a significant CAD. Thus, angina had a low predictive value for CAD, whereas the negative predictive value for CAD of angina alone was 88%. When a risk score was calculated, using multivariate logistic regression for angina, age, and sex, the negative predictive value increased further to 95%. Both CAD and non-CAD patients had similar grades of angina, with 12% having grade 1; 59%, grade 2; 23%, grade 3; and 6%, grade 4.

In cases of severe aortic valvular stenosis, coronary arteriography can only be omitted for men aged younger-than 40 years and for women aged younger than 50 years who have no angina pectoris. For all other patients, coronary arteriography is warranted. Whether missing 5% of CAD is permissible still remains a debatable point.

▶ It is significant that all the men in this series with severe coronary artery disease were aged 45 or more years and all the women were aged 53 or more years. As indicated in the comments above (Abstract 3–8), I agree with the authors that coronary arteriography can only be omitted in patients with severe aortic stenosis if they have no symptoms of myocardial ischemia, have no risk factors to increase its incidence, and are men aged younger than 40 or women aged younger than 50 years. The next article is from the same institution but looks at the authors' experience with patients with aortic regurgitation.— R.C. Schlant, M.D.

Angina Pectoris and Coronary Artery Disease in Severe Aortic Regurgitation
Timmermans P, Willems JL, Piessens J, De Geest H (Univ Hosp Gasthuisberg, Leuven, Belgium)
Am J Cardiol 61:826–829, April 1988   3–10

Patients with aortic regurgitation often have angina pectoris. However, there is controversy over the prevalence of angina and coronary artery disease in this population and over the need for coronary arteriography. To determine the prevalence of angiographically significant coronary artery disease, data on 198 patients with isolated, severe aortic regurgitation were retrospectively reviewed.

Significant coronary artery disease was detected in 28 patients, 16 of whom had typical angina pectoris. Angina alone had a sensitivity of 57% to detect coronary artery disease. However, 19 patients without coronary artery disease also had angina, giving a specificity of 89%. Angina had a positive predictive value of 46% for this population. Absence of angina correctly predicted absence of coronary artery disease in 93% of patients.

These data indicate that coronary arteriography can be safely avoided in many severe aortic regurgitation patients who do not have symptoms or risk factors of ischemic heart disease.

▶ This study is one of the largest available in which the value of coronary arteriography in patients with aortic regurgitation has been critically evaluated. The authors conclude that coronary arteriography can be safely omitted if the patients have no symptoms of myocardial ischemia and have no risk factors known to increase its incidence. At present, most of our patients requiring elective surgery for aortic regurgitation have cardiac catheterization and have coronary arteriography at that time because it entails minimal risk or morbidity and may detect unexpected disease or variation. Additional, larger studies are needed before one can omit coronary arteriography at the time of cardiac catheterization. The next article documents 1 factor in the production of angina pectoris and other manifestations of myocardial ischemia in patients with aortic regurgitation but without evidence of coronary artery disease, a diminished coronary flow reserve.— R.C. Schlant, M.D.

Long-Term Vasodilator Therapy of Chronic Aortic Insufficiency: A Randomized Double-Blinded, Placebo-Controlled Clinical Trial
Greenberg B, Massie B, Bristow JD, Cheitlin M, Siemienczuk D, Topic N, Wilson RA, Szlachcic J, Thomas D (Oregon Health Sciences Univ, Portland; San Francisco VA Med Ctr; Univ of California, San Francisco)
Circulation 78:92–103, July 1988   3–11

Previous studies have shown that vasodilator drugs acutely reduce regurgitation and improve cardiac performance in patients with aortic insufficiency. These findings raise the possibility that long-term therapy may chronically reduce the volume overload to the left ventricle. However, the long-term effects of vasodilator drugs on left ventricular size and function have not yet been assessed.

Of 80 minimally symptomatic or asymptomatic patients with moderate-to-severe aortic insufficiency, 35 were randomly assigned to treatment with placebo, whereas the other 45 patients were treated with hydralazine in dosages titrated up to 150 to 300 mg per day, or an average dosage of 216 mg per day. Ten patients discontinued drug treatment early in the study, and 6 patients dropped out before their first radionuclide angiographic (RNA) evaluation at 3 months after randomization. Fifty-six of the remaining 64 patients were available at the 12-month RNA study, and 37 were available at the 24-month RNA evaluation, including 16 who were taking placebo and 21 who were receiving hydralazine. Overall, 13 of the 31 (42%) placebo patients who were available for follow-up examination stopped taking the study drug during the trial period. Thirteen of the 39 (33%) patients randomized to hydralazine who were available for follow-up discontinued use of the study drug.

Placebo-treated patients had only minimal changes in the mean left ventricular end-diastolic volume index (LVEDVI) after 24 months of treatment, compared with baseline values as measured by RNA. The LVEDVI was reduced by 30 ± 38 ml/m² (18%) in the 21 patients who were maintained on hydralazine for 24 months. The left ventricular end-systolic volume index (LVESVI) in hydralazine-treated patients showed a stepwise reduction over the 24-month study period, averaging 12 ml (21%) at 12 months, and 16 ml (28%) at 24 months.

The findings of this study show that long-term treatment with hydralazine reduces the volume overload in aortic insufficiency and suggest that hydralazine may have a beneficial effect on the natural history of aortic insufficiency.

► This preliminary study using hydralazine suggests the need for a large clinical trial to document the changes noted and to determine whether or not vasodilator therapy delays the deterioration of ventricular function and the need for surgery. Angiotensin-converting enzyme inhibitors and calcium antagonists may be even more effective.— R.C. Schlant, M.D.

Coronary Flow and Resistance Reserve in Patients With Chronic Aortic Regurgitation, Angina Pectoris, and Normal Coronary Arteries
Nitenberg A, Foult J-M, Antony I, Blanchet F, Rahali M (Centre Hospitalier Universitaire Xavier Bichat, Paris)
J Am Coll Cardiol 11:478–486, March 1988   3–12

In patients with chronic aortic regurgitation, the left ventricle can adapt to increased workload through myocardial hypertrophy. However,

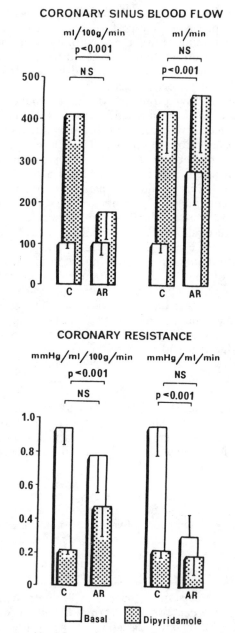

Fig 3–5.—Coronary sinus blood flow and coronary resistance in controls *(C)* and in patients with aortic regurgitation *(AR)* before and after intravenous administration of dipyridamole (0.14 mg/kg per minute × 4 minutes). (Courtesy of Nitenberg A, Foult J-M, Antony I, et al: *J Am Coll Cardiol* 11:478–486, March 1988.)

this hypertrophy has been associated with a reduction of coronary vascular reserve, which could be responsible for myocardial ischemic episodes. To examine this issue, coronary sinus blood flow and coronary resistance were measured before and after intravenous administration of dipyridamole, 0.14 mg/kg per minute for 4 minutes in 8 patients with aortic regurgitation, exertional angina, and normal coronary arteriograms, and in 8 controls.

By comparing basal and dipyridamole values, coronary flow reserve was significantly reduced in patients with aortic regurgitation compared with controls (1.67 ± 0.40 vs. 4.03 ± 0.52). Coronary resistance reserve was significantly reduced in patients with aortic regurgitation compared with controls (1.71 ± 0.50 vs. 4.38 ± 0.88). Basal coronary sinus blood flow was significantly higher in patients than in controls (276 ± 81 vs. 105 ± 24 ml per minute). Basal coronary resistance in patients was significantly lower than in controls (0.31 ± 0.13 vs. 0.95 ± 0.17 mm Hg/ml per minute). Coronary blood flow and resistance did not differ significantly between the 2 groups after administration of dipyridamole (Fig 3–5).

Coronary reserve appears to be reduced in patients with chronic left ventricular hypertrophy caused by aortic regurgitation. This reduction may contribute to stress-induced angina pectoris and could induce ischemic episodes that contribute to the progressive decline in left ventricular function seen in these patients.

▶ The mechanism of the reduction of coronary flow reserve may be failure of growth of the coronary circulation or restricted vasodilator capacity in the hypertrophied left ventricle or both. A marked decrease in the left coronary driving pressure may occasionally contribute. Unfortunately, the present study did not include patients with aortic regurgitation and left ventricular hypertrophy who did not have angina pectoris.—R.C. Schlant, M.D.

Transesophageal Two-Dimensional Echocardiography and Color Doppler Flow Velocity Mapping in the Evaluation of Cardiac Valve Prostheses
Nellessen U, Schnittger I, Appleton CP, Masuyama T, Bolger A, Fischell TA, Tye T, Popp RL (Stanford University)
Circulation 78:848–855, October 1988   3–13

Although transthoracic 2-dimensional and Doppler echocardiography are often useful in assessing prosthetic heart valves, various problems occasionally arise that may be obviated by using transesophageal echocardiography. A prospective study was therefore undertaken to compare the diagnostic accuracy of these techniques in the evaluation of cardiac prosthesis malfunction.

Over a 12-month period, 118 patients with prosthetic cardiac valves were studied with conventional techniques, including 52 patients suspected of prosthesis malfunction. Of these 52 patients, 26 had poor transthoracic echo signal quality and were studied by transesophageal echocardiography and color Doppler flow velocity mapping (color Doppler). Fourteen of the 26 patients with suspected prosthetic malfunction subsequently underwent left ventricular angiography or surgery or both. All 14 patients had had mitral valve replacement, 5 also had had aortic valve replacement, and 1 had had mitral, aortic, and tricuspid valve replacements. Eleven of the 14 patients had bioprostheses.

Transesophageal studies were well tolerated in all patients. In 4 of the 14 patients studied by angiography or at surgery, transesophageal 2-dimensional imaging gave added reliable information to that obtained from the transthoracic approach, including visualization of 3 flail leaflets and a vegetation confirmed by surgery. In 7 patients, transesophageal testing gave no additional information to that found from transthoracic studies. Neither approach permitted visualization of a mitral leaflet tear in 2 patients, a flail leaflet in 1 patient, and an anulus dehiscence in 1 patient. When 13 patients were graded as to valvular regurgitation by both transthoracic and transesophageal approaches, left ventricular angiography resulted in grading that corresponded to the transesophageal echocardiographic grading in 12 patients. The transesophageal approach may not, however, be superior to the transthoracic in the evaluation of aortic prostheses.

These data suggest that, for patients with suspected malfunction of mitral valve prostheses, transesophageal ultrasound can provide additional information to that available from the transthoracic approach. Although this additional information may help avoid further tests and allow more timely surgery, it causes discomfort and is not entirely risk free. Its use is recommended only for patients with transthoracic echocardiograms that are suboptimal in quality or do not correspond to the clinical findings (new murmur, shortness of breath, congestion, etc.) and in whom transesophageal results might alter management decisions.

► This study documents the value of transesophageal echocardiography and color Doppler flow velocity mapping in patients with mitral valve bioprostheses in the estimation of the severity of mitral regurgitation and the identification of flail leaflets or vegetations. Hopefully, the technique of transesophageal echocardiography will soon become easier, more available, and more established and the transducers will become smaller and less expensive. This is especially pertinent with the growing number of patients with mitral bioprostheses that have been in enough years to begin to develop structural defects due to primary tissue valve failure.

In the meantime, most of us will continue to rely heavily upon left ventricular angiography and the clinical presentation (new murmur, worsening heart failure, etc.) to help make decisions regarding the need for mitral prosthetic valve replacement when transthoracic ultrasound studies are either not satisfactory or do not fit the clinical picture. Indeed, one suspects that may have been done in this series. It is noteworthy that transesophageal echocardiography may be inferior to transthoracic echocardiography in the assessment of aortic valve prostheses. An excellent review of technique and usefulness of transesophageal echocardiography is that of J.B. Sewart et al. (1). See also Abstract 1–40.—R.C. Schlant, M.D.

Reference

1. Seward JB, Khanderia BK, Oh JK, et al: Transesophageal echocardiography: Technique, anatomic correlations, implementation, and clinical applications. *Mayo Clin Proc* 63:649–680, 1988.

Prevalence, Morphologic Types, and Evolution of Cardiac Valvular Disease in Systemic Lupus Erythematosus
Galve E, Candell-Riera J, Pigrau C, Permanyer-Miralda G, Garcia-Del-Castillo H, Soler-Soler J (Hosp Gen Vall d'Hebron, Barcelona, Spain)
N Engl J Med 319:817–823, Sept 29, 1988   3–14

Although autopsy studies show endocardial disease in 13% to 50% of people with systemic lupus erythematosus, its prevalence in living patients had not been established. To investigate this issue, a prospective study was performed in patients with systemic lupus. Seventy-four patients without history of rheumatic fever or infective endocarditis were subject to 2-dimensional echocardiography. All but 2 patients were followed up approximately 5 years later, with a second echocardiographic recording and Doppler echocardiography.

Initial findings resulted in grouping of patients according to valvular involvement. Group 1 comprised 7 patients with Libman-Sacks endocarditis; group 2, 6 patients with valvular thickening or deformity with valvular dysfunction; group 3, 5 patients with miscellaneous findings but no valvular dysfunction; and group 4, 56 patients with no valvular involvement. Overall, there was an 18% prevalence of clinically important valvular disease. Patients in group 1 were younger, had a shorter duration of lupus, and had received smaller cumulative doses of steroids than those in group 2. Follow-up showed that 1 patient in group 1 and 5 of 6 in group 2 required valvular surgery. No valvular dysfunction developed in group 3, but 5 patients in group 4 required reclassification to group 2 or 3.

This work shows a relatively high overall prevalence of valvular lesions (18%) in patients with systemic lupus, both in 59 outpatients without active lupus (15% prevalence) in 15 inpatients with active disease (26% prevalence). Echocardiography identified valvular thickening and dysfunction that frequently led to a requirement for mitral or aortic valve surgery.

▶ This study documents the frequency and importance in patients with systemic lupus erythematosus and involvement of the mitral and aortic valves with the production of either stenosis or regurgitation of either valve. Interestingly, only 1 of 7 patients in group 1 with echocardiographic evidence of verrucous (Libman-Sacks) endocarditis progressed from mild to severe mitral regurgitation requiring valve replacement. Other common cardiovascular manifestations of lupus include the effects of anemia and systemic hypertension. Pericarditis is frequent and myocarditis may occur in about 10%. Coronary arteritis or vasculitis, as well as accelerated atherosclerosis due to long-term corticosteroid therapy, may also occur (1).—R.C. Schlant, M.D.

Reference

1. Stevens MB: Lupus carditis. *N Engl J Med* 319:861–862, 1988.

Color Doppler Evaluation of Valvular Regurgitation in Normal Subjects
Yoshida K, Yoshikawa J, Shakudo M, Akasaka T, Jyo Y, Takao S, Shiratori K, Koizumi K, Okumachi F, Kato H, Fukaya T (Kobe Gen Hosp, Kobe, Japan)
Circulation 78:840–847, October 1988   3–15

The presently available color Doppler techniques accurately detect regurgitation of all cardiac valves, even when very mild. Recent studies reported regurgitant turbulent flow signals in otherwise normal subjects. This prospective study was done to determine the prevalence of valvular regurgitation in normal subjects.

The study population consisted of 211 apparently healthy volunteers, including 40 aged 6–9 years, 47 aged 10–19 years, 44 aged 20–29 years, 41 aged 30–39 years, and 39 aged 40–49 years. None of the subjects had a history of cardiovascular disease. Each study subject was examined with a color Doppler flow imaging system for the presence of mitral, aortic, tricuspid, or pulmonic regurgitant flow signals.

The prevalence rate of mitral regurgitation was 38% to 45% in each age group. In all but 2 subjects, the mitral regurgitant jets came from the posteromedial commissure. None of the subjects had aortic regurgitant flow signals. Tricuspid regurgitation was found in 15% to 77% in each age group, and pulmonary regurgitation, in 28% to 88%. The prevalence rate of tricuspid and pulmonary regurgitation was age dependent and tended to be lower among subjects aged 30 years and older. In these subjects, tricuspid and pulmonary regurgitant jets came from the center of the coaptation of each valve. The area of regurgitant jet signals in normal subjects was significantly smaller than that in patients with confirmed organic valve disease.

This study confirms that a large proportion of otherwise normal individuals aged younger than 50 show regurgitant signals of the mitral, tricuspid, and pulmonary valves on color Doppler examination that have no clinical significance.

▶ This study indicates that insignificant valvular regurgitation is present in many normal individuals and can be detected with color Doppler echocardiography. At present, the long-term significance of such regurgitation is unknown, as is whether or not such individuals have an increased risk of endocarditis. As the authors emphasize, it is important to avoid "iatrogenic heart disease." It is interesting that a previous study from the same group (1), in which pulsed Doppler echocardiography was employed in subjects aged 40 to

90 years, demonstrated the appearance of regurgitation in the 50s and an increase with advancing age until it was present in all aged older than 80. Using pulsed Doppler echocardiography, they found no mitral regurgitation in 33 normal subjects aged between 40 and 49 years, whereas in the present study, which employed color Doppler, 38% of normal subjects in this same age group had mitral regurgitation (see table). To complicate matters, Smith et al. (2) found acceptable intraobserver and interobserver reproducibility for mitral regurgitant jet area with color Doppler echocardiography but that there were significant observer differences with aortic regurgitant jet areas.—R.C. Schlant, M.D.

References

1. Akasaka T, Yoshikawa J, Yoshida K, et al: Age-related valvular regurgitation: A study to pulsed Doppler echocardiography. *Circulation* 76:262–265, 1987.
2. Smith MD, Grayburn PA, Spain MG, et al: Observer variability in the quantitation of Doppler color flow jet areas for mitral and aortic regurgitation. *J Am Coll Cardiol* 11:579–584, 1988.

Myocardial Diseases

Demonstration of Restrictive Ventricular Physiology by Doppler Echocardiography
Appleton CP, Hatle LK, Popp RL (Stanford Univ)
J Am Coll Cardiol 11:757–768, April 1988   3–16

It would be useful to have a noninvasive means of recognizing restrictive cardiac filling in patients with cardiomyopathy. The effectiveness of Doppler echocardiography in demonstrating mitral and tricuspid flow velocity patterns was evaluated in 14 symptomatic patients with various restrictive myocardial processes. Symptoms of congestive failure and elevated jugular venous pressure were noted, with typical hemodynamic features of restrictive/constrictive physiology but no obvious congenital, valvular, or pericardial disease. Ventricular diastolic chamber dimensions were normal. Forty healthy subjects also were examined.

Right and left ventricular end-diastolic pressures were elevated in patients with restrictive physiology. Rapid filling waves were large and nearly equal. The most common finding on endomyocardial biopsy was nonspecific fibrosis or hypertrophy or both. Flow velocity recordings showed shortened deceleration times across both valves, indicating premature cessation of filling and a diastolic dip-plateau contour of ventricular pressure. In addition, there were abnormal central venous flow velocity reversals on inspiration (Fig 3–6). Diastolic mitral and tricuspid regurgitation were frequently noted.

Doppler echocardiography is able to demonstrate the restrictive/constrictive hemodynamic pattern characteristic of symptomatic adults having restricted cardiac filling. The abnormalities include shortened mitral and tricuspid deceleration times, diastolic regurgitation, and in-

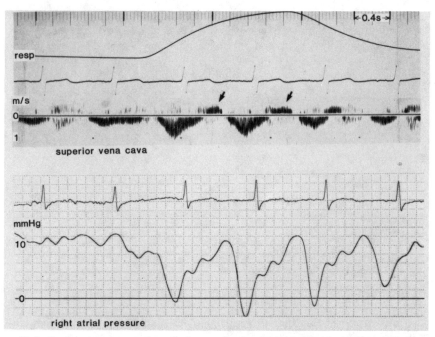

Fig 3–6.—Superior vena cava flow velocity recording *(upper panel)* and right atrial pressure recording *(lower panel)* from patient with restrictive disease with mild tricuspid regurgitation and near normal right ventricular end-diastolic pressure. Note abnormal systolic flow reversals *(arrows)* and right atrial pressure overshoots with inspiration, suggesting restriction to right heart filling. *resp*, respiration. (Courtesy of Appleton CP, Hatle LK, Popp RL: *J Am Coll Cardiol* 11:757–768, April 1988.)

creased flow reversal on inspiration in central venous flow velocity recordings.

▶ It is perhaps significant that in this study from Stanford of restrictive cardiomyopathy, which is usually idiopathic or produced by amyloid heart disease, 6 of 14 patients were cardiac transplant recipients. As with most echocardiographic diagnoses, the diagnostic accuracy is related to the presence of a combination of echocardiographic features rather than any single finding or measurement. The findings of this study, when confirmed, should enable one to make the proper diagnosis in many patients with this very difficult to diagnose (or treat) clinical syndrome.—R.C. Schlant, M.D.

Doppler Echocardiographic Determination of the Pressure Gradient in Hypertrophic Cardiomyopathy

Sasson Z, Yock PG, Hatle LK, Alderman EL, Popp RL (Stanford Univ)
J Am Coll Cardiol 11:752–756, April 1988   3–17

The continuous-wave Doppler ultrasound signal across the left ventricular outflow tract has a typical pattern in hypertrophic cardiomyopathy (Fig 3–7). The value of this method for measuring peak pressure gradi-

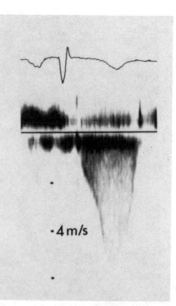

Fig 3–7.—Spectral recording of continuous wave Doppler ultrasound signal from left ventricular outflow tract in patient with hypertrophic cardiomyopathy and associated pressure gradient. Transducer is at cardiac apex. Note characteristic midsystolic acceleration and late systolic peak of maximal flow velocity contour across outflow tract displayed below *solid black horizontal baseline.* Electrocardiogram is above ultrasound signal. (Courtesy of Sasson Z, Yock PG, Hatle LK, et al: *J Am Coll Cardiol* 11:752–756, April 1988.)

ents was examined in 5 consecutive patients. Ultrasonography was done simultaneously with dual catheter pressure recordings across the left ventricular outflow tract. The gradient was altered by the Valsalva maneuver, catheter-induced ventricular extrasystoles, amyl nitrite inhalation, or intravenous isoproterenol.

Doppler-derived gradients accurately predicted measured catheter gradients over a wide range, both at rest and during provocative maneuvers (Fig 3–8). The timing of the catheter pressure gradient and its magnitude and contour all were accurately reflected by the Doppler spectral envelope. Some of the more marked interobserver differences were caused by contamination of the left ventricular outflow tract signal by a superimposed mitral regurgitation signal.

Continuous-wave Doppler echocardiography can accurately estimate the peak systolic pressure gradient across the left ventricular outflow tract in patients with hypertrophic cardiomyopathy, as long as mitral regurgitation is not present. The pressure drop is generated over a relatively short distance.

► Accurate, continuous-wave Doppler ultrasound measurements of the left ventricular outflow tract pressure gradient should be of significant value both in the management of patients with hypertrophic cardiomyopathy and in the study of its natural history. Although the findings indicate that the pressure

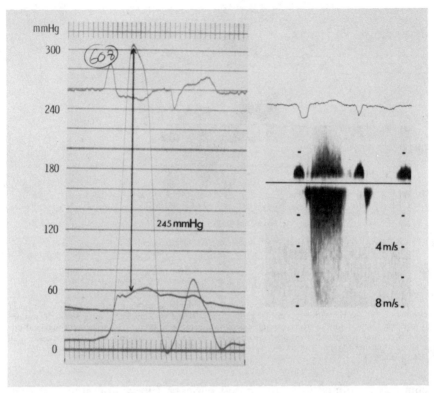

Fig 3-8.—Simultaneous Doppler ultrasound and catheter tracings during catheter-induced ventricular bigeminy in patient with hypertrophic cardiomyopathy. In postextrasystolic beat, peak Doppler flow velocity was 8.0 m/sec, corresponding to Doppler gradient of 256 mm Hg. This correlates well with measured catheter gradient of 245 mm Hg. (Courtesy of Sasson 2, Yock PG, Hatle LK, et al: *J Am Coll Cardiol* 11:752–756, April 1988.)

drop occurs over a relatively short distance, they unfortunately do not greatly clarify the mechanisms or significance of the pressure gradient. Come et al. (1) also studied 5 patients by continuous-wave Doppler echocardiography and confirmed dynamic obstruction.—R.C. Schlant, M.D.

Reference

1. Come PC, Riley MF, Carl LV, et al: Doppler evidence that true left ventricular-to-aortic pressure gradients exist in hypertrophic cardiomyopathy. *Am Heart J* 116:1253–1261, 1988.

Myocarditis Presenting as Acute Myocardial Infarction
Miklozek CL, Crumpacker CS, Royal HD, Come PC, Sullivan JL, Abelmann WH
(Beth Israel Hosp, Boston; Harvard Univ; Univ of Massachusetts, Worcester)
Am Heart J 115:768–776, April 1988   3–18

Ten patients who had signs of acute myocardial infarction were found to have acute viral myocarditis. This diagnosis was confirmed by isolation of virus, an increase in viral antibody titers, positive evidence of inflammatory filtrates, or positive pyrophosphate or gallium scans.

All patients had symptoms of viral infection. Seven had laboratory evidence of acute viral infection. The acute cardiac findings were chest pain in 9 patients, compatible electrocardiograms and elevated creatine kinase levels in 10, positive MB fractions in 8, and regional wall motion abnormalities in 8. In 6 patients, the left ventricular ejection fraction was less than 55%; 5 patients had ventricular ectopy; 4 had bundle-branch block; 3 had transient junctional escape rhythm; and 3 had congestive heart failure. Among the 9 patients who were followed for 1–14 months, there was 1 death, persistent wall motion abnormality in 4 patients, and ejection fraction of less than 55% in 3.

It appears that clinical myocardial infarction resulted from the viral myocarditis. Therefore, acute viral myocarditis should be considered in patients with impaired regional wall function simulating acute myocardial infarction. Patients who have the clinical syndrome of acute myocardial infarction and normal coronary angiograms should be considered for endomyocardial biopsy.

▶ This report of 10 patients who were aged 18 to 39 years clearly documents that viral myocarditis can produce chest pain, regional wall motion abnormalities, and focal pyrophosphate scans mimicking acute myocardial infarction. The mechanisms of the myocardial injury in myocarditis is unknown. Possibilities include diffuse, direct injury to the myocytes by the virus itself as well as potentially regional arteritis and thrombus formation, coronary artery spasm, and even coronary artery embolus from a left ventricular thrombus. The value of an endomyocardial biopsy to help establish the diagnosis of viral myocarditis will be even greater when we have an effective therapy, hopefully in the near future. The next article (Abstract 3–19) discusses a course of myocarditis that is, unfortunately, becoming more common: AIDS.—R.C. Schlant, M.D.

Prevalent Myocarditis at Necropsy in the Acquired Immunodeficiency Syndrome

Anderson DW, Virmani R, Reilly JM, O'Leary T, Cunnion RE, Robinowitz M, Macher AM, Punja U, Villaflor ST, Parrillo JE, Roberts WC (United States Food and Drug Administration, Bethesda, Md; Armed Forces Inst of Pathology, Washington, DC; Washington Hosp Ctr, District of Columbia Gen Hosp, Washington, DC)
J Am Coll Cardiol 11:792–799, April 1988   3–19

Because focal myocarditis was recently found in 2 patients with acquired immunodeficiency syndrome (AIDS) who had findings of dilated cardiomyopathy, the prevalence of myocarditis was retrospectively determined in 71 consecutive autopsies of AIDS patients encountered in 1982–1986. Fifty-eight patients had participated in National Institutes of Health trials of interferon, interleukin-2, chemotherapy, or experimental antiviral agents.

Myocarditis was found in 37 (52%) of 71 patients. All 7 patients with biventricular dilation at autopsy had myocarditis; fatal congestive failure occurred in 4 of these. Seven patients with myocarditis had viral, protozoan, bacterial, fungal, or mycobacterial opportunistic pathogens, but the cause of myocarditis was unclear in most patients. The usual finding was focal mild myocarditis, which could not be related to duration of disease or to drug treatment.

Heart failure associated with biventricular dilation and myocarditis is an infrequent finding in AIDS. However, morbidity and mortality from cardiac disease may increase as pulmonary disease is more effectively treated in patients with AIDS. Myocarditis in patients with AIDS may reflect microvascular spasm or altered immune regulation.

▶ In this series, only 4 (6%) of the 71 patients died of heart failure although 37 (52%) had microscopic evidence of myocarditis. The course of the myocarditis may be the human immunodeficiency virus, Coxsackie B virus, cytomegalovirus, or other clinically implicated viruses. Viral cultures of myocardium were carried out in only 6 cases in this study and were all negative. The clinical course of 58 of the 71 patients was reported in a separate communication from the same group (1). They found that clinical cardiac abnormalities in critically ill patients who die of AIDS were frequently associated with evidence of myocarditis at postmortem examination. Baroldi et al. (2) found lymphocytic myocarditis in 9 of 26 fatal cases, intramyocardial lymphocytic infiltrates without necrosis in 7 and epicardial lymphocytic infiltrates in 4. No patients in this series had congestive heart failure although echocardiography revealed functional abnormalities in some.

In the future, it is likely that myocarditis and heart failure will be a more important aspect of the medical care of patients with AIDS, particularly as we improve the treatment of their pulmonary infections.—R.C. Schlant, M.D.

References

1. Reilly JM, Cunnion RE, Anderson DW, et al: Frequency of myocarditis, left ventricular dysfunction and ventricular tachycardia in the acquired immune deficiency syndrome. *Am J Cardiol* 62:789–793, 1988.
2. Baroldi G, Corallo S, Moroni M, et al: Focal lymphocytic myocarditis in acquired immunodeficiency syndrome (AIDS): A correlative morphologic and clinical study in 26 consecutive fatal cases. *J Am Coll Cardiol* 12:463–469, 1988.

Detection of Myocarditis During the First Year After Discovery of a Dilated Cardiomyopathy by Endomyocardial Biopsy and Gallium-67 Myocardial Scintigraphy: Prospective Multicentre French Study of 91 Patients
Bouhour JB, Helias J, de Lajartre AY, Petitier H, Komajda M, Leger A, Delcourt A, Sacrez A, Bareiss P, Constantinesco A, Bellocq JP, Ferriere M, Chevalier·C, Baldet P, Cassagnes J, Peycelon P, Kantelip B, Geslin P, Pezard P, Saint-Andre JP (Hôpital G et R Laënnec, Nantes, France)
Eur Heart J 9:520–528, May 1988   3–20

Both endomyocardial biopsy and myocardial scanning with gallium 67 have been used to assess the frequency of myocardial inflammatory lesions in patients with dilated cardiomyopathy. The results of the 2 techniques were compared. Endomyocardial biopsy was performed on 91 patients with dilatation and hypokinesia of the left ventricle, and scintigraphy of the precordial region was performed 48–72 hours after injection of ^{67}Ga.

Scanning yielded positive findings in 14% of the patients; results were doubtful in 21% and negative in 65%. On biopsy, myocarditis with mild fibrosis was found in only 4 patients. There was no correlation between the 2 methods. Difficulty in identifying lymphocytes on pathologic examination and subjectivity in choosing the criterion for positivity on scanning were problems.

Despite its limitations in the search for focal lesions, endomyocardial biopsy remains the reference method for detecting interstitial inflammation. The value of ^{67}Ga scanning in detecting lymphocytic infiltrates was not demonstrated. Both techniques suggest that cellular infiltrates are minimal and infrequent in patients with dilated cardiomyopathy.

▶ The clinician's enthusiasm for myocardial biopsy in patients with possible myocarditis will be much greater when there is reasonable evidence that therapy affects the development of chronic cardiomyopathy or the subsequent 5-year mortality or both. At present, we do not have evidence that the available therapy of myocarditis is really beneficial. Hopefully, the results of ongoing clinical trials will be positive. The next paper reports a possible therapy in specialized cases.—R.C. Schlant, M.D.

Prevention of Murine Coxsackie B3 Viral Myocarditis and Associated Lymphoid Organ Atrophy With Recombinant Human Leucocyte Interferon αA/D

Kishimoto C, Crumpacker CS, Abelmann WH (Beth Israel Hosp, Boston; Harvard Univ)
Cardiovasc Res 22:732–738, October 1988   3–21

Although natural human interferon preparations do not show significant activity in murine cells, a recombinant human leukocyte interferon subtype αD, and the hybrid interferon-αA/D have shown relatively much antiviral activity in murine cell cultures and in vivo. Acute viral myocarditis is increasingly recognized as an important cause of morbidity and mortality. Because the Coxsackie B viruses are the most common agents associated with acute infectious myocarditis, a study was done to assess the effect of recombinant human leukocyte interferon-αA/D on experimentally induced Coxsackie B3 (CB3) viral myocarditis.

Three-week-old mice were inoculated intraperitoneally with CB3 virus. Two different dosages of interferon-αA/D were administered subcutaneously once daily to 2 groups of 10 mice each, starting 1 day before virus inoculation. The greater dose was also administered once daily to a third group of 10 mice, starting on the same day as virus inoculation. A control group of 10 mice was injected with saline. All animals were killed on day 5 for evaluation.

Administration of human leukocyte interferon-αA/D starting 1 day before or on the same day as inoculation with CB3 virus inhibited multiplication of virus in the heart and protected against myocarditis developing in the mice. Interferon-αA/D in either the greater or the smaller dose effectively reduced the inflammatory response, myocardial damage, and calcification when treatment was started before or simultaneously with CB3 inoculation.

The findings of this study are of little clinical importance, as interferon-αA/D was administered before or simultaneously with CB3 virus inoculation. Similar previous studies had already shown that administration of interferon at a later stage of myocarditis is ineffective. However, under conditions of sporadic outbreak or laboratory infection with a cardiotropic virus, consideration of therapy with interferon-αA/D may well be justified.

▶ This study suggests that interferon may be useful in the very early therapy of coxsackie B myocarditis but that such treatment would have to be given very early to be effective. The next paper describes a patient in whom a cardiomyopathy may have developed from a different interferon-α given for metastatic renal cell carcinoma.—R.C. Schlant, M.D.

Recombinant Alpha$_2$ Interferon-Related Cardiomyopathy
Cohen MC, Huberman MS, Nesto RW (New England Deaconess Hosp, Boston)
Am J Med 85:549–550, October 1988   3–22

Recombinant interferon-α has been used with some success in the treatment of advanced renal cell carcinoma and other malignancies. Almost all patients experience some toxicity during therapy that may involve flulike symptoms, transient leukopenia, increased hepatic transaminase levels, and other side effects. Cardiovascular toxicity consisting mainly of mild to moderate hypotension and tachycardia has also been reported.

Woman, 62, with metastatic renal cell carcinoma was treated with recombinant interferon-α_2 and subsequently had congestive heart failure of rapid onset caused by a dilated cardiomyopathy. The patient had a history of well-controlled hypertension and incomplete right bundle branch block, but no evidence of prior cardiac symptoms or abnormal cardiac findings before treatment with interferon-α_2 was initiated. She was given interferon-α_2 at a dose of 3 million units per day for 3 days, after which the dose was increased to 9 million units per day. Two days after the increase in dosage, she started to complain of shortness of breath, weakness, confusion, anorexia, and insomnia. Interferon-α_2 administration was discontinued, but she required hospitalization 3 days later because of progression of symptoms.

Because the patient showed signs and symptoms consistent with congestive heart failure, she was treated with isosorbide, captopril, furosemide, and digoxin.

She was discharged after improving with medical management, but she died less than 1 year later owing to progression of her pulmonary disease. Postmortem examination revealed no coronary artery disease, fibrosis, amyloidosis, or morphological changes in myocardial cells. These findings were consistent with a drug-related cardiomyopathy.

The authors believe that this is the first case report of interferon-α_2-related cardiomyopathy.

▶ This report raises the possibility that interferon-α_2 administered to treat metastatic renal cell carcinoma may produce a toxic cardiomyopathy. Previous reports had suggested that it may produce arrhythmia or myocardial infarction. For the present, it would probably be well to monitor patients receiving interferon-α_2.— R.C. Schlant, M.D.

Pericardial Diseases

Tuberculosis Pericarditis: Ten Year Experience With A Prospective Protocol for Diagnosis and Treatment
Sagristà-Sauleda J, Permanyer-Miralda G, Soler-Soler J (Hosp Gen Vall d'Hebron, Barcelona, Spain)
J Am Coll Cardiol 11:724–728, April 1988 3–23

The diagnosis of tuberculosis in a prospective group of patients with acute pericardial disease using a systematic protocol is described. The criteria for diagnosis were identification of tubercle bacilli in fluid or tissue and the identification of caseating granulomas.

Of the 294 patients, 13 had tuberculosis pericarditis. Their diagnoses were based on sputum culture, pericardial fluid culture, pericardial, lymph node, and pleural biopsy specimens. Four patients had an acute self-limiting disease course. One patient had relapsing tamponade, and 4 had tamponade that was effectively treated with pericardiocentesis. Four patients had toxic symptoms with fever. The time that elapsed from hospital admission to diagnosis was 1–14 weeks. Constrictive pericarditis developed in 6 patients, and effusive-constrictive pericarditis developed in 1. All of these patients required pericardiectomy; none of the patients died.

Tuberculosis pericarditis has a variable clinical presentation. It should be considered in all patients with acute pericarditis. Diagnosis should be based on a systematic protocol. In patients with acute pericarditis lasting longer than 1 week, 3 samples of sputum or gastric aspirate should be cultured. In patients with pleural effusion, adenosine deaminase activity should be assayed in the pleural fluid. If this activity is greater than 45 units/L, invasive cardiac studies may be justified. Pericardiocentesis should be performed when necessary, and pericardial biopsy should be performed when significant disease persists after 3 weeks or when there is a strong suspicion of tuberculosis. This approach should identify tuberculosis pericarditis when present, while avoiding invasive studies in patients with idiopathic pericarditis.

▶ The diagnostic protocol used by the authors makes very good sense and is very close to our current diagnostic plan. Interestingly, sputum or gastric aspirate study disclosed tubercle bacilli in 6 of 11 patients (by culture in all) and in 4 patients, the sputum/aspirate test first described the diagnosis. Unfortunately, an early definitive diagnosis is still difficult to achieve and still often time-consuming because of the time to grow tubercle bacilli.— R.C. Schlant, M.D.

Disturbances of Cardiac Rhythm and Conduction

Late Clinical Outcome in Patients With Early Ventricular Fibrillation After Myocardial Infarction

Nicod P, Gilpin E, Dittrich H, Wright M, Engler R, Rittlemeyer J, Henning H, Ross J Jr (Univ of California, San Diego; Univ of British Columbia)
J Am Coll Cardiol 11:464–470, March 1988   3–24

The implications of ventricular fibrillation that occurs within 48 hours after acute infarction remain incompletely understood. Of 2,088 patients admitted in a 5-year period with acute myocardial infarction, 147 (7%) had at least 1 episode of ventricular fibrillation within 48 hours of admis-

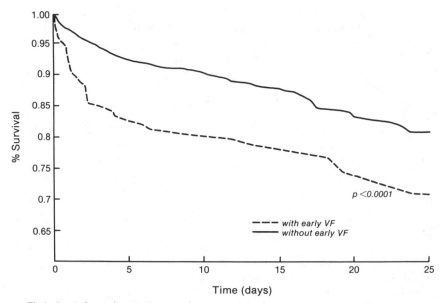

Fig 3–9.—In-hospital survival curves of patients with and without early ventricular fibrillation *(VF)*. Only cardiac deaths were analyzed in these curves. Patients with early ventricular fibrillation (within 48 hours of admission) had significantly lower in-hospital survival rate. (Courtesy of Nicod P, Gilpin E, Dittrich H, et al: *J Am Coll Cardiol* 11:464–470, March 1988.)

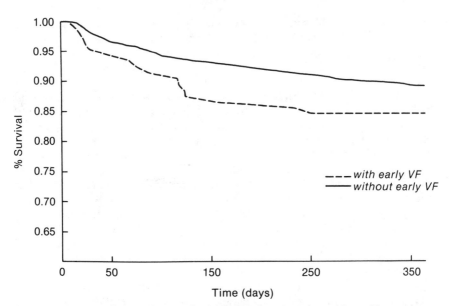

Fig 3–10.—One-year survival curves after hospital discharge in patients with or without early ventricular fibrillation *(VF)*. Only cardiac deaths were analyzed in these curves. Difference in survival between patient groups was not significant (*P* < .128), although there was trend toward increased survival in group without early ventricular fibrillation. (Courtesy of Nicod P, Gilpin E, Dittrich H, et al: *J Am Coll Cardiol* 11:464–470, March 1988.)

sion. Left ventricular failure was more prominent in these patients. A history of congestive failure was more frequent, and peak serum creatine kinase levels were higher in patients with early fibrillation.

Hospital mortality was higher in patients with early ventricular fibrillation (Fig 3–9). Left ventricular failure was a more frequent cause of death in patients with fibrillation. No important differences in physical findings or in the frequency of complex ventricular arrhythmias were noted. The difference in mortality rates at 1 year were not significant (Fig 3–10). Early fibrillation remained an independent prognostic factor in hospital mortality after controlling for left ventricular failure and other significant prognostic variables.

Patients having ventricular fibrillation within 48 hours after acute infarction have increased hospital mortality, mostly because of left ventricular failure. However, 1-year mortality for hospital survivors is not compromised.

► This study confirms several other studies that indicated that primary ventricular fibrillation in early acute myocardial infarction is not as benign as some early studies suggested. Other studies have indicated that patients with primary ventricular fibrillation after acute myocardial infarction have both an increased in-hospital mortality and an increased 1- or 5-year mortality.—R.C. Schlant, M.D.

Electrophysiologic Effects of Intravenous and Oral Sotalol for Sustained Ventricular Tachycardia Secondary to Coronary Artery Disease

Kopelman HA, Woosley RL, Lee JT, Roden DM, Echt DS (Vanderbilt Univ)
Am J Cardiol 61:1006–1011, May 1, 1988   3–25

Sotalol is a β-blocker that prolongs repolarization and refractoriness in Purkinje fibers and ventricular muscle. The electrophysiologic effects of intravenous and oral sotalol were studied in a prospective series of 16 patients having electrophysiologic studies for sustained ventricular tachycardia secondary to coronary artery disease. An intravenous dose of 1.5 mg/kg was followed by a maintenance dose of 0.008 mg/kg. The mean oral dose was 583 mg daily. A majority of the patients had marked left ventricular dysfunction.

Reductions in mean arterial pressure were not significant. Both intravenous and oral sotalol increased the sinus cycle length, atrio-His interval, and atrioventricular node relative and functional refractory periods. Oral sotalol prolonged the corrected sinus node recovery time. Sotalol prolonged the QT interval, atrial effective refractory period, and right ventricular effective refractory period by both routes. Intravenous sotalol prevented induction of ventricular tachycardia in 2 of 9 patients, whereas oral sotalol was effective in 2 of 11 patients.

Intravenous and oral sotalol exert similar electrophysiologic effects on patients having sustained ventricular tachycardia secondary to coronary artery disease. However, specific quantitative effects may differ in individual patients.

▶ This study documents the qualitatively similar efficacy of intravenous and oral sotalol in the treatment of sustained ventricular tachycardia in patients with coronary artery disease. The electrophysiologic effects of sotalol are those of a class III antiarrhythmia drug and are significantly different from those of propranolol. Sotalol appears to be effective acutely in eliminating inducibility in 18% to 22% of patients with ventricular tachycardia. It is also useful in patients with supraventricular tachycardia and premature ventricular contractions.—R.C. Schlant, M.D.

Frequency of ST-Segment Depression Produced by Mental Stress in Stable Angina Pectoris From Coronary Artery Disease

Barry J, Selwyn AP, Nabel EG, Rocco MB, Mead K, Campbell S, Rebecca G (Harvard Univ)
Am J Cardiol 61:989–993, May 1, 1988   3–26

Mental stress, as well as physical exertion, can cause myocardial ischemia in patients with coronary artery disease. The relationship of perceived mental stress to ischemia was studied in 28 patients with confirmed coronary disease during ambulatory ECG monitoring. The ECG records were analyzed separately from diaries of physical activity and perceived mental state.

There were 372 episodes of ST-segment depression in 912 hours of ECG monitoring. Twenty-six percent of episodes occurred during increased physical activity with usual mental activities. Another 22% of ischemic events occurred during usual or high levels of mental stress but low levels of physical activity. In 36% of instances, both physical and mental activities were at usual levels. Ten percent of episodes occurred during sleep. Increasing physical or mental activity was associated with an increasing duration of ischemia per unit of recording time.

The intensity of both physical activity and perceived mental stress influences myocardial ischemia during daily activities in patients with coronary disease. The findings support attempts to modify these external influences in order to lessen ischemic heart disease activity.

▶ This study presents evidence that periods of either heavy exercise or perceived high levels of mental stress are associated with increased incidence and duration of ST-segment depression in some patients with coronary artery disease. Selwyn and colleagues have previously reported that mental arithmetic activity in patients with coronary artery disease may produce evidence of regional disturbances of myocardial perfusion on positron tomography with 82RG, often without ST-segment changes (1). Much work is needed to determine the mechanisms involved and the significance of the changes before specific therapeutic recommendations can be made.

Rozanski et al. (2) found wall-motion abnormalities in 59% and a fall in ejection fraction of more than 4% in 36% of patients with coronary artery disease during periods of mental stress. M.J. Follick et al. (3) have reported a relationship between self-reported levels of psychosocial stress and premature ventricular complexes in patients who survived myocardial infarction.— R.C. Schlant, M.D.

References

1. Deanfield JE, Kensett M, Wilson RA, et al: Silent myocardial ischemia due to mental stress. *Lancet* 2:1001–1004, 1984.
2. Rozanski A, Bairey CN, Krantz DS, et al: Mental stress and the induction of silent myocardial ischemia in patients with coronary artery disease. *N Engl J Med* 318:1005–1012, 1988.
3. Follick MJ, Gorkin L, Capone RJ, et al: Psychosocial distress as a predictor of ventricular arrhythmias in a post-myocardial infarction population. *Am Heart J* 116:32–36, 1988.

Reentry as a Cause of Ventricular Tachycardia in Patients With Chronic Ischemic Heart Disease: Electrophysiologic and Anatomic Correlation

de Bakker JMT, van Capelle FJL, Janse MJ, Wilde AAM, Coronel R, Becker AE, Dingemans KP, van Hemel NM, Hauer RNW (Academic Med Ctr, Amsterdam; Antonius Hosp, Nieuwegein; Univ Hosp, Utrecht, the Netherlands)
Circulation 77:589–606, March 1988   3–27

To elucidate the mechanism of ventricular tachycardia during the chronic phase of myocardial infarction, electrophysiologic and histologic

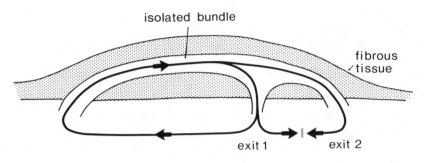

isolated bundle

fibrous tissue

exit 1   exit 2

subendocardial muscle

Fig 3–11.—Possible reentrant pathway, partly through bundles of surviving myocardial fibers embedded in fibrous tissue. Main bundle bifurcates and gives rise to 2 exits toward larger subendocardial muscle mass. If activation uses only 1 branch of bifurcation, 1 site of origin will appear; if activation leaves bundle at random, sometimes through exit 1 and sometimes through exit 2, site of origin will alternate. (Courtesy of de Bakker JMT, van Capelle FJL, Janse MJ, et al: *Circulation* 77:589–606, March 1988.)

data were obtained from 64 endocardial recording sites in 72 patients during tachycardia by microelectrode recording in 20 resected endocardial preparations and by mapping in 2 isolated perfused hearts.

During operation, 139 tachycardias were induced, 105 of which seemed to arise at focal areas of less than 1.4 cm^2. Macroreentry around the infarction scar was detected in only 3 patients. In 21 tachycardias with focal origins, presystolic activity preceded subendocardial activation. This presystolic activity was detected at several sites in 3 tachycardias, which permitted reconstruction of the route of activation. The histology of 1 of these patients demonstrated separate zones of viable myocardial fibers located intramurally and subendocardially, in which presystolic activity was recorded. This supports the hypothesis that reentry occurs through isolated bundles of surviving myocytes on the border of the infarct and the subendocardial muscle mass. The conduction velocity through these isolated bundles was approximately 25 cm per second.

The focal origin of reentrant tachycardias occurring during the chronic phase of myocardial infarction is actually caused in some patients by exit from a pathway consisting of a tract of viable myocardial fibers on the edge of the infarction and the remaining subendocardial mass (Fig 3–11). All such exits must be removed to prevent recurrence of tachycardia. Endocardial resection should not be restricted to removal of a small area at the focal origin of the tachycardia.

▶ This careful study presents strong evidence that the mechanisms of sustained ventricular tachycardia in patients after myocardial infarction is macroreentry through 1 or more isolated pathways or exits. To prevent recurrent ventricular tachycardias, it is important that endocardial resection (or ablation techniques) include all such exits.—R.C. Schlant, M.D.

Maximal Exercise Testing and Gas Exchange in Patients With Chronic Atrial Fibrillation

Atwood JE, Myers J, Sullivan M, Forbes S, Friis R, Pewen W, Callaham P, Hall
P, Froelicher V (VA Med Ctr, Long Beach, Calif)
J Am Coll Cardiol 11:508–513, March 1988   3–28

Chronic atrial fibrillation is a common arrhythmia, but it remains
poorly understood. The typical atrial fibrillation study population is heterogeneous in terms of underlying heart disease. The hemodynamic and
gas exchange response to maximal exercise of 21 men with atrial fibrillation alone was compared with that in 29 age- and sex-matched patients
with atrial fibrillation and underlying heart disease.

Patients with atrial fibrillation without underlying heart disease had
normal exercise capacity. Patients who also had underlying heart disease
had significantly diminished capacity for exercise. The maximal heart
rate in patients with atrial fibrillation alone was 189 ± 32 beats per
minute, which was significantly higher than the 166 ± 24 beats per
minute of patients with underlying heart disease. Stepwise regression
analysis indicated that maximal systolic blood pressure represented 19%
of the variance in maximal oxygen uptake, suggesting that systolic function is an important determinant of performance during exercise in patients with atrial fibrillation.

The response to exercise of patients with atrial fibrillation without underlying heart disease is different from that of a typical heterogeneous
study population. Patients with atrial fibrillation alone had a higher maximal heart rate than those with underlying heart disease. Heart rate in
patients with atrial fibrillation was directly related to total oxygen body
demand. Exercise capacity in patients with atrial fibrillation was limited
by existing underlying heart disease, but was not limited by atrial fibrillation itself.

▶ The authors suggest that the increased heart rate in atrial fibrillation may be
a compensatory mechanism for subjects to maintain functional capacity. Interestingly only 41 of the 50 patients were taking digoxin, and the mean digoxin
doses were not different between the 2 groups. It would be interesting to
know the responses in patients in whom the dose of digoxin was individually
adjusted by both the resting and exercise ventricular heart rates, which is the
technique we usually recommend. I am surprised that 4 of 21 men without apparent heart disease and that 5 of 29 men with underlying heart disease were
not on digoxin, because most patients with acquired atrial fibrillation require
digoxin to control the ventricular response rate unless they have underlying
conduction system disease.—R.C. Schlant, M.D.

The Automatic Implantable Cardioverter-Defibrillator: Clinical Experience, Complications, and Follow-up in 25 Patients

Borbola J, Denes P, Ezri MD, Hauser RG, Serry C, Goldin MD (Rush-Presbyterian-St Luke's Med Ctr, Chicago)
Arch Intern Med 148:70–76, January 1988   3–29

The automatic implantable cardioverter-defibrillator (AICD) may dramatically reduce the incidence of sudden cardiac death among patients with recurrent, drug-resistant, sustained ventricular tachyarrhythmias. However, many complications are associated with the use of this device. The results of AICD implantation in 25 patients with recurrent ventricular tachyarrhythmias were reviewed.

Patients were followed for an average of 11 months. Before implantation, these patients had survived at least 1 cardiac arrest and 2–3 episodes of syncope, and had received 5–7 antiarrhythmic drugs. After implantation, complications included 2 deaths, 1 reoperation, 1 myocardial infarction, 1 sensing failure, 5 infections, 2 pocket seromas, 4 device failures, 1 device deactivation, and 2 inappropriate discharges. In 7 patients, the device discharged appropriately. The energy required by the device was related to the type of arrhythmia induced. Ventricular tachycardia acceleration occurred in 10 patients. There were no significant changes in electrocardiogram size or cardioversion threshold after AICD implantation. By life-table analysis, there was a 1-year survival rate of 86% and an arrhythmic death survival rate of 100%.

Despite these significant complications, survival was improved in these high-risk patients with recurrent ventricular tachyarrhythmias who received AICDs. The morbidity involved in implantation of this device should be lowered by future improvements in the leads and pulse generator.

▶ This report adds to the growing success of the control of recurrent ventricular tachyarrhythmias by implantation of an automatic implantable cardioverter-defibrillator. The subsequent paper (Abstract 3–30) reports the experience at the Massachusetts General Hospital.— R.C. Schlant, M.D.

The Automatic Implantable Cardioverter-Defibrillator: Efficacy, Complications, and Survival in Patients With Malignant Ventricular Arrhythmias
Kelly PA, Cannom DS, Garan H, Mirabal GS, Harthorne JW, Hurvitz RJ, Vlahakes GJ, Jacobs ML, Ilvento JP, Buckley MJ, Ruskin JN (Massachusetts Gen Hosp, Boston; Hosp of the Good Samaritan, Los Angeles)
J Am Coll Cardiol 11:1278–1286, June 1988   3–30

Use of the automatic implantable cardioverter-defibrillator (AICD) has increased survival rates in patients with refractory ventricular arrhythmias. The safety, efficacy, and associated complications from implantation of the AICD were evaluated in 90 patients who were followed up for a mean of 17 months. The device was tested at intervals of 2–3 months during follow-up to evaluate battery status and to determine the number of discharges delivered.

In 46 patients there was at least 1 discharge of the device under circumstances suggestive of a malignant ventricular arrhythmia. There was 1 sudden death. Three patients died perioperatively, 12 had postoperative ventricular tachycardia, 8 had perioperative myocardial infarction, and

17 had device discharges for sinus tachycardia and supraventricular arrhythmias. Survival rates were 98.7% at 6 months and 95.4% at 12 months.

The AICD is an effective and relatively low-risk treatment protocol for patients with refractory life-threatening ventricular arrhythmias. For optimal results, proper device selection, scrupulous intraoperative testing, and close clinical follow-up are essential.

▶ This paper documents the current state of development and usefulness of the AICD, which was the successful dream of Mirowski, for the treatment of 90 patients with refractory recurrent ventricular tachycardia and fibrillation. Although more than 3,000 AICD pulse generators have been implanted in 2,500 patients since 1982 (1), there is a need for many additional studies including preoperative evaluation methods, surgical implantation techniques, and defibrillation threshold testing. Hopefully, the more than 200 implantation centers will provide this much needed information in the near future.

The same authors (2) reported that the probability of appropriate AICD discharge at 18 months was 86% for patients who had a sustained arrhythmia induced with 1 or 2 extrastimuli versus 15% for those requiring 3 extrastimuli for arrhythmia induction and 13% for patients without inducible sustained arrhythmias.

Tchou et al. (3) reported their experience in 70 patients who had AICD devices implanted. After a mean follow-up of 18 months, their survival was generally good; 23 patients received shocks judged to be due to recurrent ventricular arrhythmias and only 1 experienced sudden death during follow-up.— R.C. Schlant, M.D.

References

1. Troup PJ: Lessons learned from the automatic implantable cardioverter-defibrillator: Past, present and future. *J Am Coll Cardiol* 11:1287–1289, 1988.
2. Kelly PA, Cannom DS, Garan H, et al: Predictors of automatic implantable cardioverter defibrillator discharge for life-threatening ventricular arrhythmias. *Am J Cardiol* 62:83–87, 1988.
3. Tchou PJ, Kadri N, Anderson J, et al: Automatic implantable cardioverter defibrillators and survival of patients with left ventricular dysfunction and malignant ventricular arrhythmias. *Ann Intern Med* 109:529–534, 1988.

Electrocardiographic Criteria for Ventricular Tachycardia in Wide Complex Left Bundle Branch Block Morphology Tachycardias
Kindwall KE, Brown J, Josephson ME (Univ of Pennsylvania)
Am J Cardiol 61:1279–1283, June 1, 1988   3–31

Differentiation between supraventricular tachycardia and ventricular tachycardia is essential, as misdiagnosis can have potentially lethal consequences. Although the criteria used to distinguish SVT from VT in tachy-

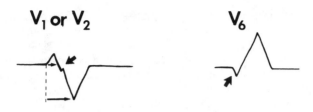

1) R in V1 or V2 >30 ms duration
2) any Q in V6
3) >60 ms from QRS onset to S nadir in V1 or V2
4) notched downstroke S wave in V1 or V2

Fig 3–12.—Four electrocardiographic criteria for ventricular tachycardia. (Courtesy of Kindwall KE, Brown J, Josephson ME: *Am J Cardiol* 61:1279–1283, June 1, 1988.)

cardias with right bundle branch block pattern have been well studied, less information is available on how to distinguish tachycardias with left bundle branch block pattern. This study was done to evaluate 4 ECG criteria for distinguishing ventricular tachycardia from supraventricular tachycardia in wide complex tachycardias with left bundle branch block pattern (Fig 3–12).

The 12-lead ECGs from 118 patients with wide complex tachycardias with left bundle branch block pattern, including 91 patients with ventricular tachycardia and 27 patients with supraventricular tachycardia, were reviewed by 3 separate readers. Interobserver differences were less than 5% and were resolved by consensus. Electrophysiologic studies to confirm the tachycardiac mechanism were performed in 113 consenting patients.

All 4 ECG criteria had very high specificities for ventricular tachycardia (Table 1). The sensitivity of each of the 4 ECG criteria for ventricular tachycardia alone was relatively low, ranging only from 30% to 64%, which limits their individual efficacy (Table 2). When criteria were grouped, however, ventricular tachycardia could be differentiated from supraventricular tachycardia with high sensitivity, specificity, and predic-

TABLE 1.—Specificity of Electrocardiographic Criteria for
Ventricular Tachycardia*

Criteria	All (n = 27)	LAD (n = 16)	Normal or RAD (n = 11)
(1) R >30 ms in V_1 or V_2 (%)	100	100	100
(2) Any Q in V_6 (%)	96	94	100
(3) >60 ms to S nadir in V_1 or V_2 (%)	96	94	100
(4) Notched downstroke S wave in V_1 or V_2 (%)	96	94	100

*LAD, left axis deviation; RAD, right axis deviation.
(Courtesy of Kindwall KE, Brown J, Josephson ME: *Am J Cardiol* 61:1279–1283, June 1, 1988.)

TABLE 2.—Sensitivity and Predictive Accuracy of Electrocardiographic Criteria for Ventricular Tachycardia*

Criteria	All LBBB (n = 91)		LAD (n = 61)		Normal or RAD (n = 30)	
	Sen	PA	Sen	PA	Sen	PA
(1) R >30 ms in V_1 or V_2 (%)	36	100	39	100	30	100
(2) Any Q in V_6 (%)	55	98	64	98	37	100
(3) >60 ms to S nadir in V_1 or V_2 (%)	63	98	64	98	60	100
(4) Notched downstroke S wave in V_1 or V_2	36	97	38	96	33	100

*LAD, left axis deviation; PA, predictive accuracy; RAD, right axis deviation; SEN, sensitivity.
(Courtesy of Kindwall KE, Brown J, Josephson ME: *Am J Cardiol* 61:1279–1283, June 1, 1988.)

tive accuracy, as the combined criteria had a sensitivity of 100%, a specificity of 89%, and a predictive accuracy of 96%.

In conclusion, systematic analysis of a 12-lead ECG alone for 4 criteria of ventricular tachycardia can be used to accurately diagnose the origin of wide complex tachycardias with left bundle branch block pattern.

▶ The differentiation between ventricular tachycardia and supraventricular tachycardia with a conduction abnormality is often difficult. This paper provides helpful guidelines for the proper diagnosis of wide complex left bundle branch morphology tachycardias, which comprise a significant fraction of such patients. Akhtar et al. (1) reviewed their experiences with 150 patients with wide QRS tachycardia, of whom 122 had ventricular tachycardia. They summarized the current, generally accepted criteria suggestive of ventricular tachycardia.—R.C. Schlant, M.D.

Reference

1. Akhtar M, Shenesa M, Jazayeri M, et al: Wide QRS complex tachycardia: Reappraisal of a common clinical problem. *Ann Intern Med* 109:905–912, 1988.

Use of the Automatic External Defibrillator in the Management of Out-of-Hospital Cardiac Arrest

Weaver WD, Hill D, Fahrenbruch CE, Copass MK, Martin JS, Cobb LA, Hallstrom AP (University of Washington)
N Engl J Med 319:661–666, Sept 15, 1988
3–32

The automatic external defibrillator is a simple device that can be used with little training by operators skilled only in first aid. Its contribution to the management of cardiac arrest in urban settings has not been definitely ascertained. To examine its efficacy, 1,287 consecutive Seattle patients with cardiac arrest were studied prospectively. Fifty-three percent were initially treated by fire fighters using automatic external defibrillators, whereas 47% received only basic cardiopulmonary resuscitation from fire fighters and awaited arrival of paramedics for defibrillation. On average, paramedics arrived 3 minutes after fire fighters did. In both groups, about 40% were found in ventricular fibrillation.

Resuscitation rates (proportion admitted to the hospital) were similar for both groups of patients. Survival rates were significantly higher for patients found in ventricular fibrillation if fire fighters used automatic external defibrillators than if defibrillation awaited arrival of paramedics. Survival was low among patients with conditions other than ventricular fibrillation. When a multivariate analysis was performed, the major benefit of the automatic defibrillator appeared to be caused by reduction in time elapsed between cardiac arrest and delivery of first shock. Other factors that were related to an enhanced survival rate included having a witness to the collapse, younger age, the presence of "course" (higher-amplitude) fibrillation, and shorter paramedic response time. Short paramedic response time contributed to survival rate independently of defibrillation by first-aid personnel.

This study suggests that early defibrillation with automatic external defibrillators enhances survival rate. Without a randomized, controlled trial, the magnitude of this enhancement is uncertain. These data support the widespread use of the automatic defibrillator although they do not address its effect on community survival rates.

▶ The results of this study suggest that the widespread use of modern external emergency defibrillator employed by minimally trained emergency personnel might save the lives of thousands of patients in the United States who otherwise might be lost to sudden cardiac death. Hopefully, such instruments will soon be widely distributed throughout the country.— R.C. Schlant, M.D.

Catheter Ablation of Accessory Pathways With a Direct Approach: Results in 35 Patients
Warin J-F, Haissaguerre M, Lemetayer P, Guillem J-P, Blanchot P (University of Bordeaux II, Bordeaux France)
Circulation 78:800–815, October 1988   3–33

Although patients with accessory pathways are sometimes successfully treated with antiarrhythmic drugs, surgery is often necessary and has a low risk with experienced teams. Recently, however, fulguration has demonstrated good early results and may be an alternative to surgery. Here, results of a study employing fulguration with a new method are presented. Thirty-five consecutive patients with an overt accessory pathway, including 33 symptomatic patients, were enrolled, and all but 2 had been unsuccessfully treated with antiarrhythmic drugs. Each was subject to attempted transcatheter ablation (fulguration) by a method employing standard bipolar catheters. The catheters were positioned on the internal surface of the right or left atrioventricular anulus, and transcatheter ca-

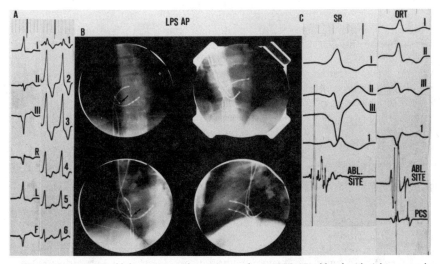

Fig 3–13.—A, ECG of left posteroseptal accessory pathway *(LPS AP)* ablated with right approach. B, location of ablation catheter *(arrow)*. Multielectrode catheter (0.5-cm interelectrode) was introduced through left subclavian vein into coronary sinus. One catheter is in His bundle region, and another is in right atrium. Ablation catheter was inserted through right subclavian vein; its tip *(arrow)* is obviously outside coronary sinus inclusive of its os. C, electrograms recorded at ablation site *(ABL SITE)* during sinus rhythm *(SR)* and orthodromic reciprocating tachycardia *(ORT)*. Ventriculoatrial time at ablation site is 90 msec (20 msec before earliest electrogram recorded in proximal coronary sinus near the os *[PCS]*). Catheter inside coronary sinus was more proximal during electrophysiologic study than during radiography performed later, just before ablation, because of instability. Note that ventricular potentials are recorded before onset of delta wave during SR in standard leads. (Courtesy of Warin J-F, Haissaguerre M, Lemetayer P, et al: *Circulation* 78:800–815, Oct 1988.)

thodic shocks were delivered to the site where the accessory pathway crosses over the atrioventricular groove.

Disappearance of conduction from the accessory pathway occurred in 32 patients with a mean follow-up of 10 months, and accessory pathways were impaired in 3 patients (Fig 3–13). These results required 1 (22 patients), 2 (9 patients), 3 (2 patients), or 4 (1 patient) sessions. Thirty-four patients were free from arrhythmias, and only 1 required antiarrhythmic drug therapy. Side effects were present, but none required that patients receive implantation of a permanent pacemaker.

Fulguration is preferable to surgery for the ablation of all right-sided accessory pathways, for left posteroseptal accessory pathways that can be ablated by shocks delivered with a right approach, and in left lateral and posterolateral accessory pathways when the foramen ovale is patent. This treatment is also recommended for Wolff-Parkinson-White syndrome. The procedure appears to be safe if the coronary sinus is not used, even with its proximal segment.

▶ These encouraging results in using the technique of right-heart catheter electrical fulguration to produce ablation of right-sided accessory pathways (and avoiding the coronary sinus) are similar to the rapidly growing experience of many laboratories. The new technique of catheter ablation using radiofrequency energy rather than electrical energy may avoid the necessity for general anesthesia and may also permit ablation of some left-sided accessory pathways though the coronary sinus (1). Also pertinent is the report of P. Tchou et al. (2), which described excellent results in 7 patients with syncope or recurrent ventricular tachycardia or both, 6 of whom had dilated cardiomyopathy, following transcatheter electrical ablation of the right bundle branch.

The proceedings of the 4th International Congress on Catheter Ablation, edited by M. Scheinman and G. Fontaine, has been published in *PACE* (3). Hopefully, this technique will continue to be more widely used in order to avoid surgical ablation, at least in some patients with accessible pathways.—R.C. Schlant, M.D.

References

1. Huang SK, Graham AR, Bharati S, et al: Short- and long-term effects of transcatheter ablation of the coronary sinus by radiofrequency energy. *Circulation* 78:416–427, 1988.
2. Tchou P, Jazayeri M, Denker S, et al: Transcatheter electrical ablation of right bundle branch: A method of treating macroreentrant ventricular tachycardia attributed to bundle branch reentry. *Circulation* 78:246–257, 1988.
3. Ashan AJ, Cunningham D, Roland E, et al: 4th International Congress on Catheter Ablation. *PACE* 12:131–267, 1989.

Prognostic Significance of Signal-Averaged ECGs During Acute Myocardial Infarction: A Preliminary Report
Grimm M, Billhardt RA, Mayerhofer KE, Denes P (Rush-Presbyterian-St Luke's Med Ctr, Chicago)
J Electrocardiol 21:283–288, August 1988   3–34

Previous studies attempted to demonstrate that the presence of late potentials as detected by body surface signal-averaged electrocardiography during acute myocardial infarction is a prognostic marker for future episodes of ventricular tachyarrhythmia or ventricular fibrillation. However, the results of these studies were inconclusive. To determine the prognostic significance of late potentials, a prospective study was done to evaluate the relationship between them and reentrant ventricular arrhythmias and sudden death from acute myocardial infarction.

The study population comprised 38 men and 14 women, with a median age of 59.6 years, admitted with acute myocardial infarctions, including 20 anterior, 24 inferior, and 8 subendocardial infarctions. On admission, 46 patients were in Killip class II or less and 6 were in classes greater than class II. Fifteen patients had previous histories of myocardial infarction. Of these 52 patients, 14 had premature ventricular complexes alone, 16 had nonsustained ventricular tachyarrhythmia, 3 had sustained ventricular tachyarrhythmia and fibrillation, and 19 had no significant arrhythmias on continuous telemetric monitoring or 24-hour Holter recording or both. Signal-averaged recordings were performed on admission and again at discharge.

Late potentials were detected on the initial signal-averaged ECG in 10 (19%) of the 52 patients, 6 of whom still had late potentials on the second recording. Three of the remaining 4 patients had no late potentials on the second recording; 1 patient died before the second recording was made. Six of the 42 patients who had no late potentials on the first recording had them on the second recording. Overall, 12 patients had late potentials on the second recording, and 9 patients changed category between the first and second recording.

Three patients in the late potential-negative group had early in-hospital sustained ventricular tachyarrhythmia and ventricular fibrillation. None of the late potential-positive patients experienced ventricular arrhythmias. Ten patients died, 7 in the hospital and 3 after discharge. Of the 7 in-hospital deaths, 2 had late potentials and 5 did not. Of the 3 postdischarge deaths, 2 had late potentials and 1 did not. Because of the small sample size, there was no significant difference in early or late mortality between the late potential-positive and the late potential-negative groups. However, there appeared to be a trend toward higher mortality in the group positive for late potentials.

Late potentials as detected by body surface signal-averaged ECG do not predict the occurrence of early in-hospital ventricular tachyarrhythmia, ventricular fibrillation, or sudden death.

▶ The results of this small, preliminary study did not demonstrate a definite value of late potentials in the identification of patients likely to have early in-hospital ventricular tachycardia, ventricular fibrillation, or sudden death. Recent studies have shown the predictive value of late potentials during mean follow-up periods of 6–12 months after infarction (1–3). There are several recent reviews of the technique. (4–6).—R.C. Schlant, M.D.

References

1. Buckingham TA, Ghosh S, Homan SM, et al: Independent value of signal-averaged electrocardiography and left ventricular function in identifying patients with sustained ventricular tachycardia with coronary artery disease. *Am J Cardiol* 59:568–572, 1987.
2. Buxton AE, Simson MB, Falcone RA, et al: Results of signal-averaged electrocardiography and electrophysiologic study in patients with nonsustained ventricular tachycardia after healing of acute myocardial infarction. *Am J Cardiol* 60:80–85, 1987.
3. Cripps T, Bennett ED, Camm AJ, et al: High gain signal averaged electrocardiogram combined with 24-hour monitoring in patients early after myocardial infarction for bedside prediction of arrhythmic events. *Br Heart J* 60:181–187, 1988.
4. Berbari E, Lazzara R: An introduction to high-resolution ECG recordings of cardiac late potentials. *Arch Intern Med* 148:1859–1863, 1988.
5. Vattertott PJ, Hammill SC, Bailey KR, et al: Signal-averaged electrocardiography: A new noninvasive test to identify patients at risk for ventricular arrhythmias. *Mayo Clin Proc* 63:931–942, 1988.

6. Hall PAX, Atwood JE, Myers J, et al: The signal-averaged surface electrocardiogram and the identification of late potentials. *Prog Cardiovasc Dis* 31:295–317, 1989.

Miscellaneous Topics

Prevalence of Patent Foramen Ovale in Patients With Stroke

Lechat P, Mas JL, Lascault G, Loron P, Theard M, Klimczac M, Drobinski G, Thomas D, Grosgogeat Y (Hôpital Pitié-Salpétrière, Paris)
N Engl J Med 318:1148–1152, May 5, 1988   3–35

In about 35% of young adults who suffer ischemic stroke, the cause is undefined. Stroke has been traced to paradoxical embolism through a patent foramen ovale in some patients, but the prevalence of this cause has not been investigated systematically. Using contrast echocardiography, the authors investigated the prevalence of patent foramen ovale in 60 young adults with ischemic stroke who had a normal cardiac examination.

Contrast echocardiography was performed with all patients at rest and during the Valsalva maneuver and a cough test. Patients also underwent standard 2-dimensional and time-motion echocardiography. Results were compared with those from a control group of 100 patients.

Forty percent of patients with stroke had patent foramen ovale as compared with 10% in controls. Patent foramen ovale was seen in 21% of 19 patients with an identifiable cause for stroke, in 40% of 15 patients with risk factor for stroke but no discernible cause, and in 54% of patients with neither identifiable cause nor risk factor.

The findings suggest that paradoxical embolism through a patent foramen ovale could account for embolic stroke more often than is usually supposed. It is suggested that patients with cerebral embolism of unknown cause should undergo contrast echocardiography. If concomitant venous thrombosis is present, anticoagulant therapy should be undertaken. If prophylactic treatment is not helpful, interruption of the vena cava or closure of the foramen ovale should be considered.

▶ This study documents the presence of a patent foramen ovale in a significant number (54%) of patients with cryptogenic stroke. The use of contrast echocardiography or, perhaps, Doppler echocardiography color flow mapping to detect a patent foramen ovale would appear to be an appropriate diagnostic procedure in many such patients, especially when the diagnosis would affect clinical management, such as the use of warfarin or aspirin (1). Transesophageal echocardiography has also been shown to be able to detect a significantly higher incidence of mitral valve prolapse in young patients with cerebral ischemic events (2).— R.C. Schlant, M.D.

References

1. Yatsu FM, Hart RG, Mohr JP, et al: Anticoagulation of embolic strokes of cardiac origin: An update. *Neurology* 38:314–316, 1988.
2. Zenker G, Erbel R, Kramer G, et al: Transesophageal two-dimensional

echocardiography in young patients with cerebral ischemic events. *Stroke* 19:345–348, 1988.

Influence on Prognosis and Morbidity of Left Ventricular Ejection Fraction With and Without Signs of Left Ventricular Failure After Acute Myocardial Infarction
Nicod P, Gilpin E, Dittrich H, Chappuis F, Ahnve S, Engler R, Henning H, Ross J Jr (Univ of California, San Diego; VA Hosp, San Diego; Naval Hosp of San Diego; Univ of British Columbia)
Am J Cardiol 61:1165–1171, June 1, 1988   3–36

Clinical signs of left ventricular failure are strong predictors of poor prognosis after acute myocardial infarction. The effect of the presence or absence of left ventricular failure on the predictive ability of normal, moderately depressed, and severely depressed left ventricular ejection fraction (LVEF) was examined. Whether heart failure occurring in the hospital is associated with an increased number of later ischemic events also was studied.

The LVEF in 972 patients was determined either by radionuclide ventriculography or angiography; left ventricular failure was also assessed, both clinically and radiographically. Patients underwent submaximal treadmill testing before hospital discharge.

The overall 1-year mortality was 11%. A high LVEF was associated with better survival, whereas the presence of clinical signs of left ventricular failure was consistently associated with poorer survival. Respective 1-year mortality rates were 8%, 19%, and 26% among patients with normal, moderately depressed, and severely depressed LVEF when clinical signs of left ventricular failure were present; when it was absent, these rates fell to 3%, 6%, and 12%. There was a similar relationship in mortality when only radiographic signs of failure were present. The incidence of new nonfatal ischemic events did not differ with the presence or absence of signs of failure.

The presence of clinical heart failure is an independent predictor that increases the risk of 1-year mortality, regardless of the LVEF. A depressed LVEF in the absence of clinical or radiographic heart failure also is predictive of increased 1-year mortality, but at a lower rate than when clinical heart failure is also present.

▶ This study indicates that both evidence of clinical heart failure (rales on physical examination, pulmonary edema on chest roentgenogram) and decreased left ventricular ejection fraction are useful predictors of prognosis in patients after myocardial infarction. These 2 variables appear to be independent variables in those patients in whom they are discordant. It would have been interesting if the authors had been able to detect any influence of medical management upon prognosis.—R.C. Schlant, M.D.

Effect of Captopril on Progressive Ventricular Dilatation After Anterior Myocardial Infarction

Pfeffer MA, Lamas GA, Vaughan DE, Parisi AF, Braunwald E (Brigham and Women's Hosp, Boston; West Roxbury VA Med Ctr, Boston; Harvard Univ) *N Engl J Med* 319:80–86, July 14, 1988   3–37

Left ventricular dilatation is the most important predictor of survival among patients with coronary artery disease. The purpose of this randomized, double-blind, placebo-controlled, parallel-group trial was to determine whether left ventricular dilatation continues during the late convalescent phase after anterior myocardial infarction, and whether long-term therapy with an angiotension-converting enzyme inhibitor alters this process.

The study population consisted of 59 patients, 54 men and 5 women, with a first anterior myocardial infarction and a radionuclide ejection fraction of 45% or less. Thirty patients with a mean age of 59 years were randomly assigned to treatment with 50 mg of captopril 3 times a day, and 29 patients with a mean age of 56 years were assigned to the placebo group. All study patients underwent cardiac catheterization 11 to 31 days after anterior myocardial infarction and 1 year after randomization to evaluate interval changes in hemodynamic function and left ventricular volume. Ambulatory follow-up visits were scheduled at 1 week and at 1, 3, 6, and 9 months. Thirty-eight men underwent quarterly maximal symptom-limited treadmill exercise tests.

Fifty-two of the 59 patients underwent repeat catheterization; 4 patients in the placebo group and 3 in the captopril group did not complete the trial. At the 1-year evaluation, the mean arterial pressure was consistently higher in the placebo group than in the captopril group. End-systolic volume did not change significantly between baseline and follow-up in either the placebo or the captopril group. However, the end-diastolic volume of the left ventricle increased by a mean of 21 ml in the placebo group, but by only 10 ml in the captopril group. Left ventricular filling pressure remained elevated with placebo but decreased with captopril. Captopril prevented further left ventricular dilatation in a subset of 36 patients who were at high risk for ventricular enlargement because of persistent occlusion of the left anterior descending coronary artery. Patients in the captopril group also showed increased exercise capacity.

The results of this preliminary study confirm that left ventricular enlargement after anterior myocardial infarction is progressive. Treatment with captopril appears to attenuate this process, reduce filling pressures, and improve exercise tolerance.

▶ This important preliminary study is currently being followed by a large multicenter trial (survival and ventricular enlargement [SAVE]), which will test the hypothesis supported by the present study that long-term captopril therapy will reduce mortality and prevent the development of congestive heart failure after myocardial infarction.—R.C. Schlant, M.D.

Antithrombotic Therapy for Patients With Cardiac Disease

Penny WJ, Chesebro JH, Heras M, Fuster V (Univ of Wales, Cardiff; Mayo Clinic; Mt Sinai Med Ctr, New York)
Curr Probl Cardiol 13:427–513, July 1988   3–38

Long-term warfarin therapy presently is recommended for patients with valvular heart disease (Table 1) to prolong the prothrombin time to 1.5 to 2 times that of control. In patients with cardiac valve prostheses, treatment (Table 2) is best started before operation.

Intravenous heparin may be started 6 hours after surgery to maintain the activated partial thromboplastin time at the upper limit of normal. Heparin then is given subcutaneously to maintain the activated partial thromboplastin time at 1.5 to 2 times the upper normal limit. If noncardiac surgery is required, anticoagulation may be stopped for 7 to 10 days. When prosthetic valve endocarditis is present, it seems reasonable to continue treatment.

Heparin infusion may reduce the occurrence of myocardial infarction in patients with unstable angina or non-Q wave infarction. Patients at risk of deep venous thrombosis and pulmonary embolism after acute myocardial infarction should receive subcutaneous heparin. Intravenous heparin is recommended for patients having a large anterior transmural infarct or an extensive transmural inferior infarct involving the apex.

Arterial thromboembolism may occur in patients with dilated cardiomyopathy. Oral anticoagulation may be used to elevate the prothrombin time, but further studies are needed. Anticoagulation also may be used to prevent reocclusion after successful thrombolytic therapy. Both heparin and platelet inhibitor therapy are used.

Platelet inhibitors are used to prevent graft occlusion following saphenous vein bypass surgery. Patients who cannot use aspirin may receive either sulfinpyrazone or heparin followed by oral anticoagulation. Heparin and aspirin are used in conjunction with balloon dilatation for coronary angioplasty. A randomized, double-blind trial of aspirin and dipyridamole for 6 months after coronary angioplasty is now in progress.

▶ Antithrombotic therapy represents a major advance in our management of

---

TABLE 1.—Valvular Heart Disease: Indications for
Anticoagulation

Atrial fibrillation (chronic or paroxysmal)
Sinus rhythm with a very large left atrium (>55 mm by
 M-mode echocardiography)
Presence of heart failure or severe left ventricular dysfunction
History of previous systemic embolism

*Prothrombin time to 1.5–2.0 times control, using rabbit brain thromboplastin (standardized international normalized ratio = 3.0–4.5).
(Courtesy of Penny WJ, Chesebro JH, Heras M, et al: *Curr Probl Cardiol* 13:427–513, July 1988.)

TABLE 2.—Antithrombotic Therapy for Prosthetic Heart Valves:
Current Recommendations*

In all patients, begin intravenous heparin‡ starting 6 hours after operation and continue until chest tubes are removed. Then use subcutaneous heparin, starting with 10,000 U every 12 hours§, for the duration of hospitalization.

Valve	Situation	Therapy
Mechanical	Routine	Warfarin¶ + Dip mg/day
	Dip side effects	Warfarin¶ + Sulf 800 mg/day
	ACRx problems (bleeding)	1. ↓ Warfarin# + Dip 400 mg/day
		2. Dip 400 mg/day + Sulf 800 mg/day
	Recurrent embolism	Consider reoperation
Bioprosthetic	AVR routine	Subcutaneous heparin for 7 to 10 days, then ASA 80 mg/day
	MVR routine	Subcutaneous heparin, warfarin¶ for 3 mo, then ASA 80 mg/day
	If LA > 55 mm or AF	Warfarin¶ long-term

*ACRx, anticoagulant therapy; AF, atrial fibrillation; ASA, aspirin; AVR, aortic valve replacement; Dip, dipyridamole; LA, left atrium; MVR, mitral valve replacement; Sulf, sulfinpyrazone.
†Approximately 600 to 700 United States Pharmacopeia units/hour; sufficient to maintain activated partial thromboplastin time at upper limit of normal.
‡Adjust dose to prolong activated partial thromboplastin time to 1.5 to 2 times upper limit of normal.
§Prolong prothrombin time to 1.5 to 2 times control, using rabbit brain thromboplastin (standardized international normalized ratio = 3.0 to 4.5).
¶Prolong prothrombin time to 1.2 to 1.5 times control, using rabbit brain thromboplastin (standardized international normalized ratio = 2.0 to 3.0).
(Courtesy of Penny WJ, Chesebro JH, Heras M, et al: Curr Probl Cardiol 13:427–513, July 1988.)

many forms of acute and chronic cardiovascular disease, including complications of atherosclerosis, prosthetic heart valves, cardiomyopathy, atrial fibrillation, and pulmonary embolism. The future will hold exiciting advances in this rapidly developing area.— R.C. Schlant, M.D.

The Value of Echocardiography in Blunt Chest Trauma

Hiatt JR, Yeatman LA Jr, Child JS (Univ of California, Los Angeles)
J Trauma 28:914–922, July 1988   3–39

Two-dimensional echocardiography was performed in all blunt trauma victims admitted to a level I trauma center in a 1-year period. In addition, levels of creatine kinase (CK) and MB isoenzymes (CK-MB) were determined serially over 24 hours, and 12-lead ECGs were recorded for the first 3 days. A total of 73 patients were evaluated.

Thirty-five patients had normal echographic and ECG findings. Sixteen others had abnormal ECGs but normal echocardiograms, whereas 14 had echographic findings of abnormal wall motion or pericardial fluid. In 8 patients echocardiography showed a nontraumatic valvular or wall motion abnormality. Patients with echographic findings of abnormal wall motion or pericardial fluid had higher CK and CK-MB values, more as-

Blunt Chest Trauma

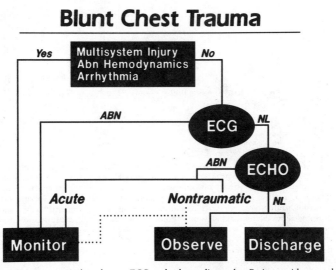

Fig 3–14.—Triage strategy based upon ECG and echocardiography. Patients with normal ECG and echocardiogram do not require cardiac monitoring; those with nontraumatic echocardiographic abnormalities are monitored selectively. (Courtesy of Hiatt JR, Yeatman LA Jr, Child JS: *J Trauma* 28:914–922, July 1988.)

sociated injuries, and higher Injury Severity Scores. Seven of them required invasive hemodynamic monitoring. No patients died.

Echocardiography is a useful means of evaluating victims of blunt chest trauma. Intensive care is not necessary for patients who have normal ECG and echocardiographic findings at admission (Fig 3–14). Hypoxemia and hypotension associated with echocardiographic abnormalities are clear indications for invasive monitoring. Monitoring is strongly considered for patients with wall motion abnormality who require general anesthesia.

▶ This study documents the very significant clinical usefulness of echocardiography in the management of chest trauma, most often due to an automobile accident. Echocardiography, which may identify wall motion abnormalities or pericardial effusion in such patients, is especially useful in helping to identify 2 groups of patients: those with no echocardiographic abnormalities who otherwise might be monitored to rule out a myocardial contusion, and those with wall motion abnormalities who should be monitored, especially during procedures requiring general anesthesia.—R.C. Schlant, M.D.

Digitalis: Mechanisms of Action and Clinical Use
Smith TW (Brigham and Women's Hosp, Boston; Harvard Univ)
N Engl J Med 318:358–365, Feb 11, 1988   3–40

Digitalis, which enhances ventricular contractility, has long been used to treat heart failure. The inotropic effect results from binding to and in-

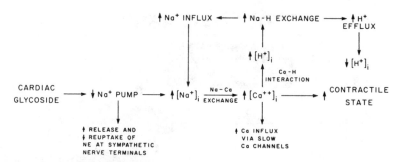

Fig 3–15.—Mechanisms of modulation of myocardial function by cardiac glycosides. In addition to horizontal sequence leading from cardiac glycoside-induced inhibition of sodium-ion pump to enhanced myocardial contractile state, 3 ancillary processes are shown: enhanced norepinephrine *(NE)* release and reduced reuptake at cardiac sympathetic-nerve terminals, which may occur in experimental circumstances but has doubtful clinical relevance; enhanced slow inward calcium current with increased calcium influx through slow calcium channels in response to an increased concentration of intracellular calcium ions over a limited range of values for these ions; and decreased intracellular pH (increased $[H+]_i$) in response to increased intracellular calcium, leading to enhanced sodium–hydrogen exchange and hence augmentation of rise in intracellular sodium ($[Na+]_i$) caused by sodium-pump inhibition. (Courtesy of Smith TW: *N Engl J Med* 318:358–365, Feb 11, 1988.)

hibition of sodium-and-potassium-activated adenosine triphosphatase (NaK-ATPase), the enzymatic equivalent of the sodium pump. Partial inhibition of NaK-ATPase in the sarcolemmal membrane of myocytes alters excitation-contraction coupling by making more calcium available to the contractile elements (Fig 3–15). Glycosides increase the availability of activator calcium to contractile proteins in the cardiac myocytes. The sodium-calcium exchanger, which mediates the transsarcolemmal movement of calcium ion in exchange for sodium, has a key role in the increase in systolic intracellular calcium ion concentration.

Cardiac glycosides slow conduction and increase the refractory period in cardiac conducting tissue while increasing conduction velocity in working heart muscle. Digitalis is demonstrably effective in patients with congestive heart failure complicated by supraventricular tachyarrhythmia. Patients with chronic congestive heart failure and sinus rhythm also have documented sustained improvement in cardiac performance. In this setting, there is little to gain from increasing the digoxin dose to a level resulting in a serum or plasma concentration greater than 1.5–2.0 ng/ml. Patients with diastolic rather than systolic dysfunction are approached by finding the underlying cause of left ventricular hypertrophy or ischemia, rather than inotropic support with glycosides.

Most toxicity from digitalis is caused, at least in part, by neurally mediated mechanisms. Disordered cardiac rhythm is due to both a direct effect on excitable cardiac cells and altered sympathetic activity and vagal tone. Serious toxicity now is effectively treated with digoxin-specific Fab fragments.

▶ This fine update on digitalis clearly defines our current knowledge of the pharmacology of digitalis and succinctly summarizes its clinical use. It is worth keeping in mind that the increased survival of patients with heart failure treated with vasodilators reported in the Veterans Administration Study (1) and CON-SENSUS (2) was noted while patients were also receiving digitalis and diuretics therapy, to which the vasodilators were added.— R.C. Schlant, M.D.

References

1. Cohn JN, Archibald DG, Ziesche S, et al: Effect of vasodilator therapy on mortality in chronic congestive heart failure: Results of a Veterans Administration Cooperative Study. *N Engl J Med* 314:1547–1552, 1986.
2. Effects of enalapril on mortality in severe congestive heart failure: Results of the Cooperative North Scandinavian Enalapril Survival Study (CONSENSUS). *N Engl J Med* 316:1429–1435, 1987.

Cocaine-Induced Supersensitivity and Arrhythmogenesis
Inoue H, Zipes DP (Indiana Univ; Roudebush VA Med Ctr, Indianapolis)
J Am Coll Cardiol 11:867–874, April 1988   3–41

Cocaine-related sudden deaths may occur after recreational drug use and may sometimes be associated with myocardial ischemia or infarction. Ventricular tachycardia has been noted sporadically. An attempt was made to determine whether cocaine potentiates (1) changes in atrioventricular nodal function after infusion or norepinephrine or sympathetic nerve stimulation and (2) the induction of ventricular tachyarrhythmia. Open-chest dogs received intravenous injections of cocaine 5 mg/kg. Norepinephrine was infused at a rate of 0.01–0.20 μg/kg minute, and frequency-response curves were recorded with stimulation of the ansae subclaviae.

Cocaine increased the responses of the sinus cycle length and AH interval to infused norepinephrine, and propranolol countered these effects. Cocaine did not influence responses to sympathetic nerve (ansae subclaviae) stimulation. Ventricular tachyarrhythmia was not induced before or after cocaine injection. However, in dogs with acute myocardial infarction, cocaine produced a supersensitive shortening of refractoriness and promoted the induction of tachyarrhythmia when given in conjunction with norepinephrine.

These findings do not explain sudden deaths in cocaine users. In this canine model, the "normal" sympathetic response is not arrhythmogenic. Cocaine potentiates the development of ventricular tachycardia in dogs given norepinephrine by infusion after acute infarction.

▶ Although cocaine did not induce a ventricular tachyarrhythmia under the conditions of this experiment, it did potentiate the effects of infused norepinephrine and potentiate the development of ventricular tachycardia by norepinephrine infusion 3.5–4 hours after acute myocardial infarction, but not in dogs without myocardial infarction. Of possible clinical interest, propranolol attenuated the cocaine-induced increased responses of sinus cycle length, AH interval, and ventricular refractory periods to infused norepinephrine. See the next paper for additional electrophysiologic studies on cocaine.—R.C. Schlant, M.D.

Acute Effects of Cocaine on Catecholamines and Cardiac Electrophysiology in the Conscious Dog

Schwartz AB, Boyle W, Janzen D, Jones RT (Univ of California, Davis; VA Med Ctr, Martinez, Calif; Univ of California, San Francisco)

Can J Cardiol 4:188–192, May 1988   3–42

The incidence of cocaine-related deaths is increasing. Sudden death during cocaine usage may occur in the absence of myocardial infarction, suggesting the possibility of serious primary cardiac electrophysiologic changes. However, the cardiac electrophysiologic effects of cocaine have not been systematically evaluated. The effects of cocaine on the sinus node, atrioventricular node, and His-Purkinje system were assessed in conscious dogs. These changes then were correlated with plasma catecholamine levels.

Fourteen nonconditioned mongrel dogs were infused with cocaine to either maximum tolerance or to at least a 15% increase in the systolic blood pressure. Plasma cocaine and catecholamine concentrations, blood pressure, and surface and intracardiac electrograms were recorded before and during the study. Programmed electrical stimulation was carried out from the right atrium.

The sinoatrial conduction time, paced PR interval, atrioventricular nodal conduction time, atrioventricular nodal effective refractory period, and blood pressure all increased after cocaine infusion. Plasma norepinephrine, epinephrine, and dopamine concentrations were increased and remained 2–3 times higher than control levels, whereas plasma cocaine levels declined throughout the study. Epinephrine levels were correlated strongly with the hemodynamic response, but plasma cocaine levels were not.

None of the dogs experienced sustained spontaneous atrial or ventricular arrhythmias after cocaine infusion. Pacing after cocaine administration induced atrial fibrillation with a slow ventricular response in only 3 of the 14 dogs. Cocaine infusion did not produce any significant changes in pacing threshold, right intra-atrial conduction time, infranodal conduction time, heart rate, QRS, or QT. No pacing-induced infranodal block occurred.

Submaximal intravenous doses of cocaine may cause neurohumoral and electrophysiologic changes. In addition to the expected increase in sympathetic tone, parasympathetic tone also increased, accounting for the predominant cardiac electrophysiologic effect. The parasympathetic nervous system may be involved in the electrophysiologic changes observed after cocaine administration.

▶ It is of interest that, in this study, cocaine did not produce spontaneous atrioventricular block, HV prolongation, or pacing-induced infranodal block. The drugs used for the treatment of cocaine toxicity include propranolol, labetalol, and calcium antagonists. Diazepam is useful for the hyperkinetic state, and chronic treatment with carbamazepine may present high-dose cocaine seizures. Lathers et al. (1) have reviewed the pathophysiology of cocaine and the treatment of cocaine arrhythmias and seizures.—R.C. Schlant, M.D.

Reference

1. Lathers CM, Tyau LSY, Spino MM, et al: Cocaine-induced seizures, arrhythmias, and sudden death. *J Clin Pharmacol* 28:584—593, 1988.

Cardiovascular Effects of Cocaine: An Autopsy Study of 40 Patients
Virmani R, Robinowitz M, Smialek JE, Smyth DF (Armed Forces Inst of Pathology, Washington, DC; Office of the Chief Med Examiner for the State of Maryland, Baltimore)
Am Heart J 115:1068—1076, May 1988   3–43

Although the clinical and pathologic findings in persons who abuse cocaine are well studied, the prevalence of myocarditis in individuals who abuse cocaine has not yet been determined. The autopsy findings in 40 patients who died of either natural or homicidal causes with cocaine detected in their body fluids were compared with those in 27 victims of sudden traumatic death in whom no cocaine was found.

The cocaine-associated group, 29 men and 11 women aged 21–47 years, included 31 patients in whom death was attributed solely to cocaine toxicity, as the rest of the autopsy findings were not found to contribute to their deaths, and 9 patients in whom cocaine was found but in whom homicide was the direct cause of death. Fourteen patients had needle tracks at autopsy; 18 were known chronic drug abusers. Causes of death in the acute trauma control group, 25 men and 2 women aged 18–48 years, were motor vehicle accidents, gunshot wounds, asphyxiation, trauma, drowning, and suicide.

In the cocaine-associated autopsy group, 1 patient had total thrombotic occlusion of the left anterior descending coronary artery overlying mild coronary atherosclerosis, whereas 8 (20%) patients had myocarditis at the time of death. In comparison, only 1 (3.7%) patient in the control group had myocarditis at the time of death.

Myocarditis occurs frequently in patients who die of cocaine abuse. Although the cause of myocarditis is still unknown, infectious agents are thought to be a possible primary or contributory factor. However, histologic examination did not show any bacteria, fungi, or viral inclusions in any of the cocaine-associated autopsies. Cocaine itself may cause myocardial necrosis and inflammation by an as yet unknown mechanism. Possible mechanisms include myocyte necrosis from high concentrations of norepinephrine, increased killer cell activity injuring myocytes, microvascular vasospasm, and hypersensitivity myocarditis.

▶ The widespread use of cocaine is now a relatively frequent cause of death from acute myocardial infarction or ventricular arrhythmia, in addition to being a frequent cause of infective endocarditis. Cocaine-induced coronary artery spasm has been assumed to be responsible for infarction in individuals with little or no fixed obstructive coronary artery disease although such spasm has not previously been demonstrated. Ascher et al. (1), have, however, recently reported the occurrence of spontaneous spasm of the infarct related artery.—R.C. Schlant, M.D.

Reference

1. Ascher EK, Stauffer J-C, Gaasch WH: Coronary artery spasm, cardiac arrest, transient electrocardiographic Q waves and stunned myocardium in cocaine associated acute myocardial infarction. *Am J Cardiol* 61:939–941, 1988.

Echocardiographic and Clinical Correlates in Drug Addicts With Infective Endocarditis: Implications of Vegetation Size

Manolis AS, Melita H (New York Med College, New York)
Arch Intern Med 148:2461–2465, November 1988   3–44

Infective endocarditis involving predominantly right-sided valves is common among drug addicts. The prognostic value of vegetation size, as determined by echocardiography, is controversial for right-sided endocarditis. To address this issue, a prospective study involving 34 drug addicts with endocarditis was undertaken, in which the prognostic value of vegetation size and its short-term changes, as determineed by 2-dimensional echocardiography (2-DE), were assessed.

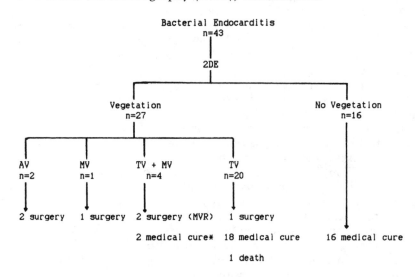

* 1 late death

Fig 3–16.—Clinical outcome of patients with and without bacterial vegetations. *2-DE*, 2-dimensional echocardiography; *AV*, aortic valve; *MV*, mitral valve; *TV*, tricuspid valve; and *MVR*, mitral valve replacement. (Courtesy of Manolis AS, Melita H: *Arch Intern Med* 148:2461–2465, November 1988.)

Forty-three separate episodes of clinically diagnosed bacterial endocarditis in 34 drug addicts were studied. *Staphylococcus aureus* was responsible for 60% of the cases. Vegetations were detected with 2-DE in 63% of the episodes. These were found in the tricuspid valve alone in 20 patients, mitral valve in 1, aortic valve in 2, and both tricuspid and mitral valves in 4. All vegetations were 1 cm or greater in size, with a mean maximum length of 1.7 cm for tricuspid valve vegetations. In all 16 patients without vegetations and in 90% of 20 patients with tricuspid valve vegetations, medical cures were effected with intravenous antibiotics. Surgery was required for the patient with mitral valve vegetation, both patients with aortic valve vegetations, 2 of the 4 patients with both tricuspid and mitral valve vegetation, and only 1 of 20 patients with tricuspid valve vegetation alone (Fig 3–16). The only death among these patients was of a patient with tricuspid valve vegetation who suffered respiratory complications. Fourteen patients were monitored with 2-DE after 1 to 8 weeks of antibiotic therapy. Changes in vegetations did not correlate with clinical outcome.

This study suggests that, although large tricuspid valve vegetations are often associated with complications and failure of medical therapy, there is little prognostic value in short-term size changes. More important predictors of outcome in drug addicts with endocarditis may include multivalve infection, left-side involvement, persistent bacteremia, polymicrobial or virulent infection, and myocardial invasion.

▶ This experience with infective endocarditis in drug addicts mirrors our own. The detection of a vegetation by 2-dimensional echocardiography does have useful clinical associations, because such patients are more likely to have persistent infection, virulent bacteria, and multivalve involvement, and are more likely to die or to require surgery, particularly when the tricuspid vegetations are large (greater than 10 mm). As the authors noted, some patients may have only detectable vegetations after the first week or 2 of hospitalization. Most of the patients in this series responded to medical therapy, whether or not they had detectable vegetations. A pertinent recent article is that of A.S. Bayer et al. (1). A proposed short-term double-antibiotic regimen for the treatment of right-sided endocarditis in drug abusers is the subject of the next article (Abstract 3–45) in which only 8 (16%) patients had unequivocal tricuspid valve vegetations by echocardiography, though another 5 patients had increased reflectance of the tricuspid valve.—R.C. Schlant, M.D.

Reference

1. Bayer AS, Blomquist IK, Bello E, et al: Tricuspid valve endocarditis due to *Staphylococcus aureus:* Correlation of two-dimensional echocardiography with clinical outcome. *Chest* 93:247–253, 1988.

Right-Sided *Staphylococcus aureus* Endocarditis in Intravenous Drug Abusers: Two-Week Combination Therapy
Chambers HF, Miller RT, Newman MD (Univ of California, San Francisco; San Francisco Gen Hosp)
Ann Intern Med 109:619–624, Oct 15, 1988   3–45

A common treatment of *Staphylococcus aureus* endocarditis in human beings is 4- to 6-week combination antibiotic therapy, but no studies have ever shown that this duration is required. The study reported here was a test of whether 2-week combination therapy would be effective in treating staphylococcal endocarditis in drug addicts, for whom a shorter treatment course would be an attractive option. Over a 4-year period, 53 consecutive admissions to a county hospital of intravenous drug abusers with relatively uncomplicated right-sided staphylococcal endocarditis were studied. All patients had blood cultures positive for *S. aureus*, and none had any other infections requiring long courses of therapy or surgery. They received 2 weeks of therapy with nafcillin, 1.5 gm intravenously every 4 hours, plus tobramycin 1 mg/kg intravenously every 8 hours. Vancomycin, 30 mg/kg/day intravenously, was given in place of nafcillin to 3 patients who were allergic to penicillin.

Forty-seven episodes (94%) were cured after 2 weeks of combination therapy with nafcillin plus tobramycin. Of the 3 failures, 2 were due to management errors. Vancomycin plus tobramycin treatment cured only 1 patient of 3 studied and was not thought to be effective.

This work shows that a 94% cure rate was achieved when treating *S. aureus* endocarditis in intravenous drug users with 2 weeks of nafcillin and tobramycin. This result is based on selection of patients with right-sided endocarditis and no complicating additional infections. Vancomycin plus tobramycin treatment appeared relatively ineffective. Future studies comparing directly 2 weeks with 4 to 6 weeks of combination therapy appear warranted.

▶ It is important to emphasize that the patients selected for short-term therapy of right-sided *Staphylococcus aureus* endocarditis in this study were very carefully selected. In particular, patients with evidence of left-sided endocarditis, other infectious complications (osteomyelitis, pericarditis, meningitis, abscess, etc.), renal insufficiency, pregnancy, or methicillin-resistant isolates were excluded. The 2-week therapy with nafcillin and tobramycin appears to be highly effective. It also results in the saving of considerable money by decreasing the length of hospitalization. Hopefully, the results of this report will soon be confirmed in larger trials.—R.C. Schlant, M.D.

Carotid Sinus Hypersensitivity in Patients With Unexplained Syncope: Clinical, Electrophysiologic, and Long-Term Follow-up Observations
Huang SKS, Ezri MD, Hauser RG, Denes P (Tucson VA Med Ctr; Univ of Arizona; Rush Med College, Chicago)
Am Heart J 116:989–996, October 1988   3–46

In some patients with unexplained syncope, electrophysiologic studies have aided diagnosis and management. In some patients with unexplained syncope, carotid sinus hypersensitivity and its association with electrophysiologic findings, 76 patients with unexplained syncope were studied. Their evaluation included carotid sinus massage during electro-

TABLE 1.—Comparison of Clinical and Electrophysiologic Findings in Patients With and Without Carotid Sinus Hypersensitivity (CSH) in Unexplained Syncope

Clinical or electrophysiologic findings	With CSH (21 patients)	Without CSH (55 patients)	p value*
Mean age (mean ± SD)	62 ± 10	57 ± 12	
Sex: Male	17/21 (81%)	40/55 (73%)	NS
Female	4/21 (19%)	15/55 (27%)	NS
Multiple syncopal episodes	16/21 (76%)	38/55 (69%)	NS
Organic heart disease	13/21 (62%)	47/55 (85%)	<0.05
Abnormal ECG	12/21 (57%)	46/55 (84%)	<0.01
Sinus node dysfunction	6/21 (29%)	12/55 (22%)	NS
AV node dysfunction	7/21 (33%)	15/55 (27%)	NS
Inducible ventricular tachycardia (≥3 beats)	2/21 (9%)	16/55 (29%)	<0.01

*With chi-square test; $P < .05$ is considered statistical significance. NS, not significant.
(Courtesy of Huang SKS, Ezri MD, Hauser RG, et al: Am Heart J 116:989–996, October 1988.)

physiologic studies. Some patients received permanent pacemakers, and the success of this treatment was assessed.

Twenty-one of the 76 patients (28%) with unexplained syncope had carotid sinus hypersensitivity. These were predominantly men (17/21), with a mean age of 62 years. Eleven had coronary artery disease, and 2 were hypertensive. Electrophysiologic findings showed that 3 patients had abnormal sinus node function, 4 had abnormal atrioventricular node function, and 3 had abnormal functions of both sinus and atrioventricular nodes (table). Eleven showed normal node function. During carotid sinus massage, 12 patients exhibited sinus arrest alone, and the other 9 patients showed combined sinus arrest and atrioventricular nodal block. Thirteen patients received permanent pacemakers. None had recurrence of syncope after follow-up averaging 42 months (range, 10 to 75 months).

These findings suggest that unexplained syncope is frequently associated with carotid sinus hypersensitivity. Generally, electrophysiologic studies gave similar results in unexplained syncope patients with or without carotid sinus hypersensitivity. In some patients, permanent pacemakers appear beneficial in avoiding recurrent syncope.

▶ The authors tested their patients for carotid sinus hypersensitivty at the end of the electrophysiologic study. If the patients are carefully selected, I think that one can frequently test for such hypersensitivity while the patient has a continuous electrocardiographic rhythm recording with minimal risk. Patients with carotid bruits or decreased carotid pulsation may have an increased risk of a cerebrovascular accident in association with carotid sinus massage, which should always be performed while either watching the electrocardiogram or listening to the heart or both. In a paper published the previous month, P. Denes et al. (1) reviewed their 9-year experience with electrophysiologic testing of 89 patients with syncope of unknown origin, many of whom were also included in this report in the *American Heart Journal*. D.L. Kuchar et al. (2) and E.S. Gang et al. (3) reported that the signal-averaged electrocardiogram can noninvasively identify most patients with unexplained syncope due to ventricular tachyarrhythmias.—R.C. Schlant, M.D.

References

1. Denes P, Uretz E, Ezri MD, et al: Clinical predictors of electrophysiologic findings in patients with syncope of unknown origin. *Arch Intern Med* 148:1922–1928, 1988.
2. Kuchar DL, Thorburn CW, Sammel NL, et al: Signal-averaged electrocardiogram for evaluation of recurrent syncope. *Am J Cardiol* 58:949–953, 1986.
3. Gang ES, Peter T, Rosenthal ME, et al: Detection of late potentials on the surface electrocardiogram in unexplained syncope. *Am J Cardiol* 58:1014–1020, 1988.

High Dose Dipyridamole-Echocardiography Test in Women: Correlation With Exercise-Electrocardiography Test and Coronary Arteriography
Masini M, Picano E, Lattanzi F, Distante A, L'Abbate A (Univ of Pisa, Italy)
J Am Coll Cardiol 12:682–685, September 1988   3–47

The exercise-electrocardiography test for noninvasive diagnosis of coronary artery disease has not proved reliable in women. Recently, the high-dose dipyridamole-echocardiography test has been shown to be a useful exercise-independent diagnostic tool, but these studies have involved predominantly men. The present work was undertaken to evaluate the use of this test in detection of coronary artery disease in women. Enrolled in the study were 83 women with a mean age of 55 years, all of whom presented with chest pain and 15 of whom had previously had a myocardial infarction. Each woman underwent both exercise-electrocardiography and 2-dimensional echocardiography during a dipyridamole infusion of 0.84 mg/kg over 10 minutes and with electrocardiographic monitoring. The tests were performed on different days and in random order. All patients also underwent coronary angiography.

When results were correlated with angiographic findings, both tests demonstrated a similar sensitivity of more than 70% and similar predictive value of approximately 70% to 80% when tests were negative. When compared with exercise-cardiography, dipyridamole-echocardiography showed significantly higher values of specificity (93% versus 52%), accuracy (87% versus 62%), and predictive value of a positive test (91% versus 57%), compared with the exercise-cardiography test. These results were independent of the presence or absence of a previous myocardial infarction. No women had significant complications during the dipyridamole-echocardiography test, although 73% of patients had mild extracardiac side effects that did not prevent completion of the test.

These findings suggest that, in women, dipyridamole-echocardiography has higher specificity, accuracy, and predictive value of a positive test than exercise-electrocardiography. Because the 2 tests have equivalent sensitivity and predictive value of a negative test, the authors propose that dipyridamole-echocardiography is the test of choice for noninvasive diagnosis of coronary artery disease in women.

▶ After the development of exercise echocardiography as a useful diagnostic procedure, it is logical that dipyridamole-echocardiography be utilized both in those patients who are unable to exercise and in patients in whom the exercise/echocardiogram is not satisfactory. The use of dipyridamole makes it easier to obtain high-quality echocardiographic studies, although not all patients can tolerate intravenous dipyridamole or large oral doses of dipyridamole. In addition, there is a slight but definite risk of an untoward reaction from the dipyridamole. It is hoped that the usefulness and limitations of this promising test, which has previously been used predominantly in male patients, will soon be further evaluated in additional and larger studies of both men and women. It would also be helpful to have good cost-benefits studies in which dipyridamole echocardiography is compared in the same patients with dipyridamole thallium scintigraphy.—R.C. Schlant, M.D.

Skeletal Muscle Metabolism During Exercise Under Ischemic Conditions in Congestive Heart Failure: Evidence for Abnormalities Unrelated to Blood Flow

Massie BM, Conway M, Rajagopalan B, Yonge R, Frostick S, Ledingham J, Sleight P, Radda G (Univ of Oxford, England; Univ of California, San Francisco)
Circulation 78:320–326, August 1988   3–48

Exercise intolerance is the main symptom of chronic congestive heart failure, but its severity is correlated poorly with hemodynamic indexes of cardiac function. Previous ^{31}P nuclear magnetic resonance studies have shown that patients with congestive heart failure often have metabolic skeletal muscle abnormalities that may play a role in determining the degree of exercise limitation in these patients. However, the mechanism for these abnormalities remains poorly understood. This study was done to determine whether these metabolic abnormalities occur as a result of impaired blood flow or impaired oxygen delivery.

The study was done in 9 patients with mild-to-moderate congestive heart failure and 9 age- and size-matched healthy controls. All study participants performed repetitive submaximal finger flexion exercise, consisting of pulling a lever at a rate of 40 pulls per minute, under aerobic and ischemic conditions. Skeletal muscle metabolism was evaluated with ^{31}P nuclear magnetic resonance studies of the flexor digitorum superficialis.

During steady-state aerobic exercise at 33% of each subject's predetermined maximum workload, patients with congestive heart failure exhibited significantly lower pH values and phosphocreatine concentrations than did the controls. Similar differences were also observed throughout ischemic exercise at the same workload. The calculated lactate production and adenosine 5′-triphosphate consumption rates in patients with congestive heart failure were significantly higher than those in controls.

Many patients with congestive heart failure have an increased glycolytic metabolism and decreased oxidative phosphorylation in exercising skeletal muscle. However, these metabolic changes cannot be explained by a reduced blood flow or impaired oxygen delivery alone and need to be further investigated.

▶ These important studies confirm that an increase in glycolytic metabolism and a decrease in oxidative phosphorylation occur in exercising skeletal muscle in many patients with congestive heart failure. The metabolic changes do not appear to be related only to reduced blood flow or impaired oxygen delivery. The results suggest that some factor or factors associated with heart failure produce intrinsic changes in skeletal muscle energetics. This may have important therapeutic implications if the mechanism(s) for such changes could be identified and blocked.— R.C. Schlant, M.D.

Hemodynamics in Humans During Conventional and Experimental Methods of Cardiopulmonary Resuscitation

Swenson RD, Weaver WD, Niskanen RA, Martin J, Dahlberg S (Univ of Washington)
Circulation 78:630–639, September 1988   3–49

Experimental animal studies of cardiopulmonary resuscitation (CPR) have shown that both aortic pressure and aortic flow can be substantially increased over the low levels obtained during conventional CPR by using alternative techniques such as simultaneous ventilation and chest compression, abdominal binding, and high-impulse manual chest compression. However, the relevance of these findings to a clinical setting is uncertain, as very few human beings have undergone hemodynamic recordings during CPR.

The hemodynamics of conventional and experimental CPR protocols were evaluated, using high-fidelity recording, in 7 men and 2 women, aged 44–83 years, who had suffered out-of-hospital cardiopulmonary arrest. The experimental protocol, which included the use of high-impulse CPR and pneumatic vest CPR, with or without simultaneous ventilation and abdominal binding, was performed after the patients had been declared dead. Because all 9 study patients died, autopsy examinations could be performed within the next 24 hours to look for evidence of traumatic visceral injuries that might have resulted from using the pneumatic vest and abdominal binder. The experimental CPR tests were done in random order.

During conventional CPR, the aortic peak pressure averaged 61 mm Hg, and the coronary perfusion gradient, 9 mm Hg. Of the various experimental CPR protocols tested, only the high-impulse CPR technique significantly elevated both the aortic peak pressure and the coronary perfusion gradient. The pneumatic vest method significantly improved the peak aortic pressure but not the coronary perfusion gradient. Simultaneous ventilation and chest compression created high end-expiratory pressures but actually lowered the coronary perfusion gradient. Abdominal binding with phasic compression had no significant hemodynamic effects. Postmortem examinations showed evidence of either sternal or rib fractures in all 9 patients, but these fractures had occurred during the clinical resuscitation attempt.

None of the experimental CPR techniques evaluated in this study offered substantial improvement over conventional CPR methods. Furthermore, simultaneous ventilation appears to be detrimental because of its negative effect on the coronary perfusion gradient.

▶ This unique study provides important data that is impossible to obtain from animal studies. That the authors were able to perform this study signifies the superb rapport they had with the patients' families, who also deserve our thanks. It is important to know that simultaneous ventilation was not helpful but may even be detrimental and that abdominal binding with phasic compression was also not helpful.—R.C. Schlant, M.D.

Prevalence of the Coexistence of Left Ventricular False Tendons and Premature Ventricular Complexes in Apparently Healthy Subjects: A Prospective Study in the General Population
Suwa M, Hirota Y, Kaku K, Yoneda Y, Nakayama A, Kawamura K, Doi K (Osaka Med College, Japan)
J Am Coll Cardiol 12:910–914, October 1988   3–50

Most false tendons in the left ventricle contain Purkinje fibers, and false tendons often are found in patients who have premature ventricular complexes without underlying heart disease. A prospective study was undertaken with 187 healthy company employees aged 21–50 years, 118 men and 69 women. Two-dimensional echocardiography was carried out in addition to 24-hour ambulatory ECG monitoring.

Left ventricular false tendons were found in 71% of the study population. False tendons and premature ventricular complexes coexisted in 40 subjects after 8 with mitral prolapse were excluded. Premature ventricular complexes occurred at a higher rate in subjects with false tendons. Six of these patients had multiform, and 4, coupled complexes, and 1 had nonsustained ventricular tachycardia. Premature ventricular complexes were most closely associated with thick rather than thin false tendons, and with longitudinal rather than diagonal or transverse structures. Premature ventricular complexes tended to decrease during exercise testing, and cardiac ischemia was not observed.

The frequent coexistence of left ventricular false tendons and premature ventricular complexes suggests that these structures may have a role in the development of ventricular arrhythmias in apparently healthy persons.

▶ Left ventricular false tendons, which have been described by many terms including *left ventricular bands, false* or *anomalous chordae tendineae,* and *moderator bands,* are present at autopsy in about one half of hearts carefully examined. This study suggests a relationship between such structures and the occurrence of ventricular ectopy in apparently healthy individuals. Darazs et al. (1) reviewed the subject and noted that such structures had also been associated with many other clinical phenomena including murmurs, thrombi, and atypical chest pain. They suggested that the vibratory systolic murmur known as Still's murmur was produced by aeolian oscillations caused by blood flow around a left ventricular false tendon or band. Undoubtedly, future studies will establish the true prevalence of these tendons or bands, as well as provide criteria for determining when they are clinically significant and when they are merely a clinical variant.—R.C. Schlant, M.D.

Reference

1. Darazs B, Taylor HR, Van Gelder AL: The relevance of left ventricular bands. *S Afr Med J* 64:68–71, 1988.

4 Coronary Artery and Other Heart Diseases, Heart Failure

Introduction

This past year has been highlighted by many outstanding clinical trials of thrombolytic therapy with or without percutaneous transluminal coronary angioplasty in the setting of acute myocardial infarction. These studies are presented in the initial section of this chapter and deserve careful review by all physicians managing patients with acute myocardial infarction. A fundamental change in management of these patients has occurred and is part of a continuum of change initiated many years ago by the work of Dr. Sam Levine and others with early ambulation of patients following myocardial infarction. While we are appropriately challenged in these days of attempts to contain costs of medical care, the studies included on thrombolytic therapy and other topics represent an excellent response, in my judgment, of a profession seeking high-quality evidence to determine what is in the best interest of our patients.

R.L. Frye, M.D.

Intervention Early After Acute Myocardial Infarction

Randomised Trial of Intravenous Streptokinase, Oral Aspirin, Both, or Neither Among 17,187 Cases of Suspected Acute Myocardial Infarction: ISIS-2

Second International Study of Infarct Survival Collaborative Group (Radcliffe Infirmary, Oxford, England)

Lancet 2:349–360, Aug 13, 1988   4–1

A large number of patients admitted to 417 hospitals within 24 hours of the onset of suspected acute myocardial infarction were entered into the Second International Study of Infarct Survival. The median duration of symptoms was 5 hours. Half the patients were assigned to receive 1.5 million units of streptokinase, whereas half received a matching placebo. Infusions were administered over 1 hour. Half of all patients received oral aspirin in enteric-coated tablets in a daily dose of 160 mg.

Both streptokinase alone and aspirin alone led to a highly significant reduction in 5-week vascular mortality (Fig 4–1). The combination of streptokinase and aspirin was better than either agent alone. Their effects on vascular mortality appeared to be additive. Streptokinase therapy was

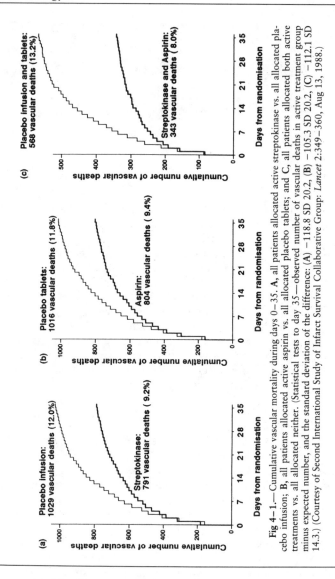

Fig 4–1.— Cumulative vascular mortality during days 0–35. A, all patients allocated active streptokinase vs. all allocated placebo infusion; B, all patients allocated active aspirin vs. all allocated placebo tablets; and C, all patients allocated both active treatments vs. all allocated neither. (Statistical tests to day 35—observed number of vascular deaths in active treatment group minus expected number, and the standard deviation of the difference: (A) −118.8 SD 20.2, (B) −105.3 SD 20.2, (C) −112.1 SD 14.3.) (Courtesy of Second International Study of Infarct Survival Collaborative Group: *Lancet* 2:349–360, Aug 13, 1988.)

associated with bleeding requiring transfusion and cerebral hemorrhage, but fewer other strokes occurred. No such excess bleeding was associated with aspirin use. An excess of nonfatal reinfarction, seen with streptokinase alone, was apparently avoided by adding aspirin. The reduction in vascular mortality has remained highly significant after a median follow-up of 15 months.

Streptokinase and aspirin are practicable and effective agents. If both are used in patients with suspected acute infarction, many deaths should be avoided.

▶ This is a landmark study that actually extends the limits of current concepts of thrombolytic therapy in that benefit was noted up to 24 hours after onset of symptoms. Entry criteria included patients with *suspected* myocardial infarction. The activation of platelets in the setting of acute myocardial infarction and with thrombolytic therapy noted in another paper (Abstract 4–2) in this section provides a basis for the demonstrated advantage of aspirin when combined with thrombolytic therapy. The powerful effect demonstrated in reducing mortality emphasizes the need for careful reassessment of relative contraindications to thrombolytic therapy, particularly in patients with a high risk of myocardial infarction mortality.—R.L. Frye, M.D.

Marked Platelet Activation In Vivo After Intravenous Streptokinase in Patients With Acute Myocardial Infarction
Fitzgerald DJ, Catella F, Roy L, FitzGerald GA (Vanderbilt Univ; Inst of Cardiology, Quebec City)
Circulation 77:142–150, January 1988   4–2

Six male patients with acute myocardial infarction who had not taken aspirin 10 days before hospitalization were given intravenous streptokinase. These patients were compared with 14 others who did not receive thrombolytic therapy. Analysis of those given streptokinase showed a notable increase of urinary 2,3-dinor-thromboxane B_2 as well as plasma

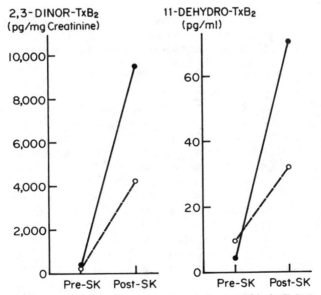

Fig 4–2.—Urinary 2,3-dinor-thromboxane *(Tx)* B_2 and plasma 11-dehydro-TxB_2 immediately before and after administration of streptokinase *(SK)* in 2 patients with acute myocardial infarction. (Courtesy of Fitzgerald DJ, Catella F, Roy L, et al: *Circulation* 77:142–150, January 1988.)

11-dehydro-thromboxane B_2 (Fig 4–2). This increase was not apparent in the patients who did not receive streptokinase.

In contrast, in 2 patients who had taken aspirin, the level of urinary 2,3-dinor-thromboxane was noticeably lowered during the 48-hour observation period. It was possible to measure urine and plasma levels in 2 patients both before and after streptokinase was administered. Again, levels showed a marked increase (see Fig 4–2).

The study suggests that streptokinase results in marked platelet activation because the platelet is the principal source of thromboxane A_2; however, the mechanism of the effect is unknown. The increase in platelet activation and thromboxane A_2 biosynthesis here observed may limit the efficacy of intravenous streptokinase in promoting the dissolution of clots and contribute to reocclusions.

▶ This is an extremely important study documenting the activation of platelets with streptokinase therapy in patients with acute myocardial infarction. The biology of thrombolysis is fascinating and will require increasing study by cardiologists. The results of ISIS-2 support the use of antiplatelet agents in combination with streptokinase.—R.L. Frye, M.D.

A Randomized Trial of Intravenous Tissue Plasminogen Activator for Acute Myocardial Infarction With Subsequent Randomization to Elective Coronary Angioplasty

Guerci AD, Gerstenblith G, Brinker JA, Chandra NC, Gottlieb SO, Bahr RD, Weiss JL, Shapiro EP, Flaherty JT, Bush DE, Chew PH, Gottlieb SH, Halperin HR, Ouyang P, Walford GD, Bell WR, Fatterpaker AK, Llewellyn M, Topol EJ, Healy B, Siu CO, Becker LC, Weisfeldt ML (Johns Hopkins Hosp, Francis Scott Key Hosp, St Agnes Hosp, Baltimore)
N Engl J Med 317:1613–1618, Dec 24, 1987   4–3

Intravenous recombinant human tissue plasminogen activator (t-PA) with elective coronary angioplasty represents an alternative approach to treatment of acute myocardial infarction. A randomized, double-blind placebo-controlled prospective study of t-PA was performed in patients presenting within 4 hours of the onset of acute myocardial infarction. Recombinant t-PA, 80–100 mg, was administered to 72 patients over 3 hours, while 66 received placebo. After coronary arteriography, patients were randomly assigned to undergo angioplasty on the third day or not to undergo angioplasty during the 10-day study period.

The patency rate of the infarct-related arteries was 66% in the t-PA group and 24% in the placebo group. There were no fatal or intracerebral hemorrhages. Bleeding requiring transfusion occurred in 9.8% of the t-PA group and 7.6% of the placebo group. Use of t-PA was associated with a higher mean ejection fraction on the tenth hospital day and a significantly improved ejection fraction during the entire study period. Use of t-PA was associated with a significant reduction in congestive heart failure, from 33% to 14%. Angioplasty improved ejection fraction response to exercise and reduced angina incidence, but did not influence the resting ejection fraction.

The administration of t-PA approximately within 4 hours of the onset of acute myocardial infarction improved left ventricular function at 10 days. Elective coronary angioplasty reduced the recurrence of ischemia and improved left ventricular function during exercise. These results support therapy with early intravenous t-PA and deferred angioplasty for patients with acute myocardial infarction.

▶ This is another extremely important trial of thrombolytic therapy and elective angioplasty in the setting of acute myocardial infarction. It supports the therapeutic benefits of thrombolytic therapy, and it documents a reduction in ischemic events in those receiving elective angioplasty. The data that are accumulating certainly favor an elective approach with angioplasty rather than urgent angioplasty in patients who can receive thrombolytic therapy.—R.L. Frye, M.D.

Thrombolysis With Tissue Plasminogen Activator in Acute Myocardial Infarction: No Additional Benefit From Immediate Percutaneous Coronary Angioplasty
Simoons ML, Arnold AER, Betriu A, de Bono DP, Col J, Dougherty FC, von Essen R, Lambertz H, Lubsen J, Meier B, Michel PL, Raynaud P, Rutsch W, Sanz GA, Schmidt W, Serruys PW, Thery C, Uebis R, Vahanian A, Van de Werf F, Willems GM, Wood D, Verstraete M (Rheinisch-Westfalische Technische Hochschule, Aachen, West Germany; Univ of Barcelona, Spain; Free Univ, Berlin; Tenon Hosp, Paris; Ziekenhuis Dijkzigt Academy, Rotterdam, the Netherlands; et al)
Lancet 1:197–203, Jan 30, 1988   4–4

It has been demonstrated that thrombolytic therapy improves survival, limits infarct size, and preserves left ventricular function in patients treated early after onset of acute myocardial infarction. A randomized trial of 367 patients was undertaken to determine whether thrombolytic therapy combined with percutaneous transluminal coronary angioplasty (PTCA) might offer improved results over thrombolytic therapy alone.

All patients received recombinant tissue-type plasminogen activator, heparin, and acetylsalicylic acid. Angiography and PTCA were performed immediately on the patients assigned to the invasive group.

Immediate PTCA reduced the percentage of stenosis in the infarct-related segment, but there was a 16% rate of transient reocclusion and a 7% rate of sustained reocclusion during the procedure. During the first 24 hours, 17% of patients also had recurrent ischemia. In the noninvasive group, only 3% of patients had recurrent ischemia within 24 hours, and there was a lower incidence of bleeding complications, hypotension, and ventricular fibrillation. Mortality at 14 days was 7% in the invasive group and 3% in the noninvasive group. There was no difference in infarct size between the treatment groups.

Because immediate PTCA does not provide additional benefit, immediate angiography and PTCA is not recommended in patients with acute myocardial infarction treated with recombinant tissue-type plasminogen activator. Delayed angiography, PTCA, or bypass surgery might be undertaken in patients with recurrent myocardial ischemia.

▶ This is an important trial, which observed a better clinical course without an invasive strategy in the setting of acute myocardial infarction (AMI). These observations combined with recent results from the TIMI Trial provide support for a noninvasive approach to patients with acute myocardial infarction if thrombolytic therapy can be given. The role of primary angioplasty without thrombolytic therapy in opening infarct-related arteries has not been settled. This is still an important question because perhaps 20% of patients with AMI may have a contraindication to thrombolytic drugs.— R.L. Frye, M.D.

Effect of Intravenous APSAC on Mortality After Acute Myocardial Infarction: Preliminary Report of a Placebo-Controlled Clinical Trial
AIMS Trial Study Group (Aberdeen Royal Infirmary, Aberdeen, Scotland; Amersham Gen Hosp; Addenbrooke's Hosp, Cambridge, England; Bangour Gen Hosp; Brook Hosp, London; et al)
Lancet 1:545–549, March 12, 1988   4–5

Anisoylated plasminogen streptokinase activator complex (APSAC) is a highly effective thrombolytic agent that achieves coronary artery reperfusion after a single intravenous injection in patients with acute myocardial infarction. An interim analysis was made of mortality data from a randomized double-blind placebo-controlled clinical trial in patients receiving a single 30-unit intravenous dose of APSAC within 6 hours of onset of infarction.

Patients were randomized to either APSAC therapy or placebo. Interim results were analyzed after 1,004 patients had been followed for at least 30 days. Intravenous heparin was begun 6 hours after treatment with APSAC or placebo; warfarin was given for at least 3 months. Data on survival and major clinical events were collected for up to 1 year.

Of 502 patients receiving placebo, 61 died within 30 days. There were only 32 deaths among the same number of APSAC-treated patients (Fig 4–3). Because this represented a 47% decrease in 30-day mortality, patient entry to the trial was ended. One-year mortality data showed a similar pattern. Decrease in the percentage of mortality with APSAC was comparable whether the drug was administered 0 to 4 hours after onset of symptoms or 4 to 6 hours after onset. Adverse events in the APSAC group included 11 occurrences of hematuria, 7 of hemoptysis, and a few cases of anaphylaxis and purpuric rash. There was no excessive gastrointestinal bleeding, hypotension, or cerebrovascular incidents in the treatment group.

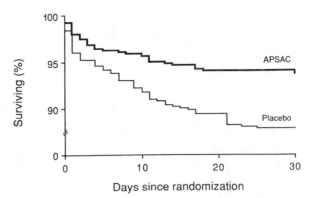

Fig 4–3.—Survival up to 30 days after dosage with APSAC or placebo (502 patients in each group). (Courtesy of the AIMS Trial Study Group: *Lancet* 1:545–549, March 12, 1988.)

These findings add to the growing body of evidence that early thrombolytic treatment after acute myocardial infarction contributes significantly to survival. There is a low risk of adverse effects with APSAC, and it has the advantage of requiring only a single dose. Further studies should determine the relative merits of APSAC compared with other thrombolytic agents.

▶ Additional clear documentation of improved survival with intravenous thrombolytic therapy. Therapy with APSAC is unique, with an important advantage of not requiring prolonged infusion because of binding properties of the complex. —R.L. Frye, M.D.

Trial of Tissue Plasminogen Activator for Mortality Reduction in Acute Myocardial Infarction: Anglo-Scandinavian Study of Early Thrombolysis (ASSET)
Wilcox RG, von der Lippe G, Olsson CG, Jensen G, Skene AM, Hampton JR (ASSET Study Group)
Lancet 2:525–530, Sept 3, 1988   4–6

Streptokinase and anistreplase, frequently used thrombolytic agents, may cause transient hypotension and a coagulation defect. Previous studies suggested that recombinant tissue-type plasminogen activator (rt-PA), which has less effect on clotting factors, might be less likely to cause bleeding and give better results than streptokinase.

In a large-scale study of patients from 52 coronary care units in Scandinavia and England the use of rt-PA was evaluated as a treatment for acute myocardial infarction. Patients with suspected acute myocardial infarction who could be treated within 5 hours after onset of symptoms entered this randomized, double-blind trial. A total of 2,512 patients received 100 mg of rt-PA plus heparin, and 2,493 were treated with heparin and a placebo.

Mortality at 1 month was 7.2% for the treatment group and 9.8% for the placebo group. Patients with a normal electrocardiogram on admission had better results: 1.6% for rt-PA and 3.0% for placebo treatment. There was a significant excess of major and minor bleeding complications in the rt-PA group. The incidence of stroke was similar in the 2 groups.

Early treatment with rt-PA reduces 1-month mortality in patients with acute myocardial infarction. These results are similar to those of trials of streptokinase. Thus rt-PA does not appear to be superior to streptokinase or to be associated with fewer bleeding episodes. However, its lack of antigenicity may prove useful in certain cases.

▶ This important trial documents clinical benefit for intravenous t-PA early after acute myocardial infarction. The reduction in early mortality seems about the same as with less expensive streptokinase as documented in prior trials. The potential advantage of a systemic fibrinolytic state was postulated by early investigators with streptokinase suggesting potential benefits unrelated to clot lysis (European Cooperative Study Group: *N Engl J Med* 301:797–802, 1979).—R.L. Frye, M.D.

Immediate vs. Delayed Catheterization and Angioplasty Following Thrombolytic Therapy for Acute Myocardial Infarction: TIMI II A Results
TIMI Research Group (Baltimore)
JAMA 260:2849–2858, Nov 18, 1988   4–7

The Thrombolysis in Myocardial Infarction (TIMI) research group undertook a trial to assess the role of percutaneous coronary angioplasty in patients given recombinant tissue-type plasminogen activator within 4 hours of the onset of acute infarction. Immediate catheterization, when appropriate, was compared with intervention 18 to 48 hours later. There were 195 patients assigned to immediate angioplasty and 194, to delayed angioplasty. Immediate procedures were done within 2 hours of the start of thrombolytic treatment.

Angioplasty was attempted in 72% of patients assigned to an immediate procedure, and 84% of attempts led to improvement. Angioplasty was attempted in 55% of the delayed group, and 93% of attempts succeeded. There were no significant group differences in ejection fraction. Bleeding was more frequent in the immediate angioplasty group, as was coronary bypass surgery. Mortality during the first 3 weeks was comparable in the 2 study groups.

Immediate catheterization and angioplasty has not led to better ventricular function in patients with acute myocardial infarction who receive plasminogen activator for thrombolysis. The risk of adverse events is higher than when catheterization is done after 18–48 hours.

▶ This is another study to document the lack of objective benefit of immediate angioplasty combined with intravenous thrombolytic therapy in patients with acute myocardial infarction as compared with angioplasty performed 18–48 hours after institution of thrombolytic therapy. Additional data have been presented from TIMI to indicate the lack of an advantage to either invasive strategy to intravenous thrombolytic therapy alone without angiography unless evidence of myocardial ischemia occurs during the subsequent course of the patient. These data will be received with great interest by all concerned with treating patients with myocardial infarction. (As a member of participating site in TIMI, my potential bias in the importance of these studies should be noted.)—R.L. Frye, M.D.

Prevention of Coronary Artery Reocclusion and Reduction in Late Coronary Artery Stenosis After Thrombolytic Therapy in Patients With Acute Myocardial Infarction: A Randomized Study of Maintenance Infusion of Recombinant Human Tissue-Type Plasminogen Activator
Johns JA, Gold HK, Leinbach RC, Yasuda T, Gimple LW, Werner W, Finkelstein D, Newell J, Ziskind AA, Collen D (Massachusetts Gen Hosp, Boston; Harvard Univ; Univ of Vermont)
Circulation 78:546–556, September 1988   4–8

Reocclusion and recurrent ischemia are problems associated with thrombolytic therapy. More successful thrombolytic agents would produce stable coronary patency and avoid the need for invasive procedures. A randomized study was designed to assess the effectiveness and safety of recombinant tissue-type plasminogen activator (rt-PA), which some trials have shown to be a more effective thrombolytic agent than streptokinase.

Sixty-eight patients with symptoms of acute myocardial infarction were treated with rt-PA within 6 hours of onset of chest pain. Fifty-two patients who had patent infarct-related arteries at 90 minutes were randomly assigned to 1 of 2 groups. Twenty-five were given a continuous infusion of heparin with a maintenance course of rt-PA, 0.8 mg/kg during 4 hours. The 27 controls received heparin alone; 1 of these patients died shortly after randomization of cardiac rupture.

None of the patients in the group given rt-PA had coronary artery reocclusion, but in 5 of the remaining 26 in the heparin-treated group reocclusion developed during the 1-hour observation period. Various ischemic events occurred at a significantly higher rate in the heparin-treated group. Residual stenosis improved in the rt-PA group within 8–14 days after infusion but was unchanged in the control group.

Treatment with rt-PA, according to the method described here, does prevent acute symptomatic coronary artery reocclusion. Furthermore, unstable angina was prevented, residual stenosis at 10 days was significantly decreased, and the need for acute angioplasty was avoided.

▶ An important observation on the problem of reocclusion of infarct-related arteries after successful thrombolysis.—R.L. Frye, M.D.

Characteristics and Outcome of Patients in Whom Reperfusion With Intravenous Tissue-Type Plasminogen Activator Fails: Results of the Thrombolysis and Angioplasty in Myocardial Infarction (TAMI) I Trial

Califf RM, Topol EJ, George BS, Boswick JM, Lee KL, Stump D, Dillon J, Abbottsmith C, Candela RJ, Kereiakes DJ, O'Neill WW, Stack RS, TAMI Study Group (Duke Univ; Univ of Michigan; Riverside Methodist Hosp, Columbus, Ohio, Christ Hosp, Cincinnati)
Circulation 77:1090–1099, May 1988   4–9

Thrombolytic therapy with tissue-type plasminogen activator (t-PA) fails in 20% to 35% of patients. Percutaneous transluminal coronary angioplasty (PTCA) has been suggested for salvaging vessel patency when pharmacologic thrombolysis fails. Ninety-six patients having occlusion after 90 minutes of t-PA therapy were reviewed. Immediate angioplasty was undertaken when the infarct vessel failed to reperfuse, unless it was technically unsuitable or the infarct was small. A comparison group of 288 patients achieved perfusion with the same protocol.

No baseline differences between the 2 patient groups was evident, but patients without perfusion had more complications during catheterization. Angioplasty achieved reperfusion with less than 50% residual stenosis in 73% of 86 attempts. Another 16% of patients had high-grade stenosis, and angioplasty failed in 11% of cases. Mortality in 9 patients with complete failure was 44% (Fig 4–4). Global ventricular function failed to improve in any group of patients.

Patients who fail to reperfuse within 90 minutes of the start of intravenous t-PA treatment have a high rate of later failure and high hospital mortality. However, immediate salvage angioplasty provides excellent long-term survival if definitive recanalization of the infarct vessel is achieved.

▶ Important data continue to be presented from the TAMI Study Group in a careful and thoughtful manner. Unfortunately, the impact of PTCA in the acute

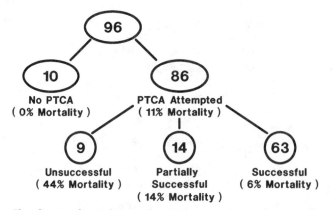

Fig 4–4.—Flow diagram of angioplasty results, reocclusion rates, and mortality in 96 patients in the t-PA failure group 90 minutes after initiation of treatment. (Courtesy of Califf RM, Topol EJ, George BS, et al: *Circulation* 77:1090–1099, May 1988.)

setting of patients with failed thrombolytic therapy is somewhat disappointing. The whole topic of failed thrombolytic therapy will require further detailed study.— R.L. Frye, M.D.

Failure of Simple Clinical Measurements to Predict Perfusion Status After Intravenous Thrombolysis
Califf RM, O'Neil W, Stack RS, Aronson L, Mark DB, Mantell S, George BS, Candela RJ, Kereiakes DJ, Abbottsmith C, Topol EJ, and TAMI Study Group (Duke Univ; Univ of Michigan; Riverside Methodist Hosp, Columbus, Ohio; Christ Hosp, Cincinnati)
Ann Intern Med 108:658–662, May 1988   4–10

Reperfusion in many patients with acute myocardial infarction fails to occur within 4–6 hours after onset of symptoms. Researchers estimate that up to 60% of patients receiving streptokinase and urokinase and from 20% to 30% of those treated with intravenous tissue plasminogen activator do not respond to treatment. Because the outlook for recovery in such patients is not favorable, a method of quickly measuring the success or failure in thrombolytic therapy would allow the clinician to prepare an appropriate backup treatment.

In this trial, 386 patients given high-dose intravenous tissue plasminogen activator were tested for infarct vessel patency by a series of angiograms. The patients rated their chest pain both before treatment and just before the 90-minute injection. Any episodes of ventricular dysrhythmia, atrioventricular block, and sinus bradycardia were monitored. Location of the infarction site was also noted.

Seventy-five percent of patients in this group achieved patency by 90 minutes. Improvement in symptoms and ST segment elevation were both associated with coronary perfusion, although arrhythmias were not. The location of the infarct was not significant. There was no relationship between the amount of time from symptom onset to treatment and the likelihood of perfusion by 90 minutes.

Unfortunately, none of the commonly used clinical methods give sufficient information for the physician to determine which patients have responded well to thrombolytic therapy and which should receive emergency angioplasty. Until a better means of evaluating the therapy or a more effective therapy is developed, all patients with acute myocardial infarction must be considered as candidates for emergency catheterization.

▶ The investigators do not justify their suggestion that emergency coronary angiography must be considered for *all* patients after thrombolytic therapy in the absence of bedside methods to assure successful reperfusion. There are no controlled studies to document the benefit of angioplasty in failed thrombolysis.— R.L. Frye, M.D.

Hemorrhagic Complications Associated With the Use of Intravenous Tissue Plasminogen Activator in Treatment of Acute Myocardial Infarction

Califf RM, Topol EJ, George BS, Boswick JM, Abbottsmith C, Sigmon KN, Candela R, Masek R, Kereiakes D, O'Neill WW, Stack RS, Stump D, Thrombolysis and Angioplasty in Myocardial Infarction Study Group (Duke Univ; Univ of Michigan; Riverside Methodist Hosp, Columbus, Ohio; Univ of Vermont; Christ Hosp, Cincinnati)

Am J Med 85:353–359, September 1988   4–11

Early studies of tissue plasminogen activator (t-PA) suggested that the rate of bleeding complications might be lower than that of older thrombolytic agents such as streptokinase and urokinase. In all, 386 patients from 5 centers were treated with t-PA for acute myocardial infarction to assess that agent's role in bleeding complications.

Beginning within 6 hours after symptoms appeared, patients were given 60 mg of t-PA intravenously in the first hour, 20 mg/hour for 2 hours, and 10 mg/hour for the next 5 hours. The last 210 patients had a weight-adjusted dosage. After t-PA therapy was initiated, patients were assigned to one of several treatment groups, based on the results of coronary angiography and left ventriculography.

Bleeding events were frequent, with 34% of patients needing transfusions. Patients treated with bypass surgery had far greater blood loss. In 45% of patients access site hematoma was the most common source of bleeding. Other risk factors included invasive procedures, female sex, smaller size, and older age. Nadir fibrinogen levels were the only laboratory parameters associated with an increase in bleeding complications.

Tissue plasminogen activator has no significant advantage over older thrombolytic agents in lowering bleeding complications or fibrinogen depletion. The clinical and hematologic risk factors for bleeding should be weighed when choosing modes of therapy. A reduction in dosage of t-PA may lower bleeding complications.

▶ This study needs careful review by all utilizing thrombolytic therapy. Although major hemorrhagic events are rare, they are devastating, particularly strokes. Clinical clues to high-risk patients are provided and must be balanced against the documented benefits of thrombolytic therapy in an individual patient.— R.L. Frye, M.D.

A Randomized Controlled Trial of Hospital Discharge Three Days After Myocardial Infarction in the Era of Reperfusion

Topol EJ, Burek K, O'Neill WW, Kewman DG, Kander NH, Shea MJ, Schork MA, Kirscht J, Juni JE, Pitt B (Univ of Michigan)

N Engl J Med 318:1083–1088, April 28, 1988   4–12

The cost increases engendered by use of reperfusion therapies after acute myocardial infarction may be justified by an increased number of lives saved, and long-term medical costs may even be reduced. Cost savings could be achieved, with or without reperfusion, if the length of hospital stay could be reduced. The feasibility and cost savings of hospital discharge 3 days after acute myocardial infarction were evaluated.

Eighty patients without complications, who had undergone early exercise testing, were randomized to early—day 3—or conventional—days 7 to 10—hospital discharge. Seventy-six of these patients had undergone coronary reperfusion therapy. Patients were followed up 1, 3, and 6 months after discharge. Patients were also evaluated using 2 psychologic measures given before randomization and at 1 and 3 months.

At 6 months, there were no deaths or new ventricular aneurysms, and the rates of readmission, reinfarctions, and patients with angina were similar in both groups. The only significant difference between groups on psychologic testing was that the early-discharge group showed a greater decline in paranoid ideation at 1 month. Patients in the early-discharge group returned to work approximately 2 weeks earlier than did those in the conventional-discharge group. Mean cumulative costs were $12,546 and $17,868 for the early- and conventional-discharge groups, respectively.

Hospital discharge is feasible after 3 days in carefully selected patients with uncomplicated myocardial infarction. Early discharge substantially reduces hospital costs. A large number of patients should be studied to determine whether this strategy can be recommended for clinical use.

▶ Intravenous thrombolytic therapy in patients with acute myocardial infarction represents a major advance in our treatment of such patients. Topol and colleagues have cautiously tested the impact of such therapy on the cost implication of acute myocardial infarction. They are appropriately cautious because large numbers of patients will require further study. We recently observed ventricular fibrillation (successfully resuscitated) 7 days after successful thrombolysis with only minimal residual stenosis in the infarct-related artery. Such patients are rare but of concern with an early discharge strategy.—R.L. Frye, M.D.

Coronary Perfusion During Acute Myocardial Infarction With a Combined Therapy of Coronary Angioplasty and High-Dose Intravenous Streptokinase

Stack RS, O'Connor CM, Mark DB, Honohara T, Phillips HR, Lee MM, Ramirez NM, O'Callaghan WG, Simonton CA, Carlson EB, Morris KG, Behar VS, Kong Y, Peter RH, Califf RM (Duke Univ; VA Med Ctr, Durham, NC)
Circulation 77:151–161, January 1988   4–13

Survival after acute myocardial infarction may be closely related to the patency of the infarct-related vessel. Thrombolytic therapy alone may not result in early reperfusion, and even if therapy is successful, patients are often left with residual stenosis and increased risk of reinfarction and limiting angina. In this study, 216 patients with acute myocardial infarction were treated with intravenously administered streptokinase and emergency percutaneous transluminal coronary angioplasty (PTCA).

Patients were treated with immediate infusion of 1.5 million units of streptokinase followed by PTCA. Repeat cardiac catheterization was performed before discharge to assess the patency of the infarct-related artery.

The infarct lesion was crossed and dilated in 99% of patients. Persistent coronary perfusion was achieved in 90%. Overall in-hospital mortality was 12%. Mortality was related to cardiogenic shock, older age, lower left ventricular ejection fraction, and female sex. Coronary reocclusion was found on repeat angiography in 11% of patients. Ninety-four percent of patients in whom infarct vessel patency was established were discharged with an open infarct artery or a bypass graft to the infarct vessel. Both the ejection fraction and regional wall motion in the infarct zone were significantly improved in patients with persistent coronary perfusion and insignificant residual stenosis at follow-up cardiac catheterization.

Patients with acute myocardial infarction treated with streptokinase, emergency PTCA, and bypass surgery when necessary have a high rate of early and sustained patency of the infarct-related vessel.

▶ This observational study from experienced investigators documents success of PTCA combined with thrombolytic therapy in providing patent infarct-related arteries. However, the lack of a "control" group is a problem. Furthermore, as noted under Abstract 4–4, the clinical advantage of combining PTCA "routinely" with early angioplasty has not been documented. It seems likely recurrent ischemia is less frequent in patients with successful angioplasty.— R.L. Frye, M.D.

Survival and Cardiac Event Rates in the First Year After Emergency Coronary Angioplasty for Acute Myocardial Infarction

Stack RS, Califf RM, Hinohara T, Phillips HR, Pryor DB, Simonton CA, Carlson EB, Morris KG, Behar VS, Kong Y, Peter RH, Hlatky MA, O'Connor CM, Mark DB (Duke Univ; VA Med Ctr, Durham, NC)
J Am Coll Cardiol 11:1141–1149, June 1988   4–14

Percutaneous transluminal coronary angioplasty is often used to overcome the limitations of thrombolytic therapy in patients with acute myocardial infarction. One-year survival and event-free survival rates were analyzed in 342 patients with acute myocardial infarction treated with early intravenous thrombolytic therapy and emergency coronary angioplasty.

Successful reperfusion was achieved in 94% of patients; perfusion was maintained by reperfusion catheter before emergency bypass surgery in 4% of the patients. The intraoperative mortality was 1.2%; total in-hospital mortality was 11%. Of surviving nonsurgical patients, 92% were discharged with an open infarct-related artery. Overall, the 1-year survival rate was 87%, and for hospital survivors, it was 98%, with an infarct-free survival rate of 94%.

An aggressive management strategy that includes early thrombolytic therapy, emergency cardiac catheterization, coronary angioplasty, and bypass surgery when necessary, can result in a high rate of infarct vessel patency. Long-term mortality and postdischarge reinfarction rates appear to be low, even in high-risk patient subgroups.

▶ The observational data from this large and carefully analyzed experience at Duke with an aggressive approach to acute myocardial infarction are of interest. However, as the investigators note, the observations are limited significantly by the lack of concurrent controls. The data are in conflict with several randomized trials showing no advantage to emergency "routine" angioplasty. There are no data to prove that routine angioplasty reduces reinfarction rates after successful thrombolytic therapy, whereas in ISIS-2 (see Abstract 4–1), aspirin therapy in combination with streptokinase clearly reduced reinfarction rates without combined angioplasty.—R.L. Frye, M.D.

Multicenter Reperfusion Trial of Intravenous Anisoylated Plasminogen Streptokinase Activator Complex (APSAC) in Acute Myocardial Infarction: Controlled Comparison With Intracoronary Streptokinase
Anderson JL, Rothbard RL, Hackworthy RA, Sorensen SG, Fitzpatrick PG, Dahl CF, Hagan AD, Browne KF, Symkoviak GP, Menlove RL, Barry WH, Eckerson HW, Marder VJ (APSAC Multicenter Investigators)
J Am Coll Cardiol 11:1153–1163, June 1988   4–15

Anisoylated plasminogen streptokinase activator complex (APSAC) is a plasminogen activator that holds promise for intravenous thrombolysis in acute myocardial infarction. It is chemically protected at its active site by an acyl group, so that nonspecific activation and fibrinogenolysis are avoided but the ability to bind to fibrin is retained. A total of 240 patients with documented coronary occlusion received either 30 units of APSAC intravenously or intracoronary streptokinase within 6 hours of the onset of symptoms of infarction. Both groups received heparin for at least 24 hours.

Reperfusion was evident in 51% of APSAC-treated patients after 90 minutes, and in 60% of patients after an hour of intracoronary streptokinase. The agent APSAC was most effective when given within 4 hours of the onset of symptoms and was generally well tolerated, although the fall in blood pressure was greater than after streptokinase. Bleeding was more frequent with APSAC, but intracranial hemorrhage did not occur. Early reocclusion was infrequent with both treatments.

Further development of APSAC for clinical use is warranted. When given within 4 hours of the onset of infarction, APSAC is associated with reperfusion similar to that achieved with intracoronary streptokinase, and of the 2 agents, APSAC is more easily administered.

▶ Here is additional data on the use of APSAC in the setting of acute myocardial infarction. Though APSAC has a theoretical advantage in terms of kinetics, this was not reflected in fewer reocclusions as compared with streptokinase.—R.L. Frye, M.D.

Balancing the Benefits, Risks, and Unknowns of Thrombolytic Therapy in Acute Myocardial Infarction
Gorlin R (Mount Sinai Med Ctr, New York)
J Am Coll Cardiol 11:1349–1354, June 1988   4–16

Thrombolysis as treatment of acute myocardial infarction has received wide exposure in the media, which will certainly lead to a clamor for its use. The Food and Drug Administration has been publicly criticized for its failure to approve recombinant tissue plasminogen activator earlier for general use. However, the appropriate doses, duration of treatment, and optimal combinations of available agents have not yet been defined. To weigh the benefits and risks of thrombolysis in everyday practice, it is necessary to assess the risk of the disease versus that of thrombolytic therapy and to evaluate the time that has elapsed between the onset of symptoms and the first opportunity to administer therapy.

A review of completed clinical trials shows that maximal benefit of thrombolytic therapy occurs in patients who are seen within the first 3 hours of symptoms, who are having their first infarction, whose infarct is anterior or multiple in site and putatively large, and who have severe left ventricular dysfunction, usually an indication of a major regional perfusion deficit. Cardiogenic shock has a mortality of more than 85% with standard therapy and should be treated with thrombolysis if direct angioplasty is not available.

To minimize the risk of thrombolytic therapy, it should not be used in patients aged older than 65, those with moderate to severe hypertension, and those with a history of cerebrovascular accident or a bleeding disorder. It is possible that long-standing diabetes with arteriopathy may also enhance risk. The judgment of the physician to do what is really best for the patient must prevail in the face of a wave of premature, unscientific endorsement of thrombolytic therapy.

▶ Doctor Gorlin provides, as usual, an excellent balanced review of the use of thrombolytic therapy in acute myocardial infarction. It should be read carefully by all engaged in these therapies.—R.L. Frye, M.D.

General Topics in Managing Acute Myocardial Infarction

Early Return to Work After Uncomplicated Myocardial Infarction: Results of a Randomized Trial
Dennis C, Houston-Miller N, Schwartz RG, Ahn DK, Kraemer HC, Gossard D, Juneau M, Barr Taylor C, DeBusk RF (Stanford Univ)
JAMA 260:214–220, July 8, 1988   4–17

Although progressive ambulation and shorter hospitalization after un-complicated myocardial infarction have become standard clinical proce-dures during recent years, the average time before return to work has not changed much over the years. A randomized trial was conducted to de-termine whether an occupational work evaluation could shorten the time between myocardial infarction and return to work.

The study population consisted of 201 employed men with a median age of 49 years recovering from uncomplicated myocardial infarction, in-cluding 102 randomly assigned to usual care and 99 who participated in an occupational work evaluation. The evaluation consisted of a symp-tom-limited treadmill test performed 23 days after myocardial infarction and a formal recommendation to both the patient and the primary phy-sician that the patient return to work within the next 2 weeks. Successful return to work was defined as 4 or more consecutive weeks of full-time employment. Two of the 99 patients receiving an occupational work evaluation subsequently withdrew from the program for personal rea-sons.

Intervention patients returned to work full-time at a median of 51 days from the date of myocardial infarction, whereas usual-care patients re-turned at a median of 75 days, representing a 32% reduction in the con-valescence period for intervention patients. At the 6-month evaluation, 91 (92%) of 99 intervention patients and 88 (86%) of 102 usual-care pa-tients were working an average of 41 hours per week. During the first 6 months after myocardial infarction, 27 patients, including 14 interven-tion and 13 usual-care patients, had 1 or more cardiac events. Earlier re-turn to work was associated with a mean salary differential of $2,102 (22%) more for intervention patients.

Objective assessment of risk and physical capacity using early postin-farction treadmill testing with explicit recommendations to patient and local physician can result in reduction of time for return to employment, with important economic consequences.

▶ This well-designed and -conducted trial provides objective data on cardiac re-habilitation efforts, specifically focusing on issues related to return to work. The beneficial effect of such programs is well documented.—R.L. Frye, M.D.

Treatment of Patients With Symptomless Left Ventricular Dysfunction Af-ter Myocardial Infarction
Sharpe N, Murphy J, Smith H, Hannan S (Univ of Auckland, New Zealand)
Lancet 1:255–259, Feb 6, 1988   4–18

Although patients with congestive heart failure who are treated with angiotensin-converting-enzyme (ACE) inhibitors have clinical improve-ment and a somewhat reduced mortality, the prognosis for most of these patients remains poor. Experimental studies in animals have shown that ACE inhibition appears to prevent progressive ventricular dysfunction and heart failure and improves survival. A randomized, double-blind, clinical trial was done to determine whether identification and early treatment with ACE inhibitors of patients with symptomless left ventricular dysfunction after acute myocardial infarction results in improved left ventricular function.

The study population consisted of 60 patients with recent Q-wave myocardial infarction who were asymptomatic and did not receive cardiac drugs before hospital discharge. Twenty patients received captopril, 25 mg 3 times daily; 20 patients received furosemide, 40 mg daily; and 20 patients were given a placebo. Left ventricular function was evaluated with cross-sectional echocardiography and Simpson's rule analysis of standardized apical views at baseline and 1, 3, 6, 9, and 12 months after initiation of treatment.

The Captopril-treated patients showed no significant change in left ventricular end-diastolic volume index, and the left ventricular end-systolic volume index was significantly reduced. Stroke volume index and ejection fraction were significantly increased at 1 month after captopril treatment was initiated and from then on. In contrast, furosemide-treated and placebo-treated patients had significant increases in ventricular volumes, no change in stroke volume index, and a slightly reduced ejection fraction.

Asymptomatic ventricular dysfunction can be improved by ACE inhibition after Q-wave myocardial infarction. The treatment effect of captopril was highly significant, and contrasted sharply with the increased dilatation that occurred with both furosemide and placebo.

▶ This extremely important study will be followed by larger trials to assess the clinical impact of improved left ventricular function with ACE inhibitors in patients with asymptomatic left ventricular dysfunction post myocardial infarction.—R.L. Frye, M.D.

Acute Myocardial Infarction Associated With Single Vessel Coronary Artery Disease: An Analysis of Clinical Outcome and the Prognostic Importance of Vessel Patency and Residual Ischemic Myocardium
Wilson WW, Gibson RS, Nygaard TW, Craddock GB Jr, Watson DD, Crampton RS, Beller GA (Univ of Virginia)
J Am Coll Cardiol 11:223–234, February 1988   4–19

Prognosis after acute myocardial infarction is related to the amount of residual ischemic myocardium. Inducible ischemia predicts a relatively poor prognosis in patients with multivessel disease, but it is not clear whether its prognostic significance is the same in patients with single-vessel disease. The prognosis and significance of residual ischemic myocardium were studied in 97 patients with single-vessel coronary artery disease and acute myocardial infarction. Coronary arteriography was performed a mean of 12 days after the myocardial infarction.

Thallium scintigraphy was performed during exercise on a treadmill approximately 11 days after onset of infarction. To assess left ventricular ejection fraction and segmental wall motion, radionuclide ventriculography as performed immediately following the delayed thallium images. Patients also underwent coronary angiography. Patients were reevaluated at 3 months and 12 months and yearly thereafter. Beginning 2 years after infarction, 58 of the 97 patients had exercise thallium scintigraphy performed at follow-up visits.

There were no deaths during follow-up. Six patients had a recurrent myocardial infarction, and 25 were hospitalized for angina. Thirty-one patients remained asymptomatic. Neither exercise-induced angina nor ST segment was predictive of a recurrent ischemic event, but the mean number of infarct zone scan segments showing thallium redistribution and the percentage of patients with infarct zone redistribution were both significantly greater in patients who had an ischemic event. The infarct-related vessel was angiographically patent in 40 patients; patency of the vessel was not related to incidence of ischemic events, but patency was associated with a greater prevalence of non–Q wave infarction, fewer persistent and more reversible infarct zone thallium defects, and a tendency toward a higher left ventricular ejection fraction.

The incidence of mortality and reinfarction is low among patients with uncomplicated myocardial infarction in single-vessel coronary artery disease. Infarct-zone thallium redistribution is predictive of a higher ischemic event rate. It is not known whether emergency angioplasty would improve survival and prevent reinfarction in these patients, but trials should be limited to those patients with inducible infarct-zone thallium redistribution.

▶ This is an important application of thallium scintigraphy in patients post myocardial infarction by a group of investigators with a large experience and commitment to high-quality radionuclide studies. This reviewer continues to have concern regarding application of thallium scanning in laboratories without similar experience and resources for quality control.—R.L. Frye, M.D.

A Computer Protocol to Predict Myocardial Infarction in Emergency Department Patients With Chest Pain
Goldman L, Cook EF, Brand DA, Lee TH, Rouan GW, Weisberg MC, Acampora D, Stasiulewicz C, Walshon J, Terranova G, Gottlieb L, Kobernick M, Goldstein-Wayne B, Copen D, Daley K, Brandt AA, Jones D, Mellors J, Jakubowski R (Harvard Univ; Yale Univ; Univ of Cincinnati; Milford Hosp, Milford, Conn; St Mary's Hosp, Waterbury, Conn; et al)
N Engl J Med 318:797–803, March 31, 1988   4–20

Clinical data from 1,379 patients at 2 hospitals participating in the Chest Pain Study were used to construct a computer protocol for predicting myocardial infarction. The protocol was tested prospectively in 4,770 patients seen at 2 university hosptials and 4 community hospitals. The computer protocol uses 9 clinical and 2 electrocardiographic factors to divide patients into 14 groups, including 6 in which the likelihood of infarction exceeded 7%.

The computer-derived protocol was significantly more specific in predicting the absence of infarction than physicians deciding whether to admit patients to coronary care. Both the protocol and physicians were 88% sensitive in detecting infarction. Protocol-based decisions would have lowered the admission rate of patients without infarction by 11.5% without impeding the admission of patients requiring intensive care for emergent complications.

Decision protocols based on the analysis of large data sets can yield better results than physicians' unaided judgments. Where appropriate, however, any computerized protocol should be overriden by a careful clinician performing in-depth evaluations of individual patients.

▶ Another provocative and excellent study by Goldman and colleagues. The influence of medical/legal risk in decision making is not addressed and undoubtedly must influence some of these decisions in emergency rooms. Unfortunately, in my own experience, atypical chest pain with initially negative electrocardiograms is still observed with evolving acute myocardial infarction.—R.L. Frye, M.D.

Intravenous Nitroglycerin Therapy to Limit Myocardial Infarct Size, Expansion, and Complications: Effect of Timing, Dosage, and Infarct Location

Jugdutt BI, Warnica JW (Univ of Alberta)
Circulation 78:906–919, October 1988   4–21

Intravenous nitroglycerin can limit infarct size and reduce the risk of complications and death, but the factors determining its effects are uncertain. A prospective study of 310 patients admitted to a coronary care unit focused on factors determining the effect of nitroglycerin in the first 48 hours on creatine kinase infarct size. Infusion of nitroglycerin in 154 cases was titrated to lower the mean blood pressure by 10% in normotensive and 30% in hypertensive patients, but not to less than 80 mm Hg. The infusion continued for 39 hours.

Earlier treatment was associated with smaller infarcts. Infarct size was less in nitroglycerin-treated than in control patients with anterior and inferior infarction. Left ventricular asynergy was less in nitroglycerin-treated patients, and ejection fraction values were higher. Major infarct-related complications occurred less often with infusion of nitroglycerin. Hospital mortality was 14% in this group and 26% in controls. After 1 year the respective mortalities were 21% and 31%.

Low-dose intravenous nitroglycerin limits infarct size in acute myocardial infarction and lowers the risk of major infarct-related events. Mortality also is lowered for up to a year after infarction. Infarct extension and cardiogenic shock are less likely to occur when nitroglycerin is administered. Early treatment is beneficial. The mean blood pressure should be kept greater than 80 mm Hg.

▶ The study clearly documents the beneficial effect of low-dose intravenous nitroglycerin in the setting of acute myocardial infarction. The importance of early institution of this intervention, like all others in the setting of acute myocardial infarction, has again been documented. However, the benefit was still noted up to 10 hours after the onset of pain. The investigators emphasize the parameters for maintenance low-dose intravenous nitroglycerin and, in particular, avoiding undue hypotension.—R.L. Frye, M.D.

The Effect of Diltiazem on Mortality and Reinfarction After Myocardial Infarction

The Multicenter Diltiazem Postinfarction Trial Research Group
N Engl J Med 319:385–392, Aug 18, 1988   4–22

Long-term diltiazem was evaluated in a total of 2,466 patients with previous myocardial infarction at 38 centers in the United States and Canada. Patients were assigned to receive 240 mg of diltiazem daily or placebo, and were followed for a mean of 25 months and as long as 52 months. The 2 groups were clinically comparable. About 70% of patients in each group had Q wave infarction.

Overall mortality was very similar in the 2 groups (Fig 4–5). Cardiac

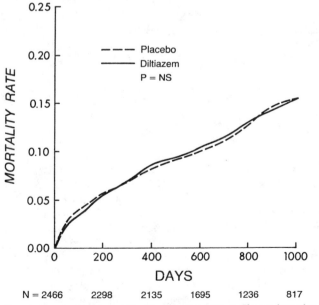

Fig 4–5.—Cumulative rate of total mortality according to treatment. The numbers of patients at risk are shown at bottom of panel. *NS*, not significant. (Courtesy of The Multicenter Diltiazem Postinfarction Trial Research Group: *N Engl J Med* 319:385–392, Aug 18, 1988.)

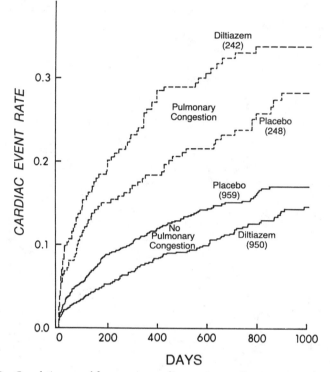

Fig 4–6.—Cumulative rate of first recurrent cardiac events, according to treatment in patients with and without pulmonary congestion. Diltiazem-treated patients with pulmonary congestion had higher rate of cardiac events than patients receiving placebo; diltiazem-treated patients without pulmonary congestion had lower rate of cardiac events than patients receiving placebo. Values in parentheses are numbers of patients. (Courtesy of the Multicenter Diltiazem Postinfarction Trial Research Group: *N Engl J Med* 319:385–392, August 18, 1988.)

deaths and nonfatal reinfarctions were 11% lower in the diltiazem group than in placebo recipients (Fig 4–6). Diltiazem therapy was associated with fewer cardiac events in 1,909 patients without pulmonary congestion, but with more events in 490 patients with pulmonary congestion. A similar pattern was evident for ejection fraction.

No significant overall effect of diltiazem on mortality or cardiac events was found in this study of patients with previous myocardial infarction. Cardiac events were, however, less frequent in patients without left ventricular dysfunction. Prospective data would be useful before drawing conclusions on the efficacy of diltiazem in this setting.

▶ Another beautifully designed and conducted trial testing the effect of a calcium channel blocker on mortality and reinfarction in patients with a previous infarction. The authors are appropriately cautious about the subgroup analysis showing differential effects based upon the presence or absence of left ventricular dysfunction. However, this study emphasizes the need for caution in the use of diltiazem in patients with congestive heart failure and depressed left ventricular function. One presumes this may relate to the negative ionotropic effects of the drug particularly in noninfarct segments of the ventricle where a compensatory increase in regional performance may be impaired by diltiazem. —R.L. Frye, M.D.

PTCA Unrelated to Acute Myocardial Infarction

Restenosis and Progression of Coronary Atherosclerosis After Coronary Angioplasty

Cequier A, Bonan R, Crépeau J, Coté G, De Guise P, Joly P, Lespérance J, Waters DD (Montreal Heart Inst; Univ of Montreal)

J Am Coll Cardiol 12:49–55, July 1988   4–23

Percutaneous transluminal coronary angioplasty (PTCA) in the treatment of obstructive coronary artery disease has short- and long-term benefits. However, restenosis remains a major limitation of PTCA. Although clinical, angiographic, and procedural risk factors associated with restenosis have been well studied, therapeutic measures to decrease restenosis rates have not been successful. To evaluate the relationship between restenosis after PTCA and the progression of coronary atherosclerosis, a prospective study was carried out in 98 patients with 110 coronary stenoses who were successfully treated with PTCA.

For 24–48 hours before angioplasty, patients were treated with aspirin, 650 mg daily; dipyridamole, 75 mg 3 times daily; and nifedipine, 10–20 mg 4 times daily; or diltiazem, 30–90 mg 4 times daily. After PTCA, patients were followed with thallium 201 treadmill exercise testing at 1, 3, and 6 months, and with angiography at 6 months. Late angiographic restudy was scheduled approximately 18 months after successful PTCA.

At the early post-PTCA angiographic evaluation, 37 patients (38%) had restenosis in 39 segments, defined as a stenosis of 50% or more of the luminal diameter or loss of 50% or more of the gain achieved by PTCA. Of 90 patients who underwent late angiography, 85 were examined for progression of atherosclerosis. Thirty-one (34%) of these 85 patients had progression of coronary atherosclerosis in 53 segments, including 9 (33%) of 27 patients with restenosis and 22 (38%) of 58 patients without restenosis. The difference was not statistically significant.

Progression of atherosclerosis in nondilated segments adjacent to dilated segments was observed in 16 (17%) of 94 dilated vessels compared with 25 (14%) of 176 nondilated vessels. The difference was not statistically significant. Restenosis developed faster than did progression of atherosclerotic disease.

Progression of coronary atherosclerosis and restenosis after PTCA apparently are dissimilar processes that progress independently.

▶ It is reassuring that in this study no new lesions were observed in segments adjacent to the dilated segments in patients undergoing coronary angioplasty. The observed independence of progression in atherosclerosis and restenosis of dilated segments may also relate to the disparity in local trauma at the dilated and nondilated segments rather than a fundamental difference in pathophysiologic mechanisms. The study is of great interest.—R.L. Frye, M.D.

Aspirin and Dipyridamole in the Prevention of Restenosis After Percutaneous Transluminal Coronary Angioplasty
Schwartz L, Bourassa MG, Lespérance J, Aldridge HT, Kazim F, Salvatori VA, Henderson M, Bonan R, David PR (Montreal Heart Inst; Toronto Gen Hosp; Boehringer Ingelheim–Canada)
N Engl J Med 318:1714–1719, June 30, 1988   4–24

Percutaneous transluminal coronary angioplasty (PTCA) is now commonly used in the treatment of coronary artery disease. However, PTCA is associated with an arterial restenosis rate of 15% to 45%. Antiplatelet agents have been used in an attempt to prevent the recurrence of arterial lesions, but no placebo-controlled study evaluating the efficacy of such treatment has as yet been published. A 3-year randomized, double-blind, placebo-controlled study was made of 376 patients who were undergoing PTCA, including 187 patients who were assigned to active drug treatment and 189 who served as controls.

Patients in the group receiving the drug were given an aspirin-dipyridamole combination 24 and 16 hours before PTCA. Eight hours before PTCA, dipyridamole given orally was replaced with dipyridamole administered intravenously at a dose of 10 mg/hour for 24 hours, whereas aspirin given orally was continued every 8 hours. Combined oral therapy was reinstituted 3 times daily at a dose of 330 mg of aspirin and 75 mg of dipyridamole per capsule and continued until follow-up angiography 4–7 months after PTCA, or earlier if symptoms developed.

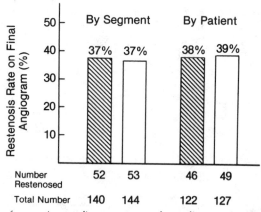

Fig 4–7.—Rate of restenosis, according to segment and according to patient, in aspirin-dipyridamole group *(hatched bars)* and placebo group *(open bars)*. (Courtesy of Schwartz L, Bourassa MG, Lespérance J, et al: *N Engl J Med* 318:1714–1719, June 30, 1988.)

The rate of restenosis was analyzed in 249 patients for whom final angiographic data were available (Fig 4–7). Restenosis in at least 1 segment occurred in 37.7% of the drug-treated patients and in 38.6% of the placebo-treated patients. The difference was not statistically significant. However, of 16 periprocedural Q-wave myocardial infarctions that occurred, 13 were in placebo-treated patients and 3, in drug-treated patients.

Although an antiplatelet regimen before and after PTCA did not reduce the rate of restenosis after successful coronary angioplasty, it markedly reduced the incidence of transmural myocardial infarction during or soon after PTCA. Therefore, the short-term use of an antiplatelet regimen in patients undergoing PTCA is recommended.

▶ The failure of aspirin and dipyridamole to improve long-term restenosis after coronary angioplasty is disappointing. On the other hand, the short-term effects in reducing postangioplasty myocardial infarction are encouraging.—R.L. Frye, M.D.

Reduction in the Rate of Early Restenosis After Coronary Angioplasty by a Diet Supplemented With n-3 Fatty Acids
Dehmer GJ, Popma JJ, van den Berg EK, Eichhorn EJ, Prewitt JB, Campbell WB, Jennings L, Willerson JT, Schmitz JM (Dallas VA Med Ctr; Univ of Texas, Dallas)
N Engl J Med 319:733–740, Sept 22, 1988   4–25

Restenosis after coronary angioplasty occurs in 25% to 40% of the dilated lesions. Conventional treatment to lower the incidence of restenosis, which consists of 1.5 gm of aspirin per day, causes gastrointestinal distress. A dietary supplement of n-3 polyunsaturated fatty acids was evaluated for its benefit in preventing early restenosis.

In a randomized unblinded trial, 82 men at relatively high risk for restenosis were studied. A control group of 39 men (53 lesions) received 325 mg of aspirin and 225 mg of dipyridamole daily. Forty-three patients (50 lesions) in the treatment group also received 3.2 gm of eicosapentaenoic acid daily. Treatment continued for 6 months after coronary angioplasty.

Restenosis occurred in 36% of lesions in the control group and in only 16% of lesions in the treatment group. Treatment with n-3 fatty acids decreased the likelihood of restenosis, and the treated patients had no important bleeding complications.

In this trial treatment with n-3 fatty acids was safe and well tolerated, and it significantly lowered the development of restenosis. Although the mechanism involved in the action of n-3 fatty acids is not defined, it is worth noting that the dietary supplement was effective with concurrent aspirin therapy and that n-3 fatty acids may work best when pretreatment is added to the postangioplasty course because the substance is incorporated over a period of time into the membrane phospholipid pool.

▶ Restenosis remains a major problem in limiting the long-term effectiveness of coronary angioplasty. These data are of great interest and suggest the need for a larger randomized trial. The intensity of the response to the initial endothelial injury associated with angioplasty has been studied carefully by Chesebro and colleagues (*J Am Coll Cardiol* 8:1380–1386, 1986), and compounds the challenge of preventing restenosis.—R.L. Frye, M.D.

Report of the Joint ISFC/WHO Task Force on Coronary Angioplasty
Bourassa MG, Alderman EL, Bertrand M, de la Fuente L, Gratsianski A, Kaltenbach M, King SB, Nobuyoshi M, Romaniuk P, Ryan TJ, Serruys PW, Smith HC, Sousa JE, Böthig S, Rapaport E
Circulation 78:780–789, September 1988   4–26

Since 1977, percutaneous transluminal coronary angioplasty (PTCA) has gained wide acceptance as a treatment for coronary artery disease. In the United States, 32,306 PTCAs were performed in 1983. During 1987, 175,680 patients underwent PTCA in this country. Data from other countries show similar trends. A task force was formed by the Council on Clinical Cardiology of the International Society and Federation of Cardiology with the World Health Organization to study and make recommendations on the use of PTCA.

The task force classifies candidates for PTCA into 3 groups: class I patients have accepted indications; class II patients have evolving indications; and class III patients have relative contraindications. Criteria for primary success and restenosis are defined in a variety of ways: angiographically (the most reliable method), hemodynamically, functionally, and symptomatically. Multivessel PTCA and multilesion PTCA are defined and distinguished from each other.

The task force also addresses the question of training requirements for those physicians performing PTCA and recommends formal training programs in angioplasty. These programs should be designed on 3 levels: clinical cardiology, cardiac catheterization and angiography, and coronary angioplasty. Guidelines for equipment are described, and the task force stresses the need for extensive operator experience.

Surgical backup for emergency situations is necessary, for various complications can be dealt with only by immediate surgical procedures. Arrangements for surgical coverage must be made before the angioplasty procedure. Postangioplasty management, including recommended medications, is also described. Future developments such as balloon devices and laser technology may overcome the current limitations found in PTCA.

▶ An excellent consensus document that deserves careful review by all cardiologists, this and other similar efforts to establish criteria for the appropriate use of this important technique should be noted (ACC/AHA Task Force Report: Guidelines for percutaneous transluminal coronary angioplasty. *J Am Coll Cardiol* 12:529–545, 1988).—R.L. Frye, M.D.

The Effect of Coronary Angioplasty on Coronary Flow Reserve

Wilson RF, Johnson MR, Marcus ML, Aylward PEG, Skorton DJ, Collins S, White CW (Univ of Iowa, Univ of Minnesota)
Circulation 77:873–885, April 1988   4–27

It has not been established that angioplasty restores normal coronary flow reserve. Availability of a small subselective coronary Doppler catheter makes it possible to study the effects of angioplasty on flow reserve both immediately and late after coronary dilation. Thirty-two studies were done just before coronary angioplasty; 32, immediately afterwards; and 31, after a mean of 7.4 months. The patients had dilation of a single discrete coronary lesion. The study employed a No. 3F coronary Doppler catheter and a maximally vasodilating dose of papaverine.

Coronary flow reserve returned to normal immediately after angioplasty in 14 of 31 patients, and improved in the others. Values were not related to angiographic variables or to the resting pressure gradient. On later study, coronary flow reserve was correlated significantly with indices of residual arterial stenosis. All patients without restenosis eventually had normal coronary flow reserve. Patients with restenosis had low coronary flow reserve at follow-up, although some had normal values immediately after angioplasty.

Coronary flow reserve became normal after angioplasty in about half these patients, and the reserve becomes normal late after the procedure when corrected for the degree of residual stenosis. Immediate postoperative estimates may not reflect how successfully angioplasty has removed a physiologically important obstruction to coronary flow. Variables from noninvasive studies of ischemia may require a time to normalize after angioplasty if maximal hyperemic flow is impaired immediately after coronary dilation.

▶ This report of quantitative angiography combined with measurement of coronary flow reserve provides new insights into the responses of the coronary circulation following coronary angioplasty. These findings are of particular importance to those who objectively assess patients early after angioplasty. The continuation of these quantitative objective methods of assessing coronary circulation is extremely important.—R.L. Frye, M.D.

Percutaneous Transluminal Coronary Angioplasty in 1985–1986 and 1977–1981

National Heart, Lung, and Blood Institute Registry (Univ of Pittsburgh)
N Engl J Med 318:265–270, Feb 4, 1988   4–28

The National Heart, Lung, and Blood Institute collected 3,248 cases of percutaneous transluminal coronary angioplasty that were performed between 1979 and 1981 to evaluate the safety and utility of the procedure. In 1985 the registry reopened to document changes in angioplasty strategy and outcome. 1,802 cases were collected between 1985 and 1986. This study compares the findings in the 2 time periods.

In both groups, only patients undergoing first-time angioplasty without evidence of acute myocardial infarction were included. Vessel disease was classified as single, double, or triple. Angioplasty was considered to be clinically successful if all lesions treated were dilated, and the patient survived in hospital without myocardial infarction or coronary-artery bypass graft surgery.

The patients in the new registry were older and had a significantly higher proportion of multivessel disease, poor left ventricular function, and previous coronary bypass surgery. The later group also had more complex coronary lesions, and more multivessel procedures were performed during angioplasty. Nevertheless, the in-hospital outcome in the new cohort was better. Success rates according to lesion increased from 67% to 88%, whereas overall success rates improved from 61% to 78%. In-hospital mortality and the nonfatal myocardial infarction rates were similar in both groups, being 1% and 4.3%, respectively.

Registry data on immediate effectiveness and short-term risk show improvement in the potential benefit of angioplasty. Follow-up is required to assess long-term efficacy, quality of life, and other relevant factors.

▶ This is an important paper for all those involved with coronary angioplasty. The National Heart, Lung, and Blood Institute Registry has been an important resource for documenting the utilization of angioplasty as well as specific features of outcome following angioplasty. This has also been an important resource for planning the BARI Trial (Bypass Angioplasty Revascularization Investigation), which began randomization August 1, 1988.—R.L. Frye, M.D.

Multiple Coronary Angioplasty: A Model to Discriminate Systemic and Procedural Factors Related to Restenosis
Lambert M, Bonan R, Côté G, Crépeau J, de Guise P, Lespérance J, David P-R, Waters DD (Montreal Heart Inst)
J Am Coll Cardiol 12:310–314, August 1988   4–29

Multivessel coronary angioplasty is now used to treat more patients, but restenosis remains the major limitation of this procedure. Medical approaches to prevention of restenosis after coronary angioplasty have been disappointing, probably because of the multiplicity of recurrence-related factors. Previous studies have shown that the balloon/artery lumen ratio, maximal inflation pressure, and stenosis after angioplasty all influence restenosis. Diabetes mellitus, unstable angina, and hyperlipidemia also appear to influence restenosis. However, the respective importance of these procedural and clinical factors remains unclear. To test the hypothesis that patient-related factors might be more common with restenosis at all sites, and that procedure-related factors might be more common with isolated restenosis, the pattern of restenosis after multiple coronary angioplasty was examined.

The study population consisted of 206 patients who had undergone a first elective coronary angioplasty of at least 2 lesions. Angioplasty was attempted on 2 sites in 148 (72%) patients, 3 sites in 45 (22%) patients, 4 sites in 11 (5%) patients, and 5 sites in only 2 (1%) patients. The procedure was clinically and angiographically successful in 185 (90%) patients. Angiographic follow-up was available for 215 lesions in 119 (64%) of the 185 patients.

Restenosis occurred in 74 (34%) of the 215 lesions. Sixty-three patients had no restenosis, 44 had at least 1 restenosis, and 12 had restenosis at all angioplasty sites. Statistical analysis of the data showed that only percent stenosis before angioplasty, diabetes mellitus, and percent stenosis after angioplasty were predictive of restenosis in the entire study group.

Patients with no restenosis and those with restenosis at all sites did not differ with respect to procedural variables, but those with restenosis at all sites differed with respect to systemic variables, such as diabetes and recent onset angina. In contrast, patients with no restenosis and those with isolated restenosis differed with respect to procedural variables, such as balloon/artery lumen ratio and maximal inflation pressure.

Procedural factors may be more related to isolated restenosis, whereas patient-related factors may be more related to multiple restenosis.

▶ This is an interesting detailed review of a major persisting problem with angioplasty, i.e., restenosis.—R.L. Frye, M.D.

Guidelines for Percutaneous Transluminal Coronary Angioplasty: A Report of the American College of Cardiology/American Heart Association Task Force on Assessment of Diagnostic and Therapeutic Cardiovascular Procedures (Subcommittee on Percutaneous Transluminal Coronary Angioplasty)
Ryan TJ, Faxon DP, Gunnar RM, Kennedy JW, King SB III, Loop FD, Peterson KL, Reeves TJ, Williams DO, Winters WL Jr
Circulation 78:486–502, August 1988   4–30

Indications for coronary angioplasty are based on the clinical profile of each patient in relation to the likelihood of successful dilation, the risk of abrupt vessel closure, and the likelihood of restenosis. Among asymptomatic or only mildly symptomatic patients with single-vessel coronary artery disease, there is general agreement that angioplasty is indicated if a significant lesion suitable for angioplasty subtends a large area of viable myocardium and severe ischemia is present. More symptomatic patients may be candidates for angioplasty if there is myocardial ischemia on medical treatment, or if angina has failed to respond adequately to treatment in the presence of lesions suitable for percutaneous transluminal coronary angioplasty (PTCA).

Patients with multivessel coronary disease who have no or mild symptoms may be candidates for angioplasty if a large area of viable myocardium is at risk, lesions suitable for PTCA are present, and severe ischemia is present during medical treatment. Patients with significant symptoms and multivessel disease may be candidates for PTCA of suitable lesions if myocardial ischemia is present on laboratory testing despite medical treatment.

Absolute contraindications to coronary angioplasty include the lack of a significant obstructing lesion, multivessel disease for which other treatment would be more effective, and significant left main coronary obstruction. Criteria for selecting lesions suitable for PTCA are provided. However, the importance of integrating the entire set of data for the individual patient is emphasized.

▶ This is an extremely important report dealing with the appropriate use of angioplasty after a thrombolytic therapy in the setting of acute myocardial infarction. From these studies and also the results of TIMI-2, immediate angioplasty did not have any clear advantage over deferred elective angioplasty of the infarct-related artery. I do remain concerned regarding the estimates for continuing experience required to maintain expertise in coronary angioplasty. Were I to require coronary angioplasty, I am sure my preference would be for a person who performed considerably more than 1 angioplasty per week.—R.L. Frye, M.D.

Silent Ischemia

Morning Increase in Platelet Aggregability: Association With Assumption of the Upright Posture

Brezinski DA, Tofler GH, Muller JE, Pohjola-Sintonen S, Willich SN, Schafer AI, Czeisler CA, Williams GH (Harvard Univ)
Circulation 78:35–40, July 1988   4–31

Platelet aggregability, like the frequencies of myocardial infarction and sudden cardiac death, increases in the morning. The specific activities associated with the increase in aggregability were studied in 16 normal subjects. Following a control day of delayed arising, subjects awakened, assumed the upright posture, and then ambulated. The subjects, males aged 20–35 years, were nonsmokers and had not taken aspirin during the previous 2 weeks.

Platelet aggregability did not increase on exposure to light and awakening but did rise after assumption of the upright posture. The effect occurred with both adenosine diphosphate and epinephrine. Platelet responsiveness was constant over time on the control day with no activity. Individual responses to being upright varied considerably. Plasma catecholamines also increased after postural change, as did the plasma renin activity and angiotensin II concentration. A small rise in hematocrit occurred with assumption of the upright posture.

Becoming upright in the morning increases platelet aggregability. Epidemiologic studies might elucidate the relations between upright posture and the onset of myocardial infarction and sudden cardiac death.

▶ Although differences in physiologic response to supine versus upright exercise have been well documented, these studies reflect a remarkable similarity of the clinical significance of a drop in blood pressure during supine exercise compared with other studies previously reported by other investigators in patients undergoing stress testing in the upright position. The lack of ST segment shifts and angina at the time of exercise even in patients with critical high-risk anatomy is noteworthy as described by the authors.—R.L. Frye, M.D.

Mental Stress and the Induction of Silent Myocardial Ischemia in Patients With Coronary Artery Disease
Rozanski A, Bairey CN, Krantz DS, Friedman J, Resser KJ, Morell M, Hilton-Chalfen S, Hestrin L, Bietendorf J, Berman DS (Univ of California, Los Angeles; Uniformed Services Univ of the Health Sciences, Bethesda, Md)
N Engl J Med 318:1005–1012, April 21, 1988 4–32

There is recent evidence that asymptomatic transient myocardial ischemia is common in patients with coronary artery disease (CAD). Although it is known that physiologic stimuli can induce transient ischemia in CAD patients, it has not yet been confirmed whether nonspecific mental arousal or emotional stress can also induce the condition. The causal relationship between acute mental stress and transient ischemia was assessed in 39 patients, 35 men and 4 women aged 39–84 years.

Thirty-three of the patients had previously confirmed CAD and 6 had a high pretest probability of CAD based on symptoms and exercise test results. The control group consisted of 11 men and 1 woman aged 28–70 years who had a low probability of CAD. Cardiac function was evaluated during a series of 4 tasks involving mental stress, including arithmetic, the Stroop color-work task, simulated public speaking, and reading. The results were compared with those induced by exercise. Radionuclide ventriculography was used to assess cardiac function.

In 29 of the 39 CAD patients wall-motion abnormalities developed during exercise, and 21 (72%) of the 29 had wall-motion abnormalities during mental stress. In 2 of the 10 CAD patients wall-motion abnormalities did not develop during exercise but did so during mental stress. Two controls also had wall-motion abnormalities, induced by exercise in 1 and by a mental task in the other.

Fourteen patients (36%) had decreases in ejection fraction of more than 5% during 22 mental tasks. Regional wall-motion abnormalities were observed during 19 (86%) of the 22 tasks that were associated with a decline in ejection fraction of more than 5%. Only 6 (23%) of the 23 patients with worsening of wall motion during mental tasks also had electrocardiographic abnormalities, and only 4 (17%) had chest pain. A personally relevant task induced more frequent and greater regional wall-motion abnormalities than did less specific cognitive tasks.

There appears to be a causal association between acute mental stress and silent myocardial transient ischemia in patients with CAD. Although electrocardiography was used in most previously reported studies, radionuclide ventriculography was much more sensitive in detecting mental-stress-induced ischemia.

▶ Additional fascinating data on the effects of emotional stress on silent myocardial ischemia.— R.L. Frye, M.D.

Epidemiology, Health Care Delivery, Primary Prevention

Ischemic Heart Disease Mortality in Hispanics, American Indians, and Non-Hispanic Whites in New Mexico, 1958–1982
Becker TM, Wiggins C, Key CR, Samet JM (Univ of New Mexico)
Circulation 78:302–309, August 1988   4–33

Although the incidence death from ischemic heart disease over the past 25 years has been well documented, it is not clear whether all racial and ethnic groups have been equally affected. Trends in mortality from ischemic heart disease in New Mexico's Hispanic, American Indian, and non-Hispanic white population between 1958 and 1982 were analyzed using data from the New Mexico Bureau of Vital Statistics. Age-adjusted and age-specific ischemic heart disease deaths in each ethnic group during the study period were calculated. Population estimates were based on census figures for each decade.

Age-adjusted mortality for ischemic heart disease for American Indians, Hispanics, and non-Hispanic white men followed nationwide patterns of rising mortality during the 1960s and declining mortality rates since then. All 3 ethnic groups in New Mexico had rates lower than the national average. American Indians had the lowest mortality among the 3 groups; Hispanics had lower rates than non-Hispanic whites.

American Indians and Hispanics in the Southwest are at decreased risk for mortality from ischemic heart disease than are whites in the Southwest or elsewhere in the United States.

▶ This paper documenting striking differences between the age-adjusted mortality for ischemic heart disease among American Indians, Hispanics, and non-Hispanic white men is of great interest. It is another example of the fascinating geographic and racial differences in coronary heart disease mortality, and the basis for these differences is not clear.— R.L. Frye, M.D.

A Prospective Randomized Trial of Outpatient Versus Inpatient Cardiac Catheterization
Block PC, Ockene I, Goldberg RJ, Butterly J, Block EH, Degon C, Beiser A, Colton T (Massachusetts Gen Hosp, Boston; Univ of Massachusetts, Worcester; Lahey Clinic, Burlington, Mass; Boston Univ)
N Engl J Med 319:1251–1255, Nov 10, 1988   4–34

Diagnostic cardiac catheterization including coronary arteriography used to be performed almost exclusively as an inpatient procedure. Recent studies reported that routine cardiac catheterization can be safely performed in stable patients on an outpatient basis. However, these studies were done in single hospital settings and did not involve randomization of patients to inpatient and outpatient settings. To compare the safety and costs of outpatient cardiac catheterizations with those of inpatient procedures, a 24-month randomized clinical trial was performed at 3 participating hospitals.

The study population consisted of 381 patients scheduled for cardiac catheterization, of whom 192 were randomly assigned to an outpatient procedure and 189 were admitted to the hospital the night before the procedure. The mean age of the outpatients was 55.7 years, and of the inpatients, 56.2 years. Only stable patients with clinical diagnoses of coronary artery disease, valvular disease, or congenital heart disease who were considered low-risk cases were included in the study.

The incidence of hematoma and myocardial infarction in the group that had cardiac catheterization on an outpatient basis was slightly greater than that in the inpatient group, but the difference was not statistically significant. For the outpatient group, the relative risk for hematoma was 1.42 and the relative risk for developing myocardial infarction within 1 week of cardiac catheterization was 2.95. None of the patients died or had a stroke. Twenty-three patients (12%) assigned to outpatient catheterization had to be hospitalized after the procedure because of complications associated with the procedure. The catheterization-related savings per outpatient averaged $679, with an average difference in total hospital-related charges of $885. Thus, performing cardiac catheterization on an outpatient basis resulted in substantial financial savings.

Elective cardiac catheterization performed as an outpatient procedure for carefully selected patients is safe and feasible. However, larger randomized trials are still needed to define the complication rate more precisely and to determine whether the financial savings justify the possibly higher complication rate.

▶ This is an important study by Block and colleagues on a controversial topic, i.e., outpatient cardiac catheterization. All accept the feasibility of outpatient cardiac catheterization, but in fact the study documents the concern of many regarding the possibility of a small increase in complication rates associated with outpatient cardiac catheterization. This occurred in spite of a very careful effort on the part of the investigators to select and monitor patients, and as they point out, additional studies are necessary to precisely estimate the complication rates and particularly the impact of the outpatient status on such complications. The investigators are to be commended for an objective scientific approach to try and judge the relative benefits and risks, particularly with the large numbers of cardiac catheterizations being performed in the United States.—R.L. Frye, M.D.

Divergence of the Recent Trends in Coronary Mortality for the Four Major Race-Sex Groups in the United States

Sempos C, Cooper R, Kovar MG, McMillen M (Natl Ctr for Health Statistics, Hyattsville, Md; Cook County Hosp, Chicago)

Am J Public Health 78:1422–1427, November 1988   4–35

Since the mid-1960s, there has been a rapid and consistent decline in mortality from coronary heart disease (CHD) in the United States. However, the rate of decline in CHD mortality has been leveling off since 1976. Previous studies have reported that changes in the prevalence of coronary risk factors among the 4 major race-sex groups of the United States are not the same.

This study was done to determine whether the changes in CHD mortality are the same for each of the 4 largest race-sex groups and whether the decline in CHD mortality has continued at the same annual rate during the 1980s. The age-adjusted and age-specific CHD mortality data for the 4 major race-sex groups were obtained from vital statistics data tabulated for 1968–1985 (Fig 4–8).

The age-adjusted absolute annual rate of decline in CHD mortality during 1968–1975 was virtually identical for white men, black men, and black women, but it was somewhat lower for white women. During 1976–1985, age-adjusted mortality from CHD continued to decline at the same annual rate for white men, but the decline was approximately half as steep for the other 3 race-sex groups.

During 1976–1985, the average annual percentage of change in age-adjusted CHD mortality for black men, black women, and white women also leveled off but it stayed the same for white men. Consequently, in 1985 more than 40,000 persons in these 3 race-sex groups died of CHD that would not have died if CHD rates would have continued to decline as they did during 1968–1975.

The factors that contributed to a continued overall decline in CHD during the past decade may not have equally affected all demographic groups in the United States. For that reason, efforts aimed at primary and secondary prevention of CHD and access to appropriate treatment should be increased for black men, black women, and white women while maintaining the gains already obtained for white men.

▶ This is a fascinating article and raises many questions regarding the distribution of health services and the impact of social status on outcomes related to coronary artery disease. This is indeed a sobering trend and merits careful study and thought by all concerned in the management of patients with cardiovascular disease. Pertinent to this topic is an observation from Sweden demonstrating the effect of socioeconomic status on coronary heart disease mortality, presumably in a system in which access to care should not be a problem (*Br Med J* 297:1497, Dec 10, 1988).—R.L. Frye, M.D.

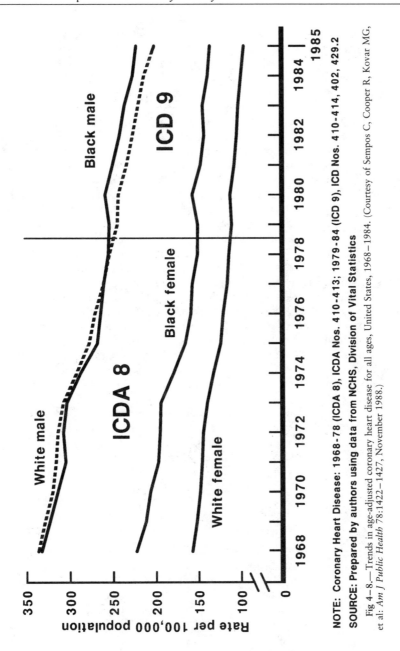

NOTE: Coronary Heart Disease: 1968-78 (ICDA 8), ICDA Nos. 410-413; 1979-84 (ICD 9), ICD Nos. 410-414, 402, 429.2

SOURCE: Prepared by authors using data from NCHS, Division of Vital Statistics

Fig 4–8.— Trends in age-adjusted coronary heart disease for all ages, United States, 1968–1984. (Courtesy of Sempos C, Cooper R, Kovar MG, et al: *Am J Public Health* 78:1422–1427, November 1988.)

Forecasting Coronary Heart Disease Incidence, Mortality, and Cost: The Coronary Heart Disease Policy Model

Weinstein MC, Coxson PG, Williams LW, Pass TM, Stason WB, Goldman L
(Harvard Univ; Brigham and Women's Hosp, Boston)
Am J Public Health 77:1417–1426, November 1987   4–36

Coronary heart disease (CHD) is presently the leading cause of death and lost life expectancy in the United States. Its annual cost in the United States exceeds $80 billion. The decline in CHD mortality during the last 2 decades has been attributed to prevention rather than treatment. To determine which interventions produce the greatest health benefit with regard to future mortality and morbidity from CHD, a computer-simulated model was developed consisting of 3 parts: a demographic-epidemiologic submodel simulating the distribution of coronary risk factors and the conditional incidence of CHD in a demographically evolving population; a "bridge" submodel to determine the outcome of an initial CHD event; and a disease history submodel for simulating subsequent CHD events in persons with a previous CHD event.

Assuming that risk factors would not change after 1980 and that the efficacy of therapies would not drastically improve after 1980, baseline projections showed that the aging of the population, especially of the post–World War II baby-boom generation, would increase CHD prevalence, annual incidence, annual mortality, and annual costs by 40% to 50% by the year 2010 (table). To offset the demographic effects on the absolute incidence of CHD, extraordinary reductions in risk factors would be required.

However, this forecast should be viewed with caution, because major changes could still occur and because baseline values could have been erroneously estimated. The model will be tested for validity by updating it with 1985 data. However, this forecast represents for now the best available projection.

▶ This is a fascinating paper by a distinguished group of investigators who have contributed importantly to our knowledge of cardiovascular disease in many areas. The findings of their current analysis are sobering from the point

Coronary Heart Disease Incidence, Prevalence, Mortality, and Cost Projections

Year	Incidence	Prevalence	Mortality	Cost*
1980	692,117	5,977,405	432,613	$31.9
1985	729,235	6,700,639	486,428	35.3
1990	759,583	7,230,904	540,557	37.8
1995	792,006	7,625,001	567,798	39.9
2000	834,522	7,973,869	596,777	42.0
2005	888,438	8,385,046	608,434	44.4
2010	953,750	8,939,816	632,304	47.4

*Billions of 1980 dollars.
(Courtesy of Weinstein MC, Coxson PG, Williams LW, et al: *Am J Pub Health* 77:1417–1426, November 1987.)

of view of the projections of cardiovascular disease in the aging population that will most likely occur in spite of major efforts at risk factor control and other preventive measures. Those who have forecast an excess of services in the future for patients with cardiovascular disease may well be wrong on the basis of these projections from the model developed by Weinstein and colleagues.— R.L. Frye, M.D.

Helsinki Heart Study: Primary-Prevention Trial With Gemfibrozil in Middle-Aged Men With Dyslipidemia: Safety of Treatment, Changes in Risk Factors, and Incidence of Coronary Heart Disease
Frick MH, Elo O, Haapa K, Heinonen OP, Heinsalmi P, Helo P, Huttunen JK, Kaitaniemi P, Koskinen P, Manninen V, Mäenpää H, Mälkönen M, Mänttäri M, Norola S, Pasternack A, Pikkarainen J, Romo M, Sjöblom T, Nikkilä EA (Univ of Helsinki; Natl Public Health Inst, Helsinki; Univ of Tampere, Finland; Finnish Railways, Posts and Telecommunications; et al)
N Engl J Med 317:1237–1245, Nov 12, 1987   4–37

Gemfibrozil reduces levels of total and low-density lipoprotein (LDL) cholesterol and triglycerides, but also raises high-density lipoprotein (HDL) cholesterol levels in both normal subjects and those with hyperlipidemia. The Helsinki Heart Study was designed to assess the effects of

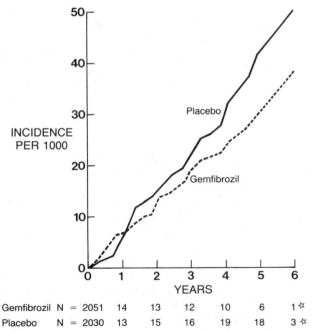

	0	1	2	3	4	5	6
Gemfibrozil N = 2051		14	13	12	10	6	1 ✫
Placebo N = 2030		13	15	16	19	18	3 ✫

Fig 4–9.—Kaplan–Meier cumulative incidence (per 1,000) and annual number of cardiac end points according to treatment group and time. (Courtesy of Frick MH, Elo O, Haapa K, et al: *N Engl J Med* 317:1237–1245, Nov 12, 1987.)

genfibrozil on the incidence of coronary heart disease in a randomized, double-blind, 5-year trial in asymptomatic middle-aged men (40 to 55 years of age) who were at high risk because of primary dyslipidemia (non-HDL cholesterol ≥200 mg/l or 5.2 mmole/L). Of 4,081 men participating, 2,051 received gemfibrozil, 600 mg, and 2,030 received placebo twice daily. Fatal and nonfatal myocardial infarction and cardiac death were the principal end points. Mean follow-up period was 60.4 months.

Gemfibrozil caused a marked increase in HDL cholesterol and persistent reductions in serum levels of total, LDL, and non-LDL cholesterol and triglycerides, whereas the placebo group had only minimal changes in serum lipid levels. The cumulative rate of cardiac end points at 5 years were 27.3 per 1,000 in the gemfibrozil group and 41.4 per 1,000 in the placebo group (Fig 4–9), for an overall reduction of 34.0% in the incidence of coronary heart disease (95% confidence interval, 8.2 to 52.6). The greatest reduction in end-point rates was noted in the group with nonfatal myocardial infarction. The decline in the incidence in the gemfibrozil group became evident in the second year of study and progressively decreased thereafter. Despite a 26% lower mortality from coronary heart disease (19 vs. 4), there were slightly more deaths overall in the gemfibrozil than in the placebo group (45 vs. 42); the difference was not significant. The groups did not differ in the number of cancer or major operations, particularly gallstone operations. Gastrointestinal side effects were reported in both groups.

Modification of lipoprotein profile with gemfibrozil reduces the incidence of coronary heart disease without any adverse side effects. These findings are in accord with those of the World Health Organization's study of clofibrate and the Pimary Lipid Research Clinic's Coronary Primary Prevention Trial of cholestyramine, and furnish additional, conclusive evidence of the role of lipid modification in preventing coronary heart diseaes.

▶ These are further impressive data on the beneficial effects of therapy in patients with "primary dyslipidemia" (non-HDL cholesterol equal to or greater than 200 mg/dl). It is interesting that no impact on total mortality occurred but there was a major reduction in the incidence of coronary heart disease-related events. Focusing aggressive lipid-lowering efforts in patients with clearly defined lipid abnormalities is important, and the efforts of the Cholesterol Education Program hopefully will enhance this effort (Abstract 4–38).—R.L. Frye, M.D.

Report of the National Cholesterol Education Program Expert Panel on Detection, Evaluation, and Treatment of High Blood Cholesterol in Adults
The Expert Panel of the National Cholesterol Education Program (National Heart, Lung, and Blood Inst, Bethesda, Md)
Arch Intern Med 148:36–69, January 1988   4–38

Previous studies have provided conclusive evidence that increased blood cholesterol levels, specifically, increased low-density lipoprotein (LDL) cholesterol levels, are causally related to an increased risk of coronary heart disease (CHD), and that lowering total and LDL cholesterol levels will reduce that risk. This report of an expert panel provides new guidelines for the treatment of hypercholesterolemia in persons aged 20 years and older.

Serum total cholesterol levels should be measured at least once every 5 years in all adults. Total serum cholesterol concentrations are defined as desirable for levels lower than 200 mg/dl, as borderline-high for levels between 200 and 239 mg/dl, and as high for levels of 240 mg/dl and higher. The risk of CHD rises sharply with cholesterol levels of 240 mg/dl and higher, corresponding to the 75th percentile for adult men and women of all ages.

Patients with desirable blood cholesterol levels should be advised to have the test repeated within 5 years and should be given educational materials on risk factors for CHD. Patients with borderline-high cholesterol levels should undergo lipoprotein analysis. Those with low LDL levels should be given dietary information and told to come back for reevaluation after 1 year. However, those who have elevated LDL levels with or without other risk factors such as male sex, hypertension, cigarette smoking, diabetes mellitus, severe obesity, or a personal or family history of CHD should undergo dietary treatment. Patients with high cholesterol levels should undergo lipoprotein analysis and dietary treatment. In those patients, drug treatment should be initiated if LDL cholesterol levels still exceed specified levels after 6 months of dietary treatment.

This report also specifies the LDL cholesterol levels at which dietary therapy should be initiated and details the recommended dietary changes.

▶ All physicians have received from multiple sources a bombardment of information regarding the importance of reducing cholesterol. I retain some skepticism toward the wholesale application of this concept to the population at large. However, the focus on those with clearly elevated levels, particularly those with vascular disease, seems important.—R.L. Frye, M.D.

Transfer of Acutely Ill Cardiac Patients for Definitive Care: Demonstrated Safety in 755 Cases
Rubenstein DG, Treister NW, Kapoor AS, Mahrer PR (Kaiser Permanente Med Ctr, Los Angeles)
JAMA 259:1695–1698, March 18, 1988   4–39

The feasibility and safety of transferring cardiac patients from community hospitals to large, regional cardiac catheterization centers have important implications for the optimal provision of this highly sophisticated medical care. To evaluate the safety of transporting acutely ill cardiac patients for cardiac catheterization, 755 consecutive patients sent by ambulance from community hospitals to a tertiary center during an 18-month period were studied.

Eighty-seven percent of 715 patients with angina pectoris and 79% of 53 patients with congestive heart failure were class III or IV on the New York Heart Association classification. Left ventricular dysfunction (ejection fraction less than 55%) was present in 40%. Forty-three percent of patients required urgent intervention such as coronary artery bypass surgery or percutaneous transluminal coronary angioplasty. Ambulance transfer time averaged 1 hour, and no patient required a physician in attendance on transfer. Majority of the patients were transported solely by paramedic ambulance. Only 1 patient died during transfer, and this patient was transferred with ongoing unevaluated pain outside the prescribed guidelines for transport and against established general medical standards. Except for this death, no other major complications occurred during transport.

Acutely ill cardiac patients can be transferred safely to a large referral center for definitive care. A single tertiary center providing immediate access to catheterization and surgical facilities can service a large population and many community hospitals.

▶ This study from the Kaiser Permanente group in southern California analyzing results of ambulance transfer of seriously ill cardiac patients to a core cardiac catheterization and cardiac surgical center is an important observation. It documents the safety of such an approach with attention to the details of the transfer and careful communication between the responsible physicians involved in the care of the patient. It is clear from this study that patients can be transferred safely, including returning patients to the initial hospital after clarification of cardiac status by invasive studies. This example of a focusing of experience and costs in 1 center for invasive study and therapy may be a model for future practice relationships.— R.L. Frye, M.D.

Other Topics of Special Interest

Aspirin, Heparin, or Both to Treat Acute Unstable Angina

Théroux P, Ouimet H, McCans J, Latour J-G, Joly P, Lévy G, Pelletier E, Juneau M, Stasiak J, deGuise P, Pelletier GB, Rinzler D, Waters DD (Montreal Heart Inst; Davis Jewish Gen Hosp, Montreal)
N Engl J Med 319:1105–1111, Oct 27, 1988   4–40

The efficacy of aspirin was compared with that of heparin and combination treatment in patients with acute unstable angina. Patients were entered into the double-blind, placebo-controlled trial a mean of 8 hours after the last episode of pain. The 479 subjects were randomized to receive 325 mg of aspirin twice daily, 1,000 units of heparin per hour by infusion, combination therapy, or placebos. The population represented 62% of all patients admitted with unstable angina.

Nearly one fourth of placebo recipients had refractory angina. Twelve percent had myocardial infarction, and 1.7% died. Heparin therapy was associated with less frequent refractory angina. Myocardial infarction was significantly reduced with all active treatments, and none of the actively treated patients died. Combined treatment was no more effective than heparin alone and caused serious bleeding more frequently. One fifth of heparin-treated patients bled, most often at catheterization puncture sites. Most serious bleeding also was related to catheterization.

This study and others suggest that heparin be given to all patients admitted with unstable angina if not contraindicated. Long-term aspirin treatment should be instituted before heparin is withdrawn. The role of fibrinolysis in unstable angina remains controversial.

▶ This carefully performed study by Theroux and colleagues provides extremely important information for the practicing cardiologist. The use of heparin has been suspected for many years to be beneficial in patients with unstable angina based on prior studies by Paul Wood and A. M. Telford in particular. This controlled clinical trial establishes the benefit of both aspirin and heparin independently and, within the limits of the study, no advantage to combined aspirin and heparin therapy. The results of trials of fibrinolytic therapy are awaited.— R.L. Frye, M.D.

Guidelines for the Interpretation of the Exercise Radionuclide Ventriculogram for Diagnosing Coronary Artery Disease
Clements IP, Gibbons RJ, Mankin HT, Zinsmeister AR, Brown ML (Mayo Clinic, Mayo Found, Rochester, Minn)
Am J Cardiol 60:1265–1268, Dec 1, 1987   4–41

This study measured the extent of suspected coronary artery disease (CAD) in 622 patients who underwent supine bicycle exercise radionuclide ventriculography and coronary arteriography. Two variables can be measured accurately and may offer valuable aid in predicting the severity of CAD: heart rate (HR) × blood pressure (BP) product and left ventricular ejection fraction (LVEF). These variables were recorded with the patients at rest and at maximal exercise.

Narrowing of the coronary arteries was viewed separately by arteriography and classified by extent in 4 categories: 0-, 1-, 2-, or 3-vessel CAD. It was found that at maximal exertion the HR × BP product and LVEF decreased as the extent of CAD increased. A high probability (70%) of 0- or 1-vessel CAD occurred when HR × BP product was ≥21,000 beats × mm Hg/minute and LVEF was 0.55 or greater at maximal exercise. Patients not achieving these levels had a high degree (72%) of 3- or 4-vessel CAD, whereas only 8% had no significant CAD.

This relatively simple analysis may predict the extent of CAD and determine the need for further testing. The study noted other possible factors that could bear upon results: the patient's ability to exercise and the effect of β-adrenergic blocking therapy. In addition, the patient group upon which the study was based had a high incidence of CAD.

▶ A carefully performed study of the use of radionuclide ventriculography in the diagnosis of CAD. The authors emphasize the nature of the study group and appropriately caution the application of these conclusions without these characteristics fully in mind.—R.L. Frye, M.D.

Prognostic Value and Limitations of Exercise Radionuclide Angiography in Medically Treated Coronary Artery Disease
Taliercio CP, Clements IP, Zinsmeister AR, Gibbons RJ (Mayo Clinic, Mayo Found, Rochester, Minn)
Mayo Clin Proc 63:573–582, June 1988   4–42

Left ventricular function and degree of major coronary artery obstruction are the 2 main factors that influence long-term survival in medically treated coronary artery disease. Several studies have found that exercise thallium 201 scintigraphy yields prognostic information in patients with coronary artery disease. Whether exercise radionuclide angiography provides additional prognostic information to that already identified by resting left ventricular function and coronary anatomy was studied in patients with medically treated coronary artery disease.

The study population consisted of 424 medically treated patients who had coronary arteriography within 3 months of exercise radionuclide angiography. All patients were followed up from 1–55 months; the median duration of follow-up was 21.7 months.

During follow-up, 16 of the 424 medically treated patients died of cardiac disease, 16 had nonfatal myocardial infarction, and 1 survived an out-of-hospital cardiac arrest. Thirty-seven patients required coronary bypass operation, and 2 patients underwent percutaneous transluminal coronary angioplasty.

Univariate analysis showed that multiple variables were associated with future cardiac events, including the number of diseased vessels, peak rest and exercise ejection fraction, history of previous myocardial infarction, and age. Multivariate Cox regression analysis showed that only 3 variables were independently associated with cardiac events at follow-up, namely, the number of diseased vessels, resting ejection fraction, and age.

In this selected sample of patients, exercise radionuclide testing does not provide additional prognostic information when a patient's age, resting ejection fraction, and the number of diseased coronary vessels are known.

▶ Another example of the importance of carefully considering the pretest characteristics of patients before engaging in additional testing of any kind.—R.L. Frye, M.D.

Potentiation of the Hemodynamic Effects of Acutely Administered Nitroglycerin by Methionine
Levy WS, Katz RJ, Ruffalo RL, Leiboff RH, Wasserman AG (George Washington Univ)
Circulation 78:640–645, September 1988   4–43

The means by which nitroglycerin achieves its hemodynamic effect is not fully understood, but the drug may bring about vasodilation through interaction with sulfhydryl groups. Methionine, an amino acid known to increase the availability of sulfhydryl, was tested for its ability to potentiate the vasodilatory effects of nitroglycerin.

Fifteen patients undergoing cardiac catheterization for suspected coronary artery disease were entered into a randomized study. Methionine-treated and control patients were similar with respect to age, sex, cardiac index, baseline mean arterial pressure (MAP), and baseline pulmonary capillary wedge pressure (PCW). Distribution of vessel involvement also was similar.

After receiving nitroglycerin to reduce MAP by 10% and PCW by 30%, patients were given either 5 gm of methionine or 5% dextrose. At baseline and after infusion of methionine or dextrose, MAP and PCW values were equal in the 2 groups. But with a second infusion of nitroglycerin, patients who received methionine required significantly less nitroglycerin to achieve the desired MAP and PCW levels. No such effect followed infusion of dextrose.

Methionine does potentiate the hemodynamic effects of nitroglycerin, the most notable response being from patients whose nitroglycerin needs were greatest. Although methionine alone has no hemodynamic effect, it appears to be a sulfhydryl donor.

▶ More data on the important topic of nitroglycerin tolerance. Sulfhydryl groups have been clearly identified as essential for the action of nitrates, and we are now seeing several approaches to replenish sulfhydryl groups, including methionine as in this study or in prior reports with *N*-acetyl-ı-cysteine.—R.L. Frye, M.D.

Clinical Implications of Internal Mammary Artery Bypass Grafts: The Coronary Artery Surgery Study Experience
Cameron A, Davis KB, Green GE, Myers WO, Pettinger M (St Luke's–Roosevelt Hosp Ctr, New York; Columbia Univ; Univ of Washington, Seattle)
Circulation 77:815–819, April 1988   4–44

Reports from single institutions have shown that the internal mammary artery bypass graft yields superior results to the saphenous vein graft. The Coronary Artery Surgery Study Registry presents an evaluation of the clinical follow-up of patients who had internal mammary artery bypass grafting at many institutions.

Data were analyzed from a group of 950 patients who had single internal mammary artery bypass graft with or without additional vein grafts and from a group of 6,027 patients who had vein grafts alone. Operative mortality was similar with all procedures and among all subgroups. Internal mammary artery grafting improved survival rates even in hospitals where the procedure was used infrequently. Survival was improved among patients with both normal and impaired ventricular function, both men and women, younger patients and those aged older than 65, and those with or without critical stenosis of the left main coronary artery. Internal mammary artery bypass grafting was an independent predictor of survival; use of this graft reduced the risk of dying by a factor of 0.64.

The internal mammary artery bypass graft is the vessel of choice for coronary artery disease. Its use should be considered for any subgroup of patients.

▶ This is another important observation on the advantage of internal mammary artery bypass grafts versus venous conduits. These data are of particular importance when one considers the observations of Loop and colleagues (*N Engl J Med* 314:1–6, 1986) and the late mortality being observed in the earlier randomized trials of coronary bypass surgery with saphenous vein bypass grafts (VA Coronary Bypass Surgery Cooperative Study: *N Engl J Med* 311:1333, 1984; and Varnowskus and the European Coronary Surgery Study group: *N Engl J Med* 319:332–337, 1988). The late mortality being reported in these studies emphasizes the need for stress testing or careful regular surveillance of patients or both after coronary artery bypass grafting.—R.L. Frye, M.D.

Randomised Trial of Prophylactic Daily Aspirin in British Male Doctors
Peto R, Gray R, Collins R, Wheatley K, Hennekens C, Jamrozik K, Warlow C, Hafner B, Thompson E, Norton S, Gilliland J, Doll R (Univ of Oxford, England)
Br Med J 296:313–316, Jan 30, 1988   4–45

By the late 1970s, randomized trials had shown that daily aspirin could definitely reduce the risk of reinfarction after recovery from a myocardial infarction. Thus, it seemed likely that prophylactic daily aspirin would also prevent some thrombotic events among apparently healthy people without an overt history of cardiac or cerebrovascular disease. A 6-year randomized trial was done among 5,139 apparently healthy male physicians to assess whether 500 mg of aspirin daily would reduce the incidence of and mortality from stroke, myocardial infarction, or other vascular conditions.

In 1978, an invitation to participate in the study was sent to all male physicians living in the United Kingdom and born during this century who had responded to a previous questionnaire about smoking habits. Almost half of the 5,139 physicians recruited were aged younger than 60 years. Treatment lasted from 1978 to 1984. Two thirds of the physicians were randomly assigned to aspirin treatment, and one third was assigned to avoid aspirin and aspirin products unless some specific indication for aspirin developed. All participants completed a questionnaire about their health and aspirin use every 6 months.

Although total mortality was 10% lower in the treated group than in the control group, this difference did not reach statistical significance and mainly involved diseases other than stroke or myocardial infarction. Also, there was no significant difference in the incidence of nonfatal myocardial infarction or stroke; disabling strokes were somewhat more common among those taking aspirin. However, the lower confidence limit for the effect of aspirin on nonfatal stroke or myocardial infarction was a substantial 25% reduction. Migraine and certain types of musculoskeletal pain were reported significantly less often in the treated group. There was no apparent decrease in the incidence of cataract in the group taking aspirin.

Although the prophylactic use of daily aspirin for secondary prevention of disease among patients at high risk for thrombotic disease has been shown to reduce the incidence of nonfatal vascular events and vascular death, this study, which was not blinded or placebo-controlled, found no definite indication that daily aspirin reduces such risk in a population of apparently healthy men with no history of cardiac or cerebrovascular disease.

▶ The lack of a clear benefit of aspirin in primary prevention of cardiovascular mortality contrasts with a widely publicized article in the *New England Journal of Medicine* (318:262–264, 1988). This discussion by Peto and colleagues of the different results in these 2 trials provides an excellent perspective for the interpretation of the conclusions on this important topic.—R.L. Frye, M.D.

Comparative Effects of Therapy With Captopril and Digoxin in Patients With Mild to Moderate Heart Failure
The Captopril-Digoxin Multicenter Research Group (Queen's Univ; VA Med Ctr, Fresno, Calif; Washington Adventist Hosp, Takoma Park, Md; Henry Ford Hosp, Detroit; New York Hosp/Cornell Med Ctr, New York; et al)
JAMA 259:539–544, Jan 22–29, 1988   4–46

Digitalis is the traditional therapy for heart failure, but some authors advocate the use of digoxin. When added to a regimen of a diuretic and digoxin, captopril, a converting-enzyme inhibitor, increases exercise performance and improves functional heart class in patients with severe heart failure. In this trial, the authors compare the effects of treatment with captopril or digoxin with those of placebo in patients with mild to moderate heart failure.

Patients maintained on diuretic therapy were randomized to groups receiving either captopril, digoxin, or placebo. Two exercise tests were performed 24 hours apart before randomization. Exercise tolerance testing was performed at 1, 3, and 6 months follow-up; the radionuclide ejection was obtained at 6 months; and ambulatory electrocardiograms were obtained at 1 and 6 months.

Captopril therapy resulted in significantly improved exercise time and improved functional class when compared with placebo, but digoxin treatment did not. Digoxin therapy increased ejection fraction compared with captopril treatment and placebo. There was a 45% decrease in the number of ventricular premature beats in the captopril group, whereas premature beats increased by 4% in the digoxin group. These patients had more than 10 premature beats per hour. Transitory hypotension occurred more frequently in patients receiving captopril. Patients receiving placebo had significantly more treatment failures, hospitalizations, and increased need for diuretic therapy than did those receiving either active treatment.

Captopril is an effective alternative to digoxin in treatment of patients with mild to moderate heart failure who are maintained on diuretic therapy. Captopril is significantly more effective than placebo in these patients.

▶ The advantages of captopril in treatment of patients with mild congestive heart failure are clearly documented in this fine multicenter trial. The lack of correlation between improvement in left ventricular ejection fraction and exercise tolerance is interesting but not clearly explained. This study provides further support for the concept that digoxin is appropriate only for a specific subset of patients with congestive heart failure.— R.L. Frye, M.D.

Prospective Evaluation of a Discriminant Function for Prediction of Recurrent Symptomatic Ventricular Tachycardia or Ventricular Fibrillation in Coronary Artery Disease Patients Receiving Amiodarone and Having Inducible Ventricular Tachycardia at Electrophysiologic Study
Klein LS, Fineberg N, Heger JJ, Miles WM, Kammerling JM, Chang M-S, Zipes DP, Prystowsky EN (Indiana Univ; Roudebush VA Med Ctr, Indianapolis)
Am J Cardiol 61:1024–1030, May 1988   4–47

Induction of ventricular tachycardia (VT) during electrophysiologic testing in patients on long-term amiodarone therapy for recurrent sustained ventricular tachyarrhythmias is a poor predictor of outcome. Because factors other than VT induction might be useful in determining outcome for patients taking amiodarone, a discriminant function was developed from retrospective data that appeared to identify high-risk patients. The validity of this discriminant function as a predictor of outcome was prospectively assessed in 60 patients, 53 men and 7 women with a mean age of 61 years, with documented coronary artery disease and a history of ventricular fibrillation or sustained VT.

All patients were taking amiodarone, with or without other antiarrhythmic agents, because sustained VT or ventricular fibrillation was inducible during electrophysiologic study. During a mean follow-up period of 16 months, 47 patients remained asymptomatic and 13 had symptomatic recurrent arrhythmia, resulting in sudden death in 8 patients and sustained VT in 5 patients. Ventricular effective refractory period, corrected QT interval, and presence of a repetitive ventricular response, all of which were parameters of the proposed discriminant function, failed to distinguish symptomatic from asymptomatic patients.

Of 16 patients who had an easier mode of VT induction (MOI), 9 (56%) had a recurrence, and 7 (44%) remained asymptomatic. Because 9 (69%) of the 13 patients who experienced a recurrence of symptomatic arrhythmia were in the easier MOI group, easier MOI during electrophysiologic testing was considered highly predictive of outcome. In contrast, only 4 (9%) of the 44 patients who had either the same or a harder MOI had a recurrence of symptomatic arrhythmia.

Determination of discriminant function various electrophysiologic variables in patients who are on amiodarone maintenance therapy has no prognostic significance for recurrence of symptomatic arrhythmic events, but easier induction of VT during electrophysiologic testing on amiodarone is highly predictive of adverse outcome.

▶ The clinical value of electrophysiologic testing is finding increased support as documented in this study by Rozanski and colleagues as well as other settings as recently reported by Wilbur et al. (*N Engl J Med* 218:19–24, 1988).—R.L. Frye, M.D.

Double-Blind Placebo-Controlled Comparison of Digoxin and Xamoterol in Chronic Heart Failure
German and Austrian Xamoterol Study Group
Lancet 1:489–493, March 5, 1988   4–48

Xamoterol is a partial β_1-adrenoceptor agonist that stabilizes the cardiac response to sympathetic drive. It increases ventricular contractility and improves diastolic function. A study compared xamoterol and digoxin in a double-blind design with 433 patients having mild to moderate heart failure. Patients were randomized to receive 200 mg of xamoterol twice daily, 0.125 mg of digoxin twice daily, or placebo. The median patient age was 62 years.

Three hundred subjects completed the trial and had valid exercise tests. Xamoterol significantly increased bicycle work and decreased breathlessness and tiredness during daily activities. Digoxin, in contrast, was not significantly better than placebo except on the Likert symptom scale. Exercise performance was better with xamoterol than with digoxin. Adverse effects leading to withdrawal were least frequent in the xamoterol-treated subjects.

Digoxin has, at best, a modest effect in patients with mild to moderate heart failure who are in sinus rhythm. It does not substantially improve exercise capacity. Xamoterol is a promising alternative to digoxin for use in these patients.

▶ Additional data documenting the mild benefit of digoxin in patients with normal sinus rhythm and congestive heart failure. The quest for additional inotropic drugs continues without overwhelming success.—R.L. Frye, M.D.

Coronary Heart Disease in the Medical Research Council Trial of Treatment of Mild Hypertension
Medical Research Council Working Party on Mild Hypertension
Br Heart J 59:364–378, March 1988   4–49

In the Medical Research Council trial of treatment for mild hypertension, 17,354 persons with diastolic pressures of 90 to 109 mm Hg at screening were randomized to receive bendrofluazide, propranolol, or placebo tablets and were followed up for as long as 5.5 years. The total observation time was 85,572 patient-years.

Drug treatment did not affect the rate of myocardial infarction or sudden coronary death. Event rates were much higher among smokers than among nonsmokers on placebo. Among nonsmoking men, those on propranolol had a lower event rate than placebo recipients. Bendrofluazide had no apparent effect on rates of events. The occurrence of ECG changes of silent infarction was not influenced by treatment with either active drug.

These findings, by themselves, are not very helpful in selecting drug treatment for mild hypertension. The effects of treatment on the rate of stroke are an important consideration as well.

▶ These data on treatment of patients with mild hypertension are of great interest. Although no major difference in sudden death was noted in the diuretic treatment group as compared with placebo, a trend similar to that in the Multiple Risk Factor Intervention Trial remains a concern.—R.L. Frye, M.D.

5 Cardiac Surgery

Introduction

Although the pace of scientific progress continues, as evidenced by the publications included in the cardiac surgical section, there are, at every administrative level affecting cardiac surgery, major concerns that are already causing changes in the quality and distribution of care. Financial restraints upon hospitals, mediated through the diagnosis-related groups system, have made it economically unwise to operate upon patients whose degree of illness threatens to require a longer than average stay in a hospital or intensive care unit. Pressures are being brought to bear on surgeons in private and academic institutions to avoid operating on patients who are likely to require more than average expenditure. The description "high risk" in our specialty is gradually coming to describe institutional fiscal risk as much as individual physical risk.

At the same time we observe the average cost of a cardiac surgical operation to be rising at an ever increasing rate. Although part of this cost is driven by higher fees and salaries for personnel involved in the direct care process, a substantial amount of the rising cost is related to unnecessarily complex monitoring, superfluous laboratory studies, and excessively expensive medications and treatments. Much of the expense could be reduced significantly by simplification of management, which, unfortunately, is impossible in the present atmosphere of regulation and litigation.

Rising hopes of an aging population have placed a great burden on those who care for patients having the most common final fatal illness in our society. There are certainly limits to what can and should be done to ameliorate suffering and prolong life of patients afflicted with arteriosclerotic diseases. It is sad, however, to see these limits influenced more by burdensome regulation and administrative entanglement than by the parameters of science.

The place of coronary bypass surgery has become well established in the management of coronary heart disease. Myocardial ischemia, whether symptomatic or silent, is best treated with revascularization. Whether revascularization is achieved via angioplasty or coronary bypass surgery seems to make little difference. Although angioplasty is simpler and carries far less morbidity, the mortality risk for any given class of patient appears to be somewhat higher than the risk for open operation. The probability of long-term relief of ischemia also seems to favor open surgery. Cost of angioplasty in most institutions is approximately one third to one half that for coronary bypass surgery. Because of the distressingly great need for a second angioplasty procedure within the first year after the initial manipulation, the total cost for successful angioplasty is surprisingly close to that of open surgery. Still, the morbidity difference justifies the application of angioplasty for those patients in whom a satisfactory result is reasonably likely.

Late follow-up in the excellent studies from the European Coronary Artery Surgery Study and the Coronary Artery Surgery Study (CASS) from the United States continues to show significant benefit from revascularization surgery. One question that has not been answered is whether or in what cases a second or third coronary bypass operation is justifiable.

In valve replacement surgery there has been a rekindling of interest in the use of human allograft aortic valves, spurred by the work of Mr. Mark O'Brien and associates in Brisbane as is described in this section. Early results strongly suggest that the cryopreservation process preserves viability and offers a substantial advantage in durability over allografts preserved by older techniques. We are just entering the critical period for these grafts (between 10 and 15 years after operation). Time will soon tell.

There has been no significant progress in totally implantable artificial hearts toward the solution of major problems of a power source, thromboembolic potential, or durability. The approaching era of fiscal restraint may well have a strong influence to reduce the rate of advance of artificial heart technology despite the favorable results reported with extracorporeal left and right ventricular assist devices, both as a "bridge to transplantation" and as definitive treatment for otherwise irreversible myocardial failure.

In congenital heart disease, we are seeing the development of worldwide cooperative efforts for development and evaluation of reparative operations. Cardiac transplantation in infants and neonates is a promising introduction.

For the future, the increasing burden of administrative and regulatory restriction threatens to throttle scientific progress in cardiac surgery. Whether it is possible to devise a means for continuing the widespread application of cardiac surgical treatment to an increasing aged population is uncertain. To do so will require major deviations from the directions of practice so far established.

Coronary Surgery

Time to First New Myocardial Infarction in Patients With Severe Angina and Three-Vessel Disease Comparing Medical and Early Surgical Therapy: A CASS Registry Study of Survival
Myers WO, Schaff HV, Fisher LD, Gersh BJ, Mock MB, Holmes DR, Gillispie S, Ryan TJ, Kaiser GC, CASS investigators (Marshfield Clinic, Marshfield, Wis; Mayo Clinic, Mayo Found, Rochester, Minn; Univ of Washington; Boston Univ; St Louis Univ; et al)
J Thorac Cardiovasc Surg 95:382–389, March 1988   5–1

Proof that coronary artery bypass surgery reduces the risk of subsequent myocardial infarction has been lacking. In this study, which includes the observational data base of the Coronary Artery Surgery Study (CASS), the incidence of first myocardial infarction in patients with severe angina pectoris and 3-vessel coronary artery disease is analyzed. Time to first myocardial infarction is compared in the 679 medically treated patients and 1,921 surgically treated patients in the study. Patients were stratified by left ventricular wall motion score and number of proximal coronary artery stenoses.

At 6 years 86% of surgical and 73% of medical patients remained free of new myocardial infarction. In subgroups of patients with at least 1 proximal 70% or greater stenosis in the left anterior descending artery and moderate to severe impairment of left ventricular function and in patients with 2 proximal coronary artery narrowings, the advantage of surgical treatment was even greater. On multivariate analysis early operation was the strongest predictor of freedom from new myocardial infarction.

These data strongly support the suggestion that direct coronary artery revascularization decreases the incidence of subsequent myocardial infarction in patients with severe angina pectoris and 3-vessel coronary artery disease.

Medical Versus Early Surgical Therapy in Patients With Triple-Vessel Disease and Mild Angina Pectoris: A CASS Registry Study of Survival
Myers WO, Gersh BJ, Fisher LD, Mock MB, Holmes DR, Schaff HV, Gillispie S, Ryan TJ, Kaiser GC, other CASS investigators (Coronary Artery Surgery Study)
Ann Thorac Surg 44:471–486, November 1987   5–2

The results of coronary bypass surgery were examined in 856 nonrandomized patients in the Coronary Artery Surgery Study (CASS) registry

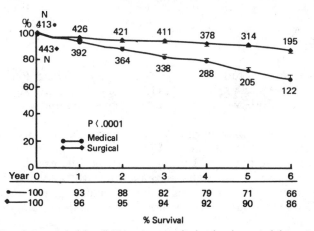

Fig 5–1.—Cumulative survival for all 856 patients (medical and early surgical therapy). Unadjusted plots. (Log rank statistic = 47.899.) All patients had 3-vessel disease and Canadian Cardiovascular Society Class I or II angina pectoris. (Courtesy of Myers WO, Gersh BJ, Fisher LD, et al: *Ann Thorac Surg* 44:471–486, November 1987.)

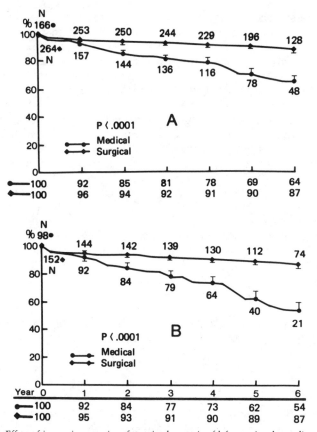

Fig 5–2.—Effect of increasing severity of proximal stenosis of left anterior descending coronary artery (LAD). All patients with LAD lesion are included, including those with 1, 2, and 3 proximal stenoses in 3-vessel disease. **A,** all patients with 70% or greater LAD stenosis. (Log rank statistic = 31.626.) **B,** same analysis limited to patients with 90% or greater LAD stenosis. (Log rank statistic = 30.682.) (Courtesy of Myers WO, Gersh BJ, Fisher LD, et al: *Ann Thorac Surg* 44:471–486, November 1987.)

having mild angina and at least 70% coronary stenosis. Early operation was done in 443 cases, whereas 413 patients were managed medically and sometimes underwent late operation. The annual rate of delayed surgery was 3.3%.

The probabilities of surviving 6 years were 66% for medically treated patients and 86% for the surgical group (Fig 5–1). Surgery was done more often as the number of proximal stenoses increased. Early surgery enhanced survival at 6 years in patients with 1 or more proximal stenoses, in contrast with those having no significant proximal coronary stenosis. Surgery promoted survival in patients with left anterior descending proximal stenosis of 70% or greater (Fig 5–2), but not if this was an isolated lesion. The incidence of surgery declined with increasingly severe left ventricular dysfunction. Early surgery had an independent prognostic effect if mild or moderate left ventricular impairment was present, but not with severely impaired function. On Cox analysis, early surgery was an independent predictor of survival.

Benefit from bypass surgery is most evident in patients with mild angina who have at least 1 proximal coronary segment with 70% stenosis in the dominant right coronary artery and mild to moderate left ventricular dysfunction. These findings complement those in the randomized CASS. Triple-vessel coronary disease is not a homogeneous category of ischemic heart disease.

Comparison of Coronary Artery Bypass Surgery and Medical Therapy in Patients With Exercise-Induced Silent Myocardial Ischemia: A Report From the Coronary Artery Surgery Study (CASS) Registry
Weiner DA, Ryan TJ, McCabe CH, Chaitman BR, Sheffield LT, Ng G, Fisher LD, Tristini FE, CASS Investigators
J Am Coll Cardiol 12:595–599, September 1988   5–3

Exercise-induced myocardial ischemia adversely affects survival, even if unaccompanied by angina. Surgical and medical approaches to silent myocardial ischemia were compared in 692 patients from the Coronary Artery Surgery Study (CASS) who had cardiac catheterization and exercise testing within a 1-month period and were followed up annually for at least 5 years. A total of 424 patients received medical treatment; 268 were operated on.

Benefit from surgery was most evident in patients having 3-vessel disease or abnormal left ventricular function. Among 75 patients with 3-vessel disease and left ventricular dysfunction, 7-year survival was 90% for those operated on and 37% for those managed medically. There was no significant difference in survival between medical and surgical patients having single-vessel or 2-vessel coronary artery disease.

Among patients with silent exercise-induced myocardial ischemia, the risk is greatest for those having marked coronary disease and abnormal left ventricular function. Coronary bypass surgery improves survival most in this group of patients.

▶ These 3 publications from the CASS, gathered from separate publications, offer cooperative evidence very useful in understanding the essence of surgical management for coronary heart disease. It is neither angina pectoris nor extent of obstructive anatomy that dictates the need for surgical intervention. Whether in patients with severe, mild, or absent angina pectoris, it is the potential for reversal of ischemia in viable myocardium that justifies myocardial revascularization surgery. The continuing follow-up and analysis of patients included in the CASS registry continue to refine our appreciation for the role of revascularization. As a general rule, active ischemia, whether symptomatic or not, is a hazard to patients with coronary obstructive disease. The larger the area of ischemia, the greater the hazard, whether the hazard be measured as death or survivable myocardial infarction.—J.J. Collins, Jr., M.D.

Twelve-Year Follow-up of Survival in the Randomized European Coronary Surgery Study

Varnauskas E, European Coronary Surgery Study Group (Sahlgrenska Hosp, Göteborg, Sweden; Edinburgh; Glasgow, Scotland; Helsinki; London; et al)
N Engl J Med 319:332–337, Aug 11, 1988   5–4

Survival was analyzed among 767 male participants in the European Coronary Surgery Study who had good left ventricular function. Data were collected 10–12 years after the men were randomly assigned to early coronary bypass surgery or medical management. The men were aged younger than 65 years and had mild or moderate angina of at least 3 months' duration at the time of entry into the study.

Cumulative survival was significantly better in patients having early surgery than in those treated medically throughout the study period. The difference was less marked after 5 years, but surgery still appeared preferable after 12 years of follow-up. Bypass surgery was done in 136 patients assigned to medical treatment, whereas 23 "surgical" patients were not operated on. Surgical benefit was greater in older patients and those with ischemia or past infarction on the resting ECG or a very ischemic response to exercise testing, but the effect was not significant.

Improved survival after surgery for coronary artery disease is less evident after 5 years of follow-up. Surgery may hold the most promise for patients with good left ventricular function whose symptoms are medically controlled but who at an increased risk of dying prematurely. In any case revascularization should not be delayed if risk factors or refractory angina or both are present despite adequate medical treatment.

▶ Late follow-up of patients included in the European Coronary Surgery Study provides further excellent data. The data clearly show that myocardial revascularization surgery exerts a substantial and significant favorable effect on survival that is most marked during the first 5 to 10 years after coronary bypass surgery, although it is still detectable even 12 years after operation. Survival curves for medically managed and surgically managed patients must eventually coincide (presuming one or the other group does not achieve immortality), and that this coincidence lies at more than 12 years after operation illustrates a major impact of surgery independent of symptom relief or any other criterion of effectiveness.—J.J. Collins, Jr., M.D.

Serum Lp(a) Level as Predictor of Vein Graft Stenosis After Coronary Artery Bypass Surgery in Patients

Hoff HF, Beck GJ, Skibinski CI, Jürgens G, O'Neil J, Kramer J, Lytle B (Cleveland Clinic Found; Univ of Graz, Austria)
Circulation 77:1238–1244, June 1988   5–5

Arterial stenosis has been related to levels of serum Lp(a), a lipoprotein fraction chemically similar to low-density lipoprotein. A cross-sectional study of the relationship between serum Lp(a) and narrowing of saphenous vein grafts was done with 167 symptomatic patients who had coronary bypass surgery. Cardiac catheterization was done as late as 14 years after bypass surgery.

The serum Lp(a) was significantly associated with the degree of saphenous vein graft stenosis. The mean level in patients with stenosis was nearly double that in patients without graft stenosis. Graft stenosis could not be related to past myocardial infarction, hypertension, diabetes, obesity, or smoking. Serum cholesterol was not markedly higher in patients with steneosis. The mean Lp(a), in contrast, increased with the degree of vein graft stenosis, and more than 90% of patients with levels as high as 32 mg/dl had graft stenosis.

Serum Lp(a) is independently associated with stenosis of saphenous vein grafts after coronary bypass surgery. Foam cells may develop in both native vessels and grafts when tissue macrophages take up low-density lipoprotein or Lp(a) that has complexes to tissue proteoglycans. Whether measures that alter the serum Lp(a) can decrease the risk of vein graft stenosis remains to be seen.

▶ The identification of a specific lipoprotein fraction associated with progressive arteriosclerotic narrowing of saphenous vein grafts provides the basis for another study of risk factor intervention. Fortunately, for experimental purposes the progression of vein graft stenosis is sufficiently rapid that a carefully controlled study should demonstrate within 5 to 10 years whether reduction of serum Lp(a) may exert a beneficial effect on vein graft patency. Results are eagerly anticipated.—J.J. Collins, Jr., M.D.

Treatment of Moderate Mitral Regurgitation and Coronary Disease by Coronary Bypass Alone

Arcidi JM Jr, Hebeler RF, Craver JM, Jones EL, Hatcher CR Jr, Guyton RA (Emory Univ)
J Thorac Cardiovasc Surg 95:951–959, June 1988   5–6

There is concern that, in patients with moderate mitral regurgitation, bypass surgery alone might be followed by functional deterioration. Fifty-eight patients with a mean age of 63 who had coronary bypass alone were compared with 20 patients with moderate mitral regurgitation who had combined valve replacement and coronary bypass surgery. Symptoms were more advanced in the latter patients. In a majority of the patients having bypass surgery only, mitral regurgitation was due to coronary disease. Two thirds of patients had some hypokinesis or akinesis.

Hospital mortality was 3.4% after bypass surgery alone. Two thirds of surviving patients were in functional class I or II after a mean follow-up of 4.5 years, and 84% of patients returned to work. No reoperations were necessary. Mortality was 25% after combined surgery. The 5-year survival was 31%, compared with 77% after bypass surgery alone.

These findings suggest a more conservative approach to mitral valve surgery in patients with moderate ischemic valve regurgitation. If symptoms of congestive failure are controlled preoperatively, functional deterioration after bypass surgery alone is rare. In addition, survival is better than after combined bypass surgery and valve replacement.

▶ This interesting retrospective study does not adequately defend a "more conservative approach" to mitral valve replacement in my opinion. It does, however, demonstrate that not all patients with "moderate" mitral regurgitation require mitral valve replacement for a satisfactory postoperative result after myocardial revascularization. The data suggest that patients in this study selected for mitral valve replacement may actually have had more severe mitral regurgitation (by symptoms) than those selected for revascularization alone. There seems little question that the presence of mitral regurgitation is a significant risk factor for diminished survival after coronary bypass. Addition of mitral valve replacement in a widespread fashion may not correct this adverse affect.—J.J. Collins, Jr., M.D.

Angina Pectoris Treated by Ventricular Plication
Gray HH, Paneth M, Gibson DG (Brompton Hosp, London)
Br Heart J 60:83–86, July 1988   5–7

Anginal pain can occur when regional abnormalities of diastolic wall motion interfere with coronary blood flow. A patient with normal coronary arteries and abnormal left ventricular wall motion underwent left ventricular plication.

Man, 59, had a 3-year history of exertional chest pain and dyspnea, and myocardial infarction was diagnosed. After several more years of disabling chest pain without ECG or enzyme abnormalities, normal coronary arteries were confirmed and left ventricular apical plication was carried out. Only very occasional episodes of left chest pain occurred during the next 5 years. Exercise tolerance improved, as did ventricular wall motion. Coronary angiography was repeatedly normal, despite frequent episodes of chest pain of presumably ischemic origin. The ventriculographic abnormalities resembled those found in patients having obstructive coronary artery disease. The patient improved markedly after ventricular plication. The rate-pressure product on exercise testing increased 80%.

It is hard to understand how a primary disturbance of coronary vasomotion is totally suppressed by localized surgery. Abnormal timing of wall motion may be a cause of angina in these cases. Many current angiographic methods take no account of asynchrony.

▶ This study of the management of angina pectoris in a patient with normal coronary arteries documents an interesting and novel approach. Whether the observed result is directly related to the surgical procedure is impossible to establish. If there is a fine balance between efficiency of myocardial contraction, localized ischemia, and angina pectoris in patients suffering the anginal syndrome without evidence of coronary obstruction, an approach such as that described by Gray and associates may not be unreasonable. Further experience is eagerly awaited.—J.J. Collins, Jr., M.D.

The Use of Autologous Pericardium for Ventricular Aneurysm Closure
Fiore AC, McKeown PP, Misbach GA, Allen MD, Ivey TD (St Louis Univ; Univ of Washington, Seattle)
Ann Thorac Surg 45:570–571, May 1988   5–8

Closure of a ventriculotomy after resection of an aneurysm may require Teflon felt strips, but any artificial tissue may serve as a site of infection. A technique was developed using autologous pericardium for ventriculotomy and aneurysm closure.

Technique.— Strips of pericardium are prepared by dissecting away fat tissue and the pleura. Heavy interrupted braided sutures are then placed in mattress fashion to incorporate the pericardium on the outer edges of the ventriculotomy. A reinforcing layer is added, using running 1-0 polypropylene sutures. The suture is run in 1 oblique direction and back in a different one in a crisscross pattern. Excess pericardium is trimmed after the ventriculotomy is closed.

The use of autologous tissue rather than Teflon felt lowers the risk of chronic infection at the repair site. This method has been used in about 20 patients, with no suture line hemorrhage or late infection. Pericardium is easy to use, readily available, and pliable enough to close the interstices. It also is strong enough to buttress the ventriculotomy sutures.

▶ Declining interest in the use of prosthetic materials for buttressing cardiac sutures has led to employment of a variety of pledget materials. There can be little argument that autologous tissue should be best. The authors' experience with pericardium for reinforcement of ventriculotomy sutures suggests that this technique may be as efficacious as the use of prosthetic felt with the advantage or avoidance of foreign materials.—J.J. Collins, Jr., M.D.

Left Thoracotomy for Reoperative Coronary Bypass
Burlingame MW, Bonchek LI, Vazales BE (Lancaster Gen Hosp, Lancaster, Penn)
J Thorac Cardiovasc Surg 95:508–510, March 1988   5–9

A left thoracotomy approach to circumflex coronary revascularization has advantages over sternotomy where there are patent internal mammary artery grafts, or patent vein grafts that might be disrupted at sternotomy. It also is useful under circumstances of past mitral valve replacement, poor coverage of the sternum, past mediastinitis or sternal wound complication, or a planned left pulmonary operation. The heart is rapidly and safely exposed during an emergency. Minimal vein length is required for grafting with this approach.

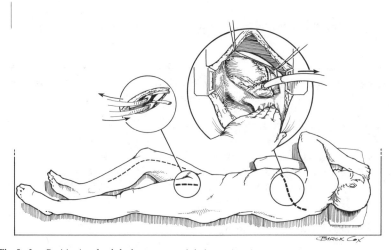

Fig 5–3.—Positioning for left thoracotomy, left femoral and atrial cannulation, and harvesting of vein from right leg. (Courtesy of Burlingame MW, Bonchek LI, Vazales BE: *J Thorac Cardiovasc Surg* 95:508–510, March 1988.)

The right femoral vessels are catheterized because the left femoral vessels are used for bypass cannulation (Fig 5–3). A posterolateral thoracotomy is made through the fourth interspace or the bed of the fifth rib. A double-lumen endotracheal tube is useful. The pericardial incision is posterior to and parallel with the phrenic nerve. No aortic cross-clamp is used during incision of the circumflex coronary artery. Anastomoses are easily made even in the beating heart (Fig 5–4). Grafts should follow an arcuate rather than a straight course to the aorta if kinking is to be avoided.

The left thoracotomy is advantageous in selected patients requiring cir-

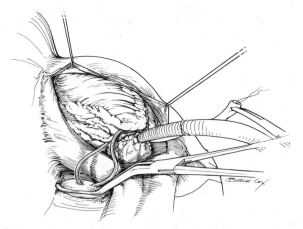

Fig 5–4.—Configuration of descending thoracic aorta to circumflex marginal coronary artery grafts. (Courtesy of Burlingame MW, Bonchek LI, Vazales BE: *J Thorac Cardiovasc Surg* 95:508–510, March 1988.)

cumflex coronary revascularization. Nevertheless, there is no access to the right ventricle or right atrium. Access to the left anterior descending artery is poor, although the proximal part of the vessel may be grafted by this approach. The ascending aorta is relatively inaccessible.

▶ The utilization of a left thoracotomy approach for coronary bypass surgery provides a technically easier access to the lateral and posterior aspects of the left ventricle. It may be remembered, however, that any limitation of exposure in coronary bypass surgery (as in other surgical operations) comes with a substantial price tag. In particular, it is important that there not be inaccessible ischemia in such patients. The authors rightly emphasize the several clinical considerations in selecting patients for left thoracotomy reoperation coronary surgery. It is a useful procedure for the surgeon's armamentarium for occasional use.—J.J. Collins, Jr., M.D.

Results of Coronary Artery Endarterectomy and Reconstruction
Brenowitz JB, Kayser KL, Johnson WD (Milwaukee Heart Surgery Associates)
J Thorac Cardiovasc Surg 95:1–10, January 1988   5–10

Of 5,005 patients having coronary bypass surgery from 1978 to 1986, 25% required 1 coronary artery endarterectomy and 25% required multiple endarterectomies. About 10% of patients required resection of a ventricular aneurysm. Triple-vessel endarterectomy and reconstruction were carried out in 144 patients.

Of all risk factor groups, patients having conventional grafts only (group A) had the lowest hospital mortality, whereas those requiring multiple endarterectomies (group C) had the highest mortality (table). Patients with multiple endarterectomies had more frequent perioperative myocardial infarction than the others. Endarterectomy did not influence early patency rates of grafts to the left anterior descending, circumflex or right coronary arteries. Late patency rates also differed little depending on whether endarterectomy was done. Comparable clinical results were obtained in all surgical groups at 5-year follow-up.

Endarterectomy did not significantly alter early or late graft patency rates in this series. Patients requiring multiple endarterectomies have increased mortality. The number of risk factors also affects survival. Marked left ventricular dysfunction is an important predictor of late mortality after coronary bypass surgery. Relief of angina is not importantly influenced by whether endarterectomy is carried out.

▶ This extensive series of patients undergoing coronary endarterectomy emphasizes the increased hazard attendant upon operations for patients with such severe coronary obstructive disease that extensive endarterectomy is a necessity. Endarterectomy itself is a surgical tour de force that may result in substantial benefit for some patients. It is, however, more difficult technically and less certain in long-term benefit and should not be performed by inexperienced or impatient operators. One may wonder whether there is perhaps a place for the

Thirty-Day Mortality for Entire Series: 308 Deaths/5,005 Patients (6.2%)

No. of risk factors	Group A		Group B		Group C		p Value
	No.	%	No.	%	No.	%	
0	6/1134	0.5	8/471	1.7	32/594	5.4	<0.001
1	31/908	3.4	27/514	5.3	45/455	9.9	<0.001
≥2	62/462	13.4	44/270	16.3	53/197	26.9	<0.001
Total	99/2504	4.0	79/1255	6.3	130/1246	10.4	

(Courtesy of Brenowitz JB, Kayser KL, Johnson WD: J Thorac Cardiovasc Surg 95:1–10, January 1988.)

return of gas endarterectomy in occasional patients. This procedure, once extolled as easy and effective, has now fallen into nearly total disuse. Perhaps better patency may be achieved using antiplatelet agents with or without anticoagulants.—J.J. Collins, Jr., M.D.

Early and Late Results in Patients With Carotid Disease Undergoing Myocardial Revascularization
Schultz RD, Sterpetti AV, Feldhaus RJ (Creighton Univ, Omaha)
Ann Thorac Surg 45:603–609, June 1988   5–11

In a series of 1,360 patients having coronary bypass graft surgery during 1975–1985, 62 with symptomatic coronary insufficiency underwent carotid endarterectomy before or at the time of coronary bypass surgery. Ninety-seven other patients with asymptomatic carotid bruits did not have endarterectomy. Fifty of the 60 patients who underwent noninvasive studies had hemodynamically significant carotid stenosis. Eighty matched patients without carotid disease and 200 unmatched patients also were evaluated. The median follow-up was 41 months.

Operative mortality among patients with proved carotid disease exceeded that among randomly selected patients without carotid disease but was similar to that of the matched group. Late neurologic deficit was most frequent among patients with carotid disease who did not undergo endarterectomy. In matched groups of patients, carotid artery disease did not significantly reduce survival.

Carotid artery disease, if asymptomatic, does not increase the risk of perioperative stroke when coronary revascularization is carried out, but the risk of late neurologic deficit is increased. Carotid disease is a sign of severe associated atherosclerosis. Patients with symptomatic carotid disease appear to benefit from carotid endarterectomy.

Stroke Following Coronary-Artery Bypass Surgery: A Case-Control Estimate of the Risk From Carotid Bruits
Reed GL III, Singer DE, Picard EH, DeSanctis RW (Harvard Univ)
N Engl J Med 319:1246–1250, Nov 10, 1988   5–12

Stroke after coronary bypass surgery often is disabling, but the causes of most such strokes are unknown. A case-control study was done to ascertain the relation of carotid bruits to postoperative stroke. Fifty-four patients having postoperative stroke or transient ischemic attacks were matched with controls who also were operated on during 1970–1984.

Carotid bruit was noted preoperatively in 13 stroke patients and 4 controls; the risk factor was 3.9. This risk remained after multiple regression analysis. Histories of stroke or transient ischemic attacks or of congestive heart failure also were associated with an increased risk, as was mitral regurgitation (table). Less prominent risk factors were postoperative atrial fibrillation, a pump time exceeding 2 hours, and past myocardial infarction. More than half the strokes occurred within 48 hours after surgery.

Carotid bruit is associated with an increased risk of stroke after coronary bypass surgery. The advisability of prophylactic carotid endarterec-

Risk Factors for Postoperative Stroke or Transient Ischemic Attack*

RISK FACTOR	CONTROLS (N = 54)	CASES (N = 54)	ODDS RATIO	95% CI
Significant				
Carotid bruits†	4	13	3.9	1.2–12.8
History of stroke or TIA	3	14	6.0	1.6–22.1
History of heart failure	4	16	5.3	1.6–17.0
Mitral regurgitation	5	16	4.3‡	1.4–12.9
Postoperative atrial fibrillation	15	29	3.0	1.4–6.7
Bypass-pump time >120 min	9	19	2.7	1.1–6.7
Previous myocardial infarction	26	37	2.3	1.1–5.1
Not significant				
Age >60	22	31	2.0	0.9–4.3
Year of surgery				
1970–1974	4	8	2.0	0.5–7.3
1975–1979	17	13	0.8	0.3–1.8
1980–1984	33	33	1.0§	—

*CI, confidence interval; TIA, transient ischemic attack.
†Preoperative data on 1 control was missing.
‡Data are missing for 2 controls and 3 cases.
§This is reference category.
(Courtesy of Reed GL III, Singer DE, Picard EH, et al: *N Engl J Med* 319:1246–1250, Nov 10, 1988.)

tomy remains an individual question, but the significance of carotid bruit must be recognized when coronary artery surgery is planned.

▶ Arteriosclerosis is fundamentally a systemic disease. For reasons that have never been well established, some persons have a principal manifestation of vascular obstructive disease in one or another organ system more severely or earlier than, or to the exclusion of, other systems. In the particular problem of carotid artery obstruction there continues controversy as to whether serial or simultaneous carotid and coronary artery operations or some other management program constitutes adequate treatment. These publications (Abstracts 5–11 and 5–12) illustrate the clinical and statistical difficulties of separating patients on the basis of measurable severity of obstruction and symptoms into groups of treatment preference. At present, it appears that simultaneous carotid endarterectomy and coronary revascularization should be reserved for those patients with symptomatic disease in both locations.—J.J. Collins, Jr., M.D.

Valvular Surgery

Long-term Results of Mitral Valve Reconstruction With Carpentier Techniques in 148 Patients With Mitral Insufficiency
Galloway AC, Colvin SB, Baumann FG, Esposito R, Vohra R, Harty S, Freedberg R, Kronzon I, Spencer FC (New York Univ)
Circulation 78(Suppl I):I-97–I-105, September 1988   5–13

Few long-term follow-up studies of the Carpentier approach to mitral insufficiency are available. The outcomes of Carpentier reconstruction were reviewed for 148 patients with mitral valve disease, most often degenerative or rheumatic in origin. Both anuloplasty with a Carpentier ring and mural leaflet resection were done in a majority of cases, but a wide range of other techniques was utilized. Surgery was done under moderate systemic hypothermia and cold blood potassium cardioplegia.

Operative mortality was 5.4% overall and was 1.2% for isolated mitral reconstruction. Freedom from cardiac death at 5 years was 90%, as was the rate of freedom from mitral valve replacement. More than 90% of patients were free of significant regurgitation at follow-up echocardiography. Ninety-five percent of patients were free of thromboembolism after 5 years without long-term warfarin therapy. The same proportion of survivors improved to New York Heart Association class I or II at follow-up. One patient had endocarditis secondary to postoperative sternal wound infection; 2 others had late endocarditis from intravenous drug abuse.

In the Carpentier approach, each pathologic defect in the valve is corrected separately. Late durability is more impressive for patients with degenerative disease than those with rheumatic disease. Even in the latter group, however, durability is comparable to that achieved with current valve prostheses.

▶ The excellent results reported by Galloway and associates using a variety of techniques for mitral valve repair are typical of what has been reported from several centers. There are still some patients who require mitral valve replacement, and the judgment necessary to differentiate between those valves that should be repaired and those that must be replaced has become perhaps more difficult.—J.J. Collins, Jr., M.D.

Left Ventricular Outflow Obstruction After Mitral Valve Repair (Carpentier's Technique): Proposed Mechanisms of Disease

Mihaileanu S, Marino JP, Chauvaud S, Perier P, Forman J, Vissoat J, Julien J, Dreyfus G, Abastado P, Carpentier A (Broussais Hosp, Paris)
Circulation 78 (Suppl I):I-78–I-84, September 1988   5–14

A review of 307 mitral valve repairs done in 1985–1986 using Carpentier's approach yielded 14 cases of left ventricular outflow tract obstruction (4.5%). The diagnosis was based on an ejection murmur and anterior motion of the mitral valve in systole. All patients had pure, severe, chronic mitral insufficiency. Angiography showed no significant mitral regurgitation postoperatively.

All 14 patients had posterior mitral prolapse, and 10 had anterior leaflet prolapse as well. Eleven patients had billowing leaflets, and 13 had ruptured posterior-leaflet chordae. Significant distention of the mitral anulus was a consistent finding. Obstruction did not occur where both leaflets had restricted motion. It also did not occur when the posterior leaflet had restricted motion, even if anterior leaflet prolapse was present.

Modifications after mitral ring placement can lead to significant anterior displacement of the posterior mitral leaflet and narrowing of the mitroaortic angle. Enhanced mobility and excessive leaflet surface then can partially block left ventricular outflow during systole. The obstruction results from a perpendicular position of the leaflets relative to ejectional flow.

Long-term Follow-Up of Patients With Left Ventricular Outflow Tract Obstruction After Carpentier Ring Mitral Valvuloplasty
Schiavone WA, Cosgrove DM, Lever HM, Stewart WJ, Salcedo EE (Cleveland Clinic Found)
Circulation 78 (Suppl I):I-60–I-65, September 1988   5–15

Dynamic left ventricular outflow tract obstruction can occur after Carpentier ring mitral valvuloplasty in patients with myxomatous valve degeneration. Of 200 such patients operated on since 1984, 12 (6%) had left ventricular outflow tract obstruction. Five patients exhibited obstruction during intraoperative echocardiography just after repair. Four of them underwent mitral replacement, and 1 had the Carpentier ring removed. The other 7 patients were followed up for a mean of 27 months.

Left ventricular outflow tract obstruction was characterized by systolic anterior motion of the mitral valve on echocardiography. The outflow tract gradient, as measured by Doppler echocardiography or by catheter, paralleled the severity of systolic anterior valve motion. Valve motion was less marked after amyl nitrite at late follow-up but was not abolished. No patient had left ventricular hypertrophy or asymmetric septal hypertrophy. All 7 patients followed up improved to New York Heart Association functional class I or II and maintained their improvement at late follow-up.

A mitral anular ring reduces the circumference of the dilated anulus in patients with myxomatous valve degeneration and regurgitation but does not allow normal mitral anular contraction. A ring having a structure reflecting the saddle shape of the anulus, with greater flexion across the line of the commissures, might allow posterior contraction of the anulus and facilitate anteroposterior compression in systole. As a result the outflow tract would be less narrowed.

▶ This potentially serious complication of mitral valvuloplasty was seen in 6% of patients in the Cleveland Clinic series (Abstract 5–15) and 4.5% in the series from Broussais Hospital in Paris (Abstract 5–14). The utilization of a rigid ring may be disadvantageous when compared with the flexible ring of Duran. Surgeons and cardiologists should be aware of this potential problem in patients having Carpentier ring anuloplasty of the mitral valve.—J.J. Collins, Jr., M.D.

Restoration of Left Ventricular Systolic Performance After Reattachment of the Mitral Chordae Tendineae: The Importance of Valvular-Ventricular Interaction
Sarris GE, Cahill PD, Hansen DE, Derby GC, Miller DC (Stanford Univ)
J Thorac Cardiovasc Surg 95:969–979, June 1988   5–16

Preservation of the chordae tendineae reportedly improves the outcome of mitral valve replacement, but it is not certain that baseline ventricular performance is returned by restoring anular-papillary continuity. An in situ isovolumic swine heart preparation was used to determine the effects of detaching all mitral chordae and then reattaching them. The slope of the peak isovolumic left ventricular pressure-volume relation and its volume intercept were determined as coronary perfusion pressure remained constant.

The slope decreased 29% after chordal detachment and returned to baseline after reattachment. The volume intercept did not change significantly at any stage. The findings suggest that the acute decline in left ventricular contractility consequent to interruption of anular-ventricular continuity can be reversed by chordal reattachment.

If these findings can be validated in the dilated human left ventricle, attempts to preserve the mitral chordae during valve replacement would be expected to optimize postoperative left ventricular function.

▶ In this well-designed study the significance of intact chordae tendineae is established beyond reasonable doubt. Where possible, maintenance of the chordae tendinae in reparative or even replacement operations involving the mitral valve probably is mechanically advantageous. In patients with severe scarring secondary to rheumatic heart disease it may well be that loss of the chordae tendineae is a less serious disadvantage than in patients with more normal subvalvular architecture.—J.J. Collins, Jr., M.D.

Aortic Valve Selection in the Elderly Patient
Borkon AM, Soule LM, Baughman KL, Baumgartner WA, Gardner TJ, Watkins L, Gott VL, Hall KA, Reitz BA (Johns Hopkins Hosp, Baltimore)
Ann Thorac Surg 46:270–277, September 1988   5–17

The importance of valve selection was examined in 141 patients aged older than 70 years who had isolated aortic valve replacement from 1970 to 1985. Sixty-eight patients received mechanical valves, and 73, bioprostheses. The most frequently used mechanical prosthesis was the Björk-Shiley valve, and the most common bioprosthesis was the Carpentier-Edwards valve. Patient follow-up averaged 4.3 years.

Hospital mortality was 18% for patients given mechanical valves and 19% for those with bioprostheses. The respective 5-year survival rates were 61% and 67%. No patient had structural valve failure or required reoperation. Anticoagulant-related bleeding was more frequent in mechanical valve recipients but did not cause death or permanent disability. Rates of freedom from all valve-related complications at 5 years were similar in the 2 groups (Fig 5–5). Thromboembolic episodes were comparably frequent. Two patients in each group had prosthetic valve endocarditis.

Use of the bioprosthesis for aortic valve replacement is less likely to cause valve-related complications, and warfarin is infrequently needed. A

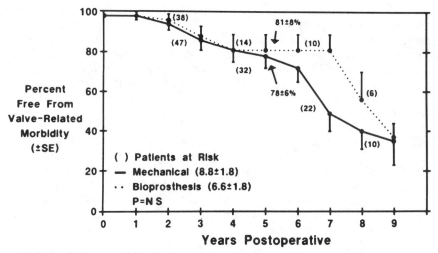

Fig 5–5.—Patient survival free from any valve-related complication. *SE,* standard error; *NS,* not significant. (Courtesy of Borkon AM, Soule LM, Baughman KL, et al: *Ann Thorac Surg* 46:270–277, September 1988.)

bioprosthesis therefore is favored for patients older than age 70 years. Structural degeneration of the bioprosthesis is limited.

▶ Although no significant disadvantage for the Carpentier-Edwards valve was found during the 5 years of follow-up in these aortic valve recipients, it is of interest that there also was found to be no significant advantage. One would have thought that, over 5 years, anticoagulation in the majority of patients would yield a significant hazard for the prosthetic valve group. If these patients are followed up between 5 and 10 years later it seems likely that a disadvantage for the Carpentier-Edwards valve group will emerge. The conclusion that porcine bioprostheses are the favored valve for patients older than 70 years is arguable.—J.J. Collins, Jr., M.D.

Balloon Closure of a Surgical Aorto-Atrial Communication
Hayward R, Kendall B, Treasure T (Middlesex Hosp, London)
Br Heart J 60:358–360, October 1988   5–18

An older woman with retrosternal pain that resulted in collapse had an extensive DeBakey type I dissection of the proximal aorta, complicated by persistent bleeding from surgical suture lines and via the false lumen. Hemorrhage was controlled by closing the aortic adventitia about the repaired aorta and creating an anastomosis between the subadventitial space and the right atrial appendage. However the aortoatrial shunt led to a marked low output state, which was corrected by percutaneously closing the fistula with a detachable balloon. Axial tomography a year afterward showed the balloon in place, although the para-aortic space persisted and communicated with the aorta.

The balloon did not totally obstruct the aortoatrial shunt at first, but later the latex surface led to thrombus formation and more complete closure. Siting of the balloon is critical because of the risk of embolism in an aortic dissection. This risk was accepted in the present case because of the adverse effects of the persistent fistula.

▶ Persistence of an aortoatrial communication following the Cabrol (1) modification of the Bentall operation would seem to be a nearly certain result when there is severe bleeding into the para-aortic lumen. That such an occurrence is apparently unusual seems surprising.—J.J. Collins, Jr., M.D.

Reference

1. Cabrol C, Gandjbakhc I, Pavie A: Surgical treatment of ascending aortic pathology. *J Cardiac Surg* 3:167–180, September 1988.

A Comparison of Aortic Valve Replacement With Viable Cryopreserved and Fresh Allograft Valves, With a Note on Chromosomal Studies
O'Brien MF, Stafford EG, Gardner MAH, Pohlner PG, McGiffin DC (Prince Charles Hosp, Brisbane, Australia)
J Thorac Cardiovasc Surg 94:812–823, December 1987   5–19

In a series of 316 aortic valve replacements in 1969–1986 the use of 124 fresh allografts stored at 4 C was compared with the use of 192 viable allografts cryopreserved in liquid nitrogen at −196 C. Patients who were given cryopreserved valves were older but less often had heart failure. More of them had degenerative aortic valve disease and more underwent concomitant coronary artery bypass grafting.

Hospital mortality was 6%. Long-term survival did not differ significantly in the 2 groups. Reoperation was necessary more often in patients who were given fresh valves. All 23 patients who had reoperation for allograft valve degeneration had received fresh valves. Thromboembolism occurred similarly frequently in the 2 groups.

Allograft valve endocarditis occurred 12 times in 230 primary isolated aortic valve replacements. Chromosomal study of a valve in place for 9 years showed that only donor cells had persisted in the leaflet tissue.

Superior results are obtained with the cryopreserved aortic valve allograft, presumably because of persistent cell viability and resultant durability. Further work is needed in valve banking to obtain maximum viability of the allograft aortic valve.

▶ The excellent results obtained by Mr. O'Brien and his associates using cryopreserved aortic allografts are most encouraging. The interval between 10 and 15 years after implantation is particularly critical in these valves. Degenerative changes may occur rather rapidly, and further follow-up at 15 years will prove or disprove the contention that viable cryopreserved valves are distinctly advantageous over valves previously implanted using alternative techniques for preservation.—J.J. Collins, Jr., M.D.

Reparative Approach for Right-Sided Endocarditis: Operative Considerations and Results of Valvuloplasty

Yee ES, Ullyot DJ (Univ of California, San Francisco)
J Thorac Cardiovasc Surg 96:133–140, July 1988   5–20

Twelve patients with medically refractory right-sided endocarditis were treated in a 5-year period with reconstructive or reparative surgery. Six were intravenous drug users, 2 had central catheters and 4 had malformations. All but 2 patients were in New York Heart Association class III or IV before operation.

Two patients with a large patulous anterior leaflet and a localized defect had débridement and pericardial patch reconstruction. Four patients with more extensive leaflet involvement had quadrant excision and simplified valvuloplasty. Three patients required more extensive reconstruction with removal of vegetations on adjacent leaflets and provision of a generous pericardial bridge between the leaflets. Additional localized anuloplasty sometimes was required to minimize tricuspid regurgitation. One patient needed an anuloplasty ring.

One patient died in hospital after a missed lesion embolized. Heart failure and renal insufficiency improved after operation. Only 2 patients had moderate tricuspid regurgitation, which did not preclude clinical improvement. All patients were clinically improved after a mean follow-up of 25 months. One patient who continued to abuse drugs and had recurrent infective endocarditis died.

Even patients with multiple leaflet involvement and anular invasion can benefit from simple reconstruction. Morbidity from a 2-stage procedure is avoided. Deeper levels of infection make adjunctive measures and pericardial or anular structural support necessary.

▶ Surgical treatment of tricuspid endocarditis is a challenging problem. The results of Yee and Ullyot suggest that a single operation with preservation of tricuspid valve function is a realistic possibility for many if not most such patients.—J.J. Collins, Jr., M.D.

Marfan's Syndrome: Combined Composite Valve Graft Replacement of the Aortic Root and Transaortic Mitral Valve Replacement

Crawford ES, Coselli JS (Baylor College of Medicine)
Ann Thorac Surg 45:296–302, March 1988   5–21

Aortic root dilation and mitral valve prolapse are important factors in death from Marfan's syndrome. Both lesions are progressive and eventually will occur in a very large proportion of patients. Six patients underwent a combined operation of valve graft replacement of the aortic root and transaortic mitral valve replacement. In the last 2 patients the aortic root was not completely excised. St Jude Medical composite valve grafts and valves were employed.

All 6 patients survived the operation and, when discharged, had normal sinus rhythm. Warfarin therapy was administered. The valves functioned normally at discharge, and all suture lines were intact. On follow-up for 1–12 months after surgery, all patients had resumed normal activities and remained in sinus rhythm. No thromboembolic events or bleeding have occurred.

This combined operative approach appears effective in young patients with Marfan's syndrome who are free of associated noncardiovascular disease. Mitral valve surgery is best done before irreversible left ventricular changes develop.

▶ Transaortic mitral valve replacement is a novel approach. The large size of the ascending aorta in Marfan's syndrome may allow this ingenious technique.—J.J. Collins, Jr., M.D.

Intermediate-Term Fate of Cryopreserved Allograft and Xenograft Valved Conduits

Kirklin JW, Blackstone EH, Maehara T, Pacifico AD, Kirklin JK, Pollock S, Stewart RW (Univ of Alabama in Birmingham)
Ann Thorac Surg 44:598–606, December 1987   5–22

The outcome of surgery was studied in 128 patients given cryopreserved allograft aortic valves and ascending aortas between a ventricle and the pulmonary artery. Another 19 patients received fresh valves and aortas. Seventy-eight earlier patients received irradiated allograft aortic valves or glutaraldehyde-preserved xenograft porcine valves incorporated into Dacron conduits.

The actuarial freedom from reoperation for obstruction was 94% at 3.5 years in the patients given allograft valved conduits. Five of 24 recatheterized patients had gradients of greater than 40 mm Hg across the conduit. All but 1% of the patients given xenograft or irradiated allograft valved conduits were free of reoperation at 3.5 years, but the rates at 5, 10, and 15 years were 95%, 59%, and 11%, respectively.

A few patients with allograft valved conduits can be expected to have postoperative gradients across the ventricle-pulmonary artery path. The pericardial valved conduit described by Horiuchi et al. deserves further study.

▶ In this rather large group of patients the time elapsed since operation for the patients having cryopreserved allografts is not long enough to demonstrate superiority. More time is necessary.—J.J. Collins, Jr., M.D.

Reconstructive Techniques for Rheumatic Aortic Valve Disease

Duran CG (Hosp Nacional "Marques de Valdecilla," Santander, Spain)
J Cardiac Surg 3:23–28, March 1988   5–23

Aortic Valvuloplasty

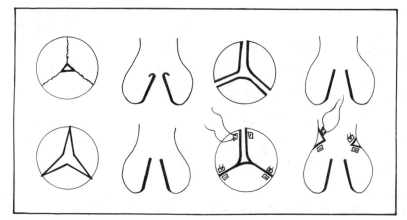

Fig 5–6.—Diagrams of 4 techniques used. Top line depicts pathology encountered; bottom line shows technique applied. From left to right: (1) commissurotomy, (2) cusp free edge unfolding, (3) commissural area anuloplasty, and (4) supra-aortic crest enlargement. (Courtesy of Duran CG: *J Cardiac Surg* 3:23–28, March 1988.)

Reconstructive techniques are available that sometimes make it possible to avoid aortic valve replacement in patients with rheumatic disease. Typically, the cusps are thickened, especially at the free edges, and there are varying degrees of commissural fusion. A central triangular rigid orifice is responsible for the regurgitation.

Satisfactory reconstruction usually requires multiple specific techniques (Fig 5–6). Each commissure is divided, regardless of the extent of fusion. Free edge unfolding is intended to increase the height of the free leaflet edge, not its length. Anuloplasty involves selectively reducing the 3 commissural areas. The supravalvular crest is enhanced by placing "U" stitches with pledgets on each sinus ridge to increase their protrusion into the aortic lumen.

Fifty patients with rheumatic valve disease had aortic valve repair from July 1974 through January 1986. Average age of the 11 male and 39 female patients was 39.5 years. All had simultaneous mitral valve surgery, and 17 had surgery on the tricuspid valve. Free edge unfolding and commissural plication were done in 39 cases; commissurotomies were done in 35; and crest enhancement was performed in 8. There were 3 hospital deaths (6%) and 3 late deaths at reoperation.

Twelve patients in all required reoperation because of failure of the mitral repair or bioprosthesis. Four patients had significant residual aortic regurgitation. Mean follow-up was 7.7 years.

The results in this group of patients show that reconstruction of the rheumatic aortic valve is feasible and yields reproducible, long-lasting results. The problems of aortic valve replacement are thereby avoided in many cases.

▶ Aortic valvuloplasty for acquired diseases of the aortic valve has had little trial by most surgeons for the past 25 years. Débridement of calcium has generally resulted in relatively short asymptomatic intervals. Conceivably with more thorough and widespread débridement better results may be obtained. The concept of surgical repair of aortic insufficiency is interesting but requires considerably longer follow-up before aortic anuloplasty for insufficiency is widely accepted.—J.J. Collins, Jr., M.D.

Long-term Performance of 555 Aortic Homografts in the Aortic Position
Matsuki O, Robles A, Gibbs S, Bodnar E, Ross DN (Natl Heart Hosp and Cardiothoracic Inst, London)
Ann Thorac Surg 46:187–191, August 1988   5–24

Because of renewed interest in aortic valve replacement with an aortic homograft, the authors reviewed the long-term results of 555 homograft operations for isolated aortic valve replacement, done from 1964 to 1986. Followup totaled 2,931 patient-years. In 5.8% of cases a previous valve had failed. Concomitant surgery was done in one third of patients.

Late mortality was 14.6% (Fig 5–7). Forty-four deaths were valve-related, the most frequent cause being primary tissue failure. This was by far the most common complication (Fig 5–8). At 20 years, 83% of patients were free of infective endocarditis. Suspected thromboembolism was reported in only 1 case. Freedom from all valve-related complications was 46% at 10 years and 9% at 20 years. Patients with aortic regurgitation had poorer outcomes than those with aortic stenosis.

The aortic homograft has advantages such as a perfect design and freedom from thromboembolic complications. The long-term results are satisfactory. Sudden and unexplained deaths are far less frequent than when mechanical prostheses are used. Primary tissue failure, the chief cause of morbidity, does not progress rapidly. The median life expectancy exceeds 20 years after valve placement. Improvements in harvesting,

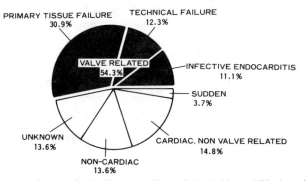

Fig 5–7.—Causes of 81 late deaths. (Courtesy of Matsuki O, Robles A, Gibbs S, et al: *Ann Thorac Surg* 46:187–191, August 1988.)

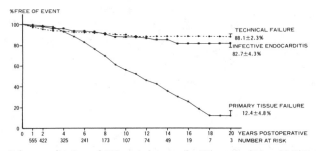

Fig 5–8.—Valve complications of 555 aortic homografts. (Courtesy of Matsuki O, Robles A, Gibbs S, et al: *Ann Thorac Surg* 46:187–191, August 1988.)

sterilizing, and storing homograft valves will provide even better results in the future.

▶ This large series of homograft aortic valve replacements from the National Heart Hospital provides important documentation of clinical results up to 20 years after operation. Although the incidence of thromboembolic complications is admirably low, the probability of significant valve failure (presumably requiring reoperation) at 10 years is 50% and becomes higher than 90% at 20 years after surgery. Therefore, the patient survival probability late after operation necessarily includes the hazard of reoperation. If one compares these results using homografts from an institution with great interest and experience in that operation, there does not appear to be a great advantage over results reported with porcine bioprostheses.—J.J. Collins, Jr., M.D.

Sutureless Aortic Valve Replacement for Periannular Abscess Due to Active Bacterial Endocarditis: A New Translocation Technique

Endo M, Nishida H, Imamura E, Koyanagi H (Tokyo Women's Med College)
Ann Thorac Surg 45:568–569, May 1988   5–25

If perianular abscess is managed by simple valve replacement, leakage may ensue. A new method of translocation was developed that yields favorable results. A composite prosthesis is prepared by direct suture of the ring prosthesis, which is separated from an intraluminal ringed graft, with a St. Jude Medical aortic valve.

Man, 51, who had closed mitral commissurotomy at age 22, had persistent fever after a rabbit bite; left ventricular failure developed. α-Hemolytic streptococcus was isolated from the blood. Echocardiography showed vegetation and a perianular abscess on the aortic valve, as well as mural thrombi in the left atrium. Aortic valve regurgitation, tricuspid regurgitation, and mitral stenosis were documented.

Under cardiopulmonary bypass with blood cardioplegia and topical hypothermia, the aortic and mitral valves were excised and the aortic anular abscess removed. Left atrial mural thrombi also were removed. A 29-mm St. Jude mitral valve was placed in the mitral position, followed by double coronary bypass

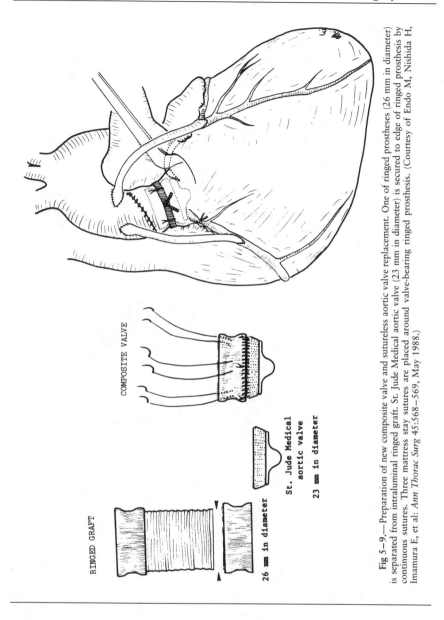

Fig 5–9.— Preparation of new composite valve and sutureless aortic valve replacement. One of ringed prostheses (26 mm in diameter) is separated from intraluminal ringed graft. St. Jude Medical aortic valve (23 mm in diameter) is secured to edge of ringed prosthesis by continuous sutures. Three mattress stay sutures are placed around valve-bearing ringed prosthesis. (Courtesy of Endo M, Nishida H, Imamura E, et al: *Ann Thorac Surg* 45:568–569, May 1988.)

grafting. A single ring prosthesis was separated from an intraluminal ringed graft and then sutured to a 23-mm St. Jude aortic valve (Fig 5–9). The composite valve was fixed to the aortic wall at 3 points by U-shaped sutures, and the aorta was bound circumferentially with Dacron tape against the groove in the ring. The patient returned to work and was in New York Heart Association functional class I after 18 months.

Previously, use of an anchoring thread from outside the aortic wall or inside the heart to the aortic anulus has been complicated by perivalvular leakage, necessitating reoperation. Treatment of 17 patients having aortic disease with an intraluminal ringed graft has been uncomplicated. This procedure can be used to replace a small aortic valve.

Aortic Valve Endocarditis With Aortic Root Abscess Cavity: Surgical Treatment With Aortic Valve Homograft
Kirklin JK, Kirklin JW, Pacifico AD (Univ of Alabama in Birmingham)
Ann Thorac Surg 45:674–677, June 1988   5–26

Aortic valve replacement with a homograft generally has been avoided because of geometric distortion of the valve. Three patients underwent homograft aortic valve replacement in the presence of aortic root abscess. A cryopreserved valve was utilized.

Technique.—After excising the infected valve (Fig 5–10), a homograft 2 to 4 mm smaller than the anulus is selected. The extent of abscess formation dictates the height of the homograft in the corresponding scalloped region (Fig 5–11). Three 4-0 polypropylene sutures are utilized (Figs 5–12 and 5–13). The homograft posts are everted and placed so as to cover the abscess cavity and leave the coronary ostia unobstructed (Fig 5–14). If the cavity encompasses much of the circumference of the anulus, it may be best to place the proximal suture line below the anular level.

All 3 patients were well after a mean of nearly 3 years, with no evidence of aortic incompetence. Because the abscess cavity usually is below the levels of the coronary ostia, it is appropriate to contour the homograftso that it can be placed below this level. This is an effective approach to at least some cases of aortic valve endocarditis with aortic root abscess.

▶ These articles (Abstracts 5–25 and 5–26) deal with the surgical dilemma of aortic root reconstruction in the presence of widespread destruction from endocarditis. The translocation technique described by Endo and his colleagues (Abstract 5–25) avoids the difficulty of valve fixation in the severely diseased subcoronary location. However, it does not solve the problem of reattachment of the aortic base to the left ventricular outflow tract, which must be accomplished in order to avoid a false aneurysm (at best) with progressive enlargement and eventual rupture.

The technique described by Kirklin and colleagues (Abstract 5–26) using a cryopreserved aortic valve homograft should produce less distortion of the base of the aorta than primary closure of the abscess orifice and avoids implantation of prosthetic material. The observation of satisfactory performance after a mean interval of nearly 3 years establishes this procedure as a reliable alter-

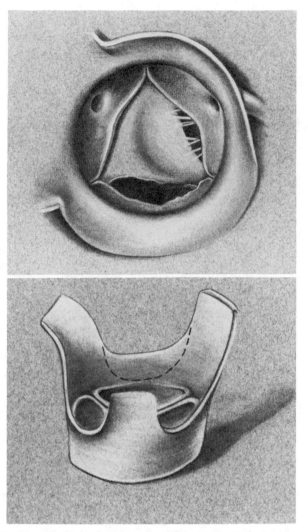

Fig 5–10, top.—Aortic valve has been excised, and abscess cavity is visualized below noncoronary sinus of Valsalva.

Fig 5–11, bottom.—In preparing homograft for standard aortic valve replacement, scalloped portions of homograft extend down into sinuses of Valsalva to within approximately 3 mm of aortic valve anulus. In presence of abscess cavity, corresponding sinus of Valsalva is left with more aortic wall. Usual extent of scalloping is indicated by *dashed line*. New height of aortic wall in scalloped area that will overlie (and exclude) abscess cavity is determined by overall extent of the abscess cavity below and above native aortic valve anulus.

(Courtesy of Kirklin JK, Kirklin JW, Pacifico AD: *Ann Thorac Surg* 45:674–677, June 1988.)

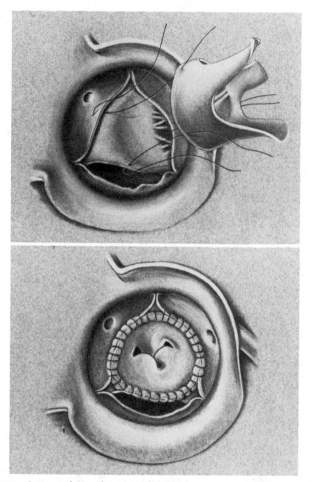

Fig 5–12, top.—In areas of normal aortic anulus, initial sutures are passed through midpoint of the anulus as usual. In sinus of Valsalva containing abscess cavity, initial suture is placed through lower extent of abscess cavity if it lies below anular level.

Fig 5–13, bottom.—Lower suture line follows lower rim of abscess cavity in involved sinus of Valsalva.

(Courtesy of Kirklin JK, Kirklin JW, Pacifico AD: *Ann Thorac Surg* 45:674–677, June 1988.)

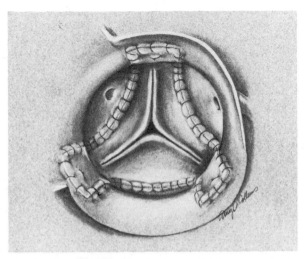

Fig 5–14.—Completed insertion of aortic valve homograft has now completely excluded abscess cavity. (Courtesy of Kirklin JK, Kirklin JW, Pacifico AD: *Ann Thorac Surg* 45:674–677, June 1988.)

native for those surgeons having access to cyropreserved homograft valves.— J.J. Collins, Jr., M.D.

Reduction in Sudden Late Death by Concomitant Revascularization With Aortic Valve Replacement
Czer LSC, Gray RJ, Stewart ME, De Robertis M, Chaux A, Matloff JM (Univ of California, Los Angeles)
J Thorac Cardiovasc Surg 95:390–401, March 1988   5–27

Coronary artery disease was present in 289 of 474 patients undergoing isolated aortic valve replacement from 1969 to 1984. Of these patients, 233 had coronary bypass grafting. The mean age of all patients was 62 years, and 89% were in New York Heart Association functional class III or IV preoperatively. Nearly two thirds of patients received a mechanical prosthesis, most often the St. Jude Medical valve, whereas 36% received a bioprosthesis, usually the Hancock valve. The mean number of bypass grafts per patient was 2.2.

Early mortality was lower in patients without coronary disease than in the others. Cardioplegia significantly lowered hospital mortality in patients having combined valve replacement and revascularization. After 10 years, actuarial survival was significantly lower in patients with coronary disease, whether or not bypass had been done (Fig 5–15). Late deaths were correlated closely with both coronary disease and depressed left ventricular function. Sudden deaths were substantially less frequent after revascularization (Fig 5–16).

Coronary atherosclerosis lessens survival after aortic valve replace-

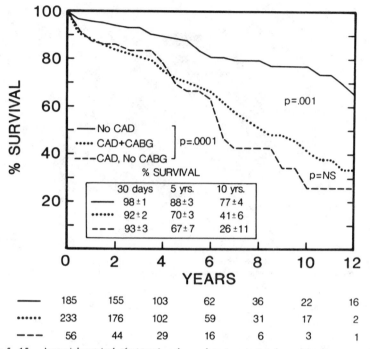

% SURVIVAL			
	30 days	5 yrs.	10 yrs.
———	98 ± 1	88 ± 3	77 ± 4
••••••	92 ± 2	70 ± 3	41 ± 6
– – –	93 ± 3	67 ± 7	26 ± 11

———	185	155	103	62	36	22	16
••••••	233	176	102	59	31	17	2
– – –	56	44	29	16	6	3	1

Fig 5–15.—Actuarial survival after aortic valve replacement in 3 cohorts of patients, stratified by presence or absence of coronary artery disease *(CAD)* and coronary artery bypass grafting *(CABG)*. Ten-year survival was significantly lower in patients with unbypassed or bypassed CAD than in patients with no CAD. *Box inset* depicts probability of survival (± standard error) at 30 days, 5 years, and 10 years. Numbers below graph indicate patients at risk during follow-up. (Courtesy of Czer LSC, Gray RJ, Steward ME, et al: *J Thorac Cardiovasc Surg* 95:390–401, March 1988.)

ment. Revascularization lessens late sudden deaths without increasing the risk of surgery. Cardioplegia will minimize the operative risk when coronary artery disease is present, as will complete revascularization.

Aortic Valve Replacement Combined With Myocardial Revascularization: Late Results and Determinants of Risk for 471 In-Hospital Survivors
Lytle BW, Cosgrove DM, Gill CC, Taylor PC, Stewart RW, Golding LA, Goormastic M, Loop FD (Cleveland Clinic Found)
J Thorac Cardiovasc Surg 95:402–414, March 1988   5–28

Five hundred patients had primary aortic valve replacement surgery combined with coronary bypass graft surgery from 1967 to 1981. Hospital mortality was 5.8%. The 471 hospital survivors were followed up for a mean of 85 months.

Survival rates were 88% at 2 years, 77% at 5 years, and 52% at 10 years (Fig 5–17). Late survival was correlated with age, New York Heart Association functional class, preoperative dyspnea, and radiographic evi-

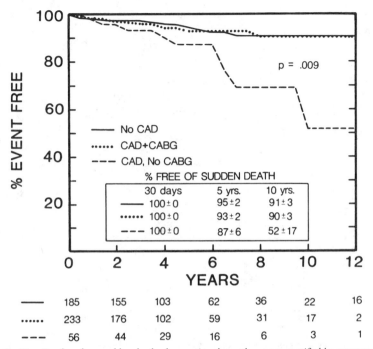

Fig 5–16.—Freedom from sudden death after aortic valve replacement, stratified by presence or absence of coronary artery disease *(CAD)* and coronary artery bypass grafting *(CABG)*. Significant protective effect of revascularization is apparent. (Courtesy of Czer LSC, Gray RJ, Stewart ME, et al: *J Thorac Cardiovasc Surg* 95:390–401, March 1988.)

dence of cardiac enlargement. A conduction defect and the extent of coronary disease also were factors. Patients given bioprostheses had better survival than those with mechanical prostheses (Fig 5–18). On multivariate analysis, age and valve type were most strongly associated with survival. Late event-free survival was decreased by moderate or severe left ventricular dysfunction, as well as by advanced age. Of 301 late survivors at the most recent follow-up, 98% were in New York Heart Association functional classes I and II.

Revascularization is indicated when patients requiring aortic valve replacement also have significant coronary artery disease. Older patients, especially those aged older than 70 years, are at the highest risk of late complications or death. Patients with bioprostheses who do not require warfarin have done better than those with mechanical prostheses. The overall outlook is quite good.

▶ These 2 publications (Abstracts 5–27 and 5–28) provide reasonable perspective on the place of coronary bypass in persons requiring aortic valve replacement. It is interesting that the beneficial effect of coronary bypass in these nonrandomized studies is not as obvious as might be expected. However, there can be little doubt that the presence of coronary artery disease is a

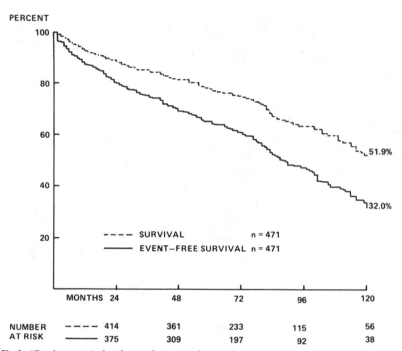

Fig 5–17.—Late survival and event-free survival curves for 471 in-hospital survivors of aortic valve replacement combined with coronary bypass grafting. Survival rates were 88%, 81%, 74%, 63%, and 52%, and event-free survival rates were 80%, 69%, 60%, 48%, and 32% at 2, 4, 6, 8, and 10 postoperative years, respectively. (Courtesy of Lytle BW, Cosgrove DM, Gill CC, et al: *J Thorac Cardiovasc Surg* 95:402–414, March 1988.).

significant risk factor in patients needing aortic valve replacement both short-term and long-term Because the principal benefit of coronary bypass is recognized in the first 5 to 8 years after surgery, it should not be surprising that there also seems to be a correlation between better survival and the utilization of porcine valves in the Cleveland Clinic Group. These data require careful study and comparison, illustrating as much as anything the difficulty of proving the obvious by retrospective analysis.—J.J. Collins, Jr., M.D.

Diseases of the Aorta

Growth of the Aortic Anastomosis in Pigs: Comparison of Continuous Absorbable Suture With Nonabsorbable Suture
Chiu I-S, Hung C-R, Chao S-F, Huang S-H, How S-W (Natl Taiwan Univ, Taipei, Taiwan)
J Thorac Cardiovasc Surg 95:112–118, January 1988   5–29

The polydioxanone used in pediatric cardiovascular surgery is rather stiff. Monofilament polyglyconate (Maxon) was evaluated in piglets undergoing primary end-to-end anastomosis of the infrarenal aorta. Both absorbable Maxon suture and nonabsorbable Prolene were employed.

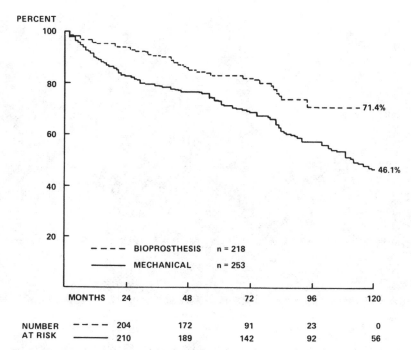

PERCENT

Fig 5–18.—Late survival curves for in-hospital survivors of aortic valve replacement combined with coronary bypass grafting according to aortic valve prosthesis type. Survival rates at 2, 5, and 8 postoperative years were 94%, 83%, and 71% for patients with biologic prostheses and 83%, 73%, and 57% for patients with mechanical valves, respectively. (Courtesy of Lytle BW, Cosgrove DM, Gill CC: *J Thorac Cardiovasc Surg* 95:402–414, March 1988.)

The animals were sacrificed 6 months after operation, and the aortas were burst-tested after radiographic evaluation.

All the anastomoses were patent, and no burst failures were seen in either suture group. Prolene sutures protruded into the lumen and were partly embedded in the aortic wall. Thrombus adhered to intraluminal Prolene in 6 of 9 animals (Fig 5–19). Growth of the anastomotic area was greater in the Maxon group, and stenosis was more frequent in the Prolene group. In both groups the distal segment was widely patent. The anastomotic site was dilated more often in the Maxon group (Fig 5–20). On histologic study, tissue reaction was more evident in the Prolene group. Maxon suture material had been completely absorbed. Neointimal hyperplasia was seen only in the Prolene suture group.

Absorbable Maxon sutures are recommended for use in cardiovascular anastomosis when suture line growth is required. Dilatation is minimal or absent if the continuity of the elastic lamina in the outer tunica media is restored before loss of tensile strength of the Maxon suture. Stenosis is the rule when nonabsorbable sutures are used in a rapidly growing host, even if the interrupted suture technique is employed.

▶ The quest continues for a technique that allows free growth at vascular

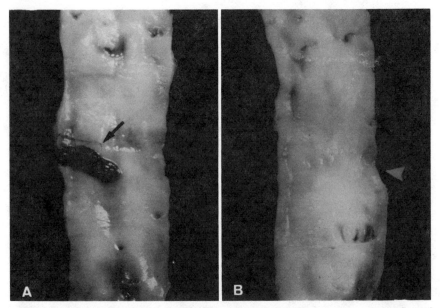

Fig 5–19.—Aorta was opened 6 months after operation. Proximal part is on top. **A,** intraluminal Prolene suture *(arrow)* was evident with thrombus adherent to it in pig P-1. **B,** smooth intima at anastomotic site of pig M-1 in Maxon suture group *(arrowhead).* No suture was visible, although slight dilatation can be seen. (Courtesy of Chiu I-S, Hung C-R, Chao S-F, et al: *J Thorac Cardiovasc Surg* 95:112–118, January 1988.)

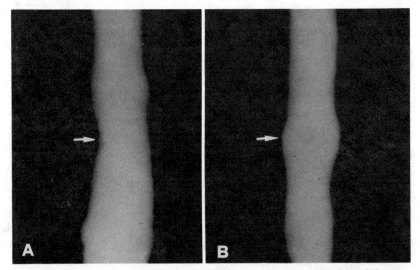

Fig 5–20.—Radiograph of abdominal aorta of pig P-6 in Prolene suture group shows slight stricture. **B,** slight dilatation of aorta of pig M-6 in Maxon suture group. Proximal part is on top. (Courtesy of Chiu I-S, Hung C-R, Chao S-F, et al: *J Thorac Cardiovasc Surg* 95:112–118, January 1988.)

anastomoses without significant weakening of the wall of the arteries. The authors' experience with a new absorbable monofilament suture is sufficiently favorable to suggest that clinical utilization of this material is probably reasonable. Would such a material also be useful for coronary artery anastomoses? An interesting observation in this study was the presence of clot at exposed suture lines where Prolene was utilized. The occurrence of significant inflammation associated with Prolene vascular sutures and the presence of clot at the suture line in some pigs emphasize the inherent hazard of nonabsorbable suture materials.—J.J. Collins, Jr., M.D.

Treatment of Extensive Aortic Aneurysms by a New Multiple-Stage Approach
Borst HG, Frank G, Schaps D (Hannover Medical School, Hannover, West Germany)
J Thorac Cardiovasc Surg 95:11–13, January 1988   5–30

Primary replacement of an extensive part of the aorta may be done to facilitate subsequent downstream surgery. When replacing the aortic arch during deep hypothermia and circulatory arrest, an appropriate length of the terminal graft is invaginated and the fold sutured end-to-end to the orifice. The invaginated portion later is advanced into the downstream aneurysm, where it is suspended freely (Fig 5–21). Air is carefully removed before tying the distal anastomotic suture, and antegrade flow is established via the arch graft. If the invaginated end of the graft is manipulated into the downstream aneurysm just before completing the distal graft-aorta connection, the aorta may be replaced in stages.

Seventeen operations were carried out in 8 patients, 4 with aneurysmal dissection and 4 with arteriosclerotic aneurysms. In 5 patients, initial replacement of the ascending aorta and arch was followed by replacement

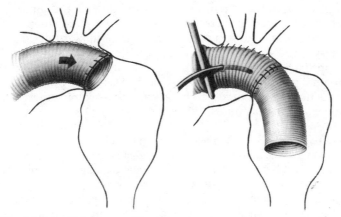

Fig 5–21.—Principle of "elephant trunk" technique in replacement of aneurysm involving ascending and arch portions of aorta preceding replacement of descending aortic aneurysm. (Courtesy of Borst HG, Frank G, Schaps D: *J Thorac Cardiovasc Surg* 95:11–13, January 1988.)

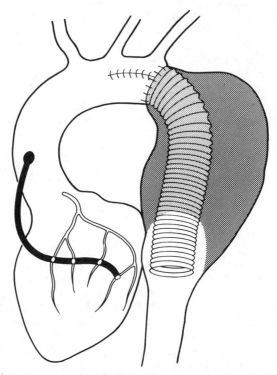

Fig 5–22.—Schematic representation of technique. In conjunction with quadruple coronary revascularization, long graft was inserted into distal aortic arch and suspended freely in descending aortic aneurysm. Aneurysm largely thrombosed around graft. (Courtesy of Borst HG, Frank G, Schaps D: *J Thorac Cardiovasc Surg 95:11–13, January 1988.*)

of the descending aorta and, in 2 instances, the thoracoabdominal segment as well. In 2 other patients, primary replacement of the proximal descending aorta preceded replacement of the thoracoabdominal portion. All patients survived. and there were no method-related complications. A good result was obtained in a patient undergoing quadruple coronary bypass surgery (Fig 5–22).

This approach facilitates second- or third-stage aortic replacement once proximal grafting is performed. The chest may be opened at the best level for further distal surgery. The aortic cross-clamp time is short because only 1 distal anastomosis is necessary.

▶ The observation by Borst and associates that an intraluminal prosthesis having only proximal attachment to the vascular wall may seek its own attachment distally is remarkably provocative. The technical difficulty and time necessary for the performance of intravascular anastomoses is sufficiently great and represents enough hazard to patients that the introduction of simple techniques to achieve protection against aneurysmal dilatation and rupture is indeed welcome. This "elephant trunk" technique deserves careful evaluation.—J.J. Collins, Jr., M.D.

Congenital Heart Surgery

Pulmonary Homograft Implantation for Ventricular Outflow Tract Reconstruction: Early Phase Results

McGrath LB, Gonzalez-Lavin L, Graf D (Univ of Medicine and Dentistry of New Jersey, New Brunswick)
Ann Thorac Surg 45:273–277, March 1988   5–31

The pulmonary valve homograft is larger in diameter than the aortic homograft and has a thinner wall and less intrinsic calcification. Eight consecutive patients with congenital cardiac defects received cryopreserved pulmonary homografts. Various disorders were present, the most common being tetralogy with pulmonary atresia. In 7 cases the homograft was placed as a valved extracardiac conduit; an orthotopic transplant was given to 1 patient with absent pulmonary valve. In 3 cases the branching pulmonary arterial part of the pulmonary homograft was utilized.

All patients survived the operations. The mean transvalvular gradient was 9 mm Hg; no valve incompetence was noted. One patient required reoperation for conduit revision because of sternal compression. The only operative complication was staphylococcal mediastinitis, which was treated effectively by irrigation and drainage.

The pulmonary homograft now is the authors' valve of choice for use in reconstruction of the ventricular outflow tract. The bifurcational part of the donor pulmonary arteries is helpful in repairing associated pulmonary arterial anomalies. The pulmonary homograft also is used for orthotopic placement in right-sided outflow tract operations.

▶ Up to now there has been no organized effort to utilize pulmonary valves and arteries for reconstruction in congenital cardiac defects. There seems no reason why the pulmonary artery with its valve should not be cryopreserved, as well as aortic valves and conduits. Gordon Danielson in his discussion of this presentation mentions satisfactory early results using cryopreserved pulmonary homografts.—J.J. Collins, Jr., M.D.

Valve Prostheses in Children: A Reassessment of Anticoagulation

Sade RM, Crawford FA Jr, Fyfe DA, Stroud MR (Med Univ of South Carolina, Charleston)
J Thorac Cardiovasc Surg 95:553–561, April 1988   5–32

Bleeding complications always have been a special problem in children requiring valve replacement. Earlier evidence is available that children receiving St. Jude Medical prostheses on the left side of the heart may not require anticoagulation. From 1979 to 1986, 48 pediatric patients had left-sided cardiac valve replacement with a St. Jude prosthesis. Five valves were replaced at reoperation. The patients received no anticoagulant therapy for a total of 122 patient-years of follow-up after valve replacement.

None of 5 early and 1 of 9 late deaths was associated with prosthetic thrombosis. The rate of thromboembolism was 5.7 events per 100 patient-years. The events were not related to patient age at surgery or the site of valve placement. Thrombotic and thromboembolic events were less frequent among 340 adults with St. Jude Medical prostheses who received warfarin therapy over 875 patient-years of follow-up.

Thromboembolism began to occur rather abruptly in the last year of this follow-up study, about 4 years after surgery. It is now preferable to reduce the risk of clotting while accepting a chance of bleeding events from anticlotting medication. A randomized trial of anticoagulation and antiplatelet therapy is in progress.

▶ This paper gives further follow-up on a previously reported group of children who were managed without anticoagulant therapy after valve replacement with St. Jude prostheses. Although early experience suggested that anticoagulants with this prosthesis might not be necessary in children this publication documents that the rate of thrombotic and thromboembolic complications eventually was greater than that observed in adults with similar prostheses who had been anticoagulated. It does not seem safe at the present time to recommend any prosthetic valve without anticoagulation in children or adults.—J.J. Collins, Jr., M.D.

Current Results of Management in Transposition of the Great Arteries, With Special Emphasis on Patients With Associated Ventricular Septal Defect

Trusler GA, Castaneda AR, Rosenthal A, Blackstone EH, Kirklin JW, Congenital Heart Surgeons Society (Hosp for Sick Children, Toronto; Children's Hosp Med Ctr, Boston; Univ of Michigan; Univ of Alabama in Birmingham)

J Am Coll Cardiol 10:1061–1071, November 1987   5–33

Because many reports on transposition of the great arteries are based on small numbers of patients, deal only with treated patients, and do not include those who died before surgical repair, the survival rate of this anomaly has been overestimated. Moreover, many reports do not include patients with associated cardiac and noncardiac congenital anomalies. The early results were reviewed of an ongoing 20-institution study of transposition of the great arteries of all types; only neonates admitted to the hospital before age 15 days were included. Follow-up is planned to extend to 1998.

From January 1985 to June 1986 245 infants with a median age of 1 day who had transposition of the great arteries, including 36 who also had a ventricular septal defect, were entered into the study. Forty-two patients died, including 14 who died before undergoing repair. A total of 154 surgical repairs have been performed to date, including 86 arterial switch repairs, 21 Mustard atrial switch repairs, and 39 Senning atrial switch repairs.

To date no differences in survival have been identified that relate to either the morphological features of the transposition or to the type of surgical repair. However, associated major cardiac and noncardiac anomalies and low birth weight did increase the risk of death.

Survival has already improved over the 16 months since the study was initiated, probably because of the improved survival with the arterial switch repair. The early results of procedures that combine repair of transposition of the great arteries with repair of ventricular septal defect indicate that the outcome is as favorable as that after simple transposition.

▶ This initial report of a cooperative study involving several of the largest children's cardiac surgical centers in the world is an important step toward establishing uniform reporting and evaluation of results in surgery for complex congenital anomalies. Such worldwide cooperation will undoubtedly become more frequent and should improve surgical results.—J.J. Collins, Jr., M.D.

Myocardial Performance After Repair of Congenital Cardiac Defects in Infants and Children: Response to Volume Loading
Burrows FA, Williams WG, Teoh KH, Wood AE, Burns J, Edmonds J, Barker GA, Trusler GA, Weisel RD (Hosp for Sick Children, Toronto)
J Thorac Cardiovasc Surg 96:548–556, October 1988   5–34

Hemodynamic responses to volume replacement were monitored in 70 infants and children within 24 hours after repair of congenital cardiac defects, in order to assess myocardial performance. The most frequent diagnoses were ventricular septal defect, transposition, and tetralogy of Fallot. Colloid solution was rapidly infused to raise the left atrial pressure 5–10 mm Hg over 20–30 minutes.

Cardiac index and left ventricular stroke work were adequate within 2 hours of cardiopulmonary bypass and increased appropriately on volume loading in all diagnostic groups. At 4 hours, patients other than those with atrial septal defect had lower cardiac and stroke work indices and a depressed response to increasing preload. Deterioration was most evident 4–12 hours after bypass; there was a tendency to recover at 24 hours (Fig 5–23). Cardiac function was most depressed in patients having repair of transposition. Myocardial performance was not predicted by bypass time, time of circulatory arrest, or the type of cardioplegia used.

In children having repair of congenital cardiac lesions, it may be best to limit volume infusion to keep the left atrial pressure less than 14 mm Hg. If necessary, afterload reduction can follow, with or without inotropic drugs. The risk of ventricular septal defect repair is greater in smaller infants.

▶ As previously reported by Kirklin and Theye (1), left ventricular contractility tends to deteriorate in most patients after intracardiac surgery, regardless of

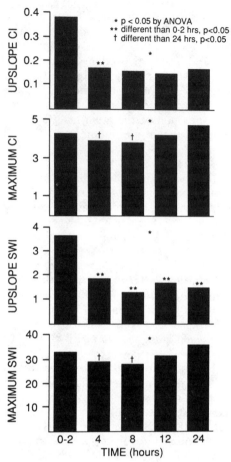

Fig 5–23.—Postoperative response to increasing preload. Average values are plotted to show trends in performance in 22 children who had additional performance curves 4–12 hours after bypass with subsequent improvement at 24 hours but persistent depression compared to 2-hour performance. (Courtesy of Burrows FA, Williams WG, Teoh KH, et al: *J Thorac Cardiovasc Surg* 96:548–556, October 1988.)

the type of surgery performed. This publication confirms that children are not exempt from this phenomenon.—J.J. Collins, Jr., M.D.

Reference

1. Kirklin JW, Theye RA: Cardiac performance after open intracardiac surgery. *Circulation* 28:1061–1070, 1963.

Preoperative Three-Dimensional Reconstruction of the Heart and Great Vessels in Patients With Congenital Heart Disease: Technique and Initial Results

Laschinger JC, Vannier MW, Gutierrez F, Gronemeyer S, Weldon CS, Spray TL, Cox JL (Washington Univ, St Louis)
J Thorac Cardiovasc Surg 96:464–473, September 1988
5–35

Magnetic resonance (MR) imaging is a noninvasive method that, unlike echocardiography, is not limited by interposed air or bone. Contiguous electrocardiographic-gated MR images from the cardiac apex to the aortic arch provide enough data to reconstruct the heart and great vessels in 3 dimensions. This was undertaken in 6 patients with congenital heart disease, using the surface reconstruction techniques developed to process computed tomographic scans. Individual scan slices first were manually edited to separate the heart and vessels from the blood within them and from extracardiac structures. Scan times ranged from 1 to 2 hours.

Reconstructions were obtained in patients having coarctation with ventricular septal defect, hypoplastic left ventricle, pulmonary artery atresia with ventricular septal defect, atrial septal defect (Fig 5–24), partial atrioventricular canal defect with anomalous pulmonary venous drainage, and tetralogy of Fallot with peripheral pulmonary artery stenosis. The anatomical findings were consistent with the 2-dimensional MR image and echocardiographic findings, cineangiography, and the intraoperative appearances. In 5 patients, additional or new diagnoses were made, and changes in management or surgical planning resulted.

Three-dimensional reconstruction can aid the interpretation of MR scan findings when surgery for congenital heart disease is planned, without sacrificing significant clinical information. The study is limited by the need for an anatomically knowledgeable operator. From 4 to 6 hours are needed to generate each set of 3-dimensional images.

▶ The concept of 3-dimensional modeling using digital reconstruction tech-

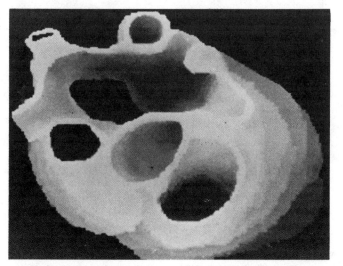

Fig 5–24.—Atrial septal defect (ASD), secundum type. Cranial-caudal cross-sectional surface view of heart and great vessels. Heart had been divided at level of midleft atrium. Note large secundum ASD with normal pulmonary venous drainage. Superior vena cava is seen entering right atrium and inferior vena cava, and coronary sinus can be seen through ASD. (Courtesy of Laschinger JC, Vannier MW, Gutierrez F, et al: *J Thorac Cardiovasc Surg* 96:464–473, September 1988.)

niques combined with magnetic resonance imaging is exciting. The authors have pioneered research in this field, and although it may not be totally practical for all units at the present time, it certainly is the way of the future.—J.J. Collins, Jr., M.D.

A New Reconstructive Operation for Ebstein's Anomaly of the Tricuspid Valve

Carpentier A, Chauvaud S, Macé L, Relland J, Mihaileanu S, Marino JP, Abry B, Guibourt P (Univ of Paris)
J Thorac Cardiovasc Surg 96:92–101, July 1988   5–36

Previous operations for Ebstein's anomaly (Fig 5–25), including repair and replacement, have given varying results. In a new operation a normal-shaped right ventricle is reconstructed and the tricuspid valve is repositioned at the normal level.

Types B and C are the most frequent types of anomaly. In these cases, after cutting fibrous bands attached to the ventricular wall and fenestrating any obliterated interchordal spaces, the right ventricle is plicated, along with the tricuspid anulus and right atrium, and the leaflets are sutured to the anulus after clockwise rotation to cover the entire orificial area. A prosthetic ring then is inserted.

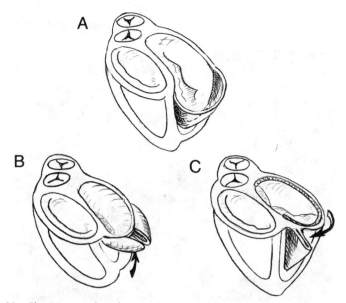

Fig 5–25.—Ebstein's anomaly and repair. **A,** anatomical features: Downward displacement of posterior and septal leaflets into right ventricle results in large atrialized chamber and tricuspid valve competence. **B,** Hunter-Lillehei-Hardy operation: transverse plication of atrialized chamber produces right ventricle that is reduced in size and distorted. **C,** proposed technique: Longitudinal plication of atrialized chamber and repositioning of tricuspid valve to normal position restores shape of right ventricle. (Courtesy of Carpentier A, Chauvaud S, Macé L, et al: *J Thorac Cardiovasc Surg* 96:92–101, July 1988.)

In type A cases the small, contractile atrialized chamber is not plicated. In type D cases the thinnest part of the ventricle is plicated longitudinally.

Of 14 patients who were operated on only 1 who had an associated atrioventricular septal defect required tricuspid valve replacement. All the others benefited from conservative surgery, although there were 2 hospital deaths. All survivors had markedly improved function, and rhythm disturbances improved.

Echocardiography and Doppler studies showed a normal-shaped right ventricle and good valve function in all patients but 1. Eight patients had no residual tricuspid valve incompetence, and none had tricuspid valve stenosis.

Ebstein's anomaly can be repaired in most of these patients by mobilization of the tricuspid valve and repositioning with longitudinal plication of the atrialized chamber. The surgery should be done before functional disability or severe arrhythmia has developed.

▶ This approach to reconstruction of the tricuspid valve in Ebstein's anomaly is another innovation from Carpentier and his associates.—J.J. Collins, Jr., M.D.

Arrhythmia Surgery

Direct Operations for the Management of Life-Threatening Ischemic Ventricular Tachycardia

Ostermeyer J, Borggrefe M, Breithardt G, Podczek A, Goldmann A, Schoenen JD, Kolvenbach R, Godehardt E, Kirklin JW, Blackstone EH, Bircks W (Univ of Düsseldorf, West Germany)
J Thorac Cardiovasc Surg 94:848–865, December 1987   5–37

The best surgical means of ablating ventricular tachycardia remains uncertain. Ninety-three consecutive patients had electrophysiologically guided operations for recurrent life-threatening ventricular tachycardia from 1978 to 1986. Most patients had other surgery as well, such as left ventricular aneurysmectomy or coronary bypass grafting. The 74 surviving patients were followed for a median of 26 months. In a majority of cases the arrhythmogenic tissue was completely or partly encircled by endocardial myotomy or subjected to endomyocardial resection.

Eighty-seven percent of survivors were free of sudden death and ventricular tachycardia a year postoperatively, and 77% were at 5 years. Recurrent arrhythmia was most likely when 3-system coronary disease was present. Survival was 70% at 5 years. Ninety percent of long-term survivors were in New York Heart Association functional class I or II at last follow-up. Both recurrent ventricular tachycardia and sudden death were more likely after endocardial resection than with encircling myotomy, but not markedly so.

Encircling endocardial myotomy is the most effective approach to malignant ventricular tachycardia. The incisions should be as limited as possible. Progressive ischemic cardiomyopathy may be a greater factor than inadequate surgery in late recurrent ventricular tachycardia. However, extensive encircling endocardial myotomy does increase the risk of early death from left ventricular pump failure. The prognosis for survival after the return of spontaneous ventricular tachycardia is poor.

▶ Surgical management of ventricular arrhythmias includes a variety of options as described by Yee and associates (1). The review of experience around the world provided by Ostermeyer in the publication above emphasizes the favorable results that may be obtained by endocardial ablation or isolation techniques combined with myocardial revascularization. The complexity of preoperative, intraoperative, and postoperative management of these patients combined with the fact that relatively few patients require such operations argues for the limitation of this specialized area of cardiac surgery to a small number of centers.—J.J. Collins, Jr., M.D.

Reference

1. Yee ES, Schienman MM, Griffin JC, et al: Surgical options for treating ventricular tachyarrhythmia and sudden death. *J Thorac Cardiovasc Surg* 94:866–873, 1987.)

Heart Failure and Artificial Heart Devices

Bridging to Cardiac Transplantation With Pulsatile Ventricular Assist Devices
Kanter KR, McBride LR, Pennington DG, Swartz MT, Ruzevich SA, Miller LW, Willman VL (St Louis Univ)
Ann Thorac Surg 46:134–140, August 1988   5–38

An increasing number of patients will require mechanical circulatory aid to "bridge" to cardiac transplantation. The concept of bridging by temporary mechanical circulatory support was introduced clinically by Cooley et al. in 1969. The first hospital survivors were reported by Reemtsma et al. in 1978. The present workers have used the Pierce-Donachy ventricular assist device (VAD) and the Novacor left ventricular assist system.

Eleven patients with a mean age of 40 years had a VAD placed since 1982. A pneumatic Pierce-Donachy pump was used in 9 patients, and an electrical Novacor pump, in 2. Six of the patients had ischemic cardiomyopathy. Two each had postpartum and idiopathic cardiomyopathy, and 1 had doxorubicin toxicity. Seven patients required left ventricular support only, whereas 4 received biventricular support. The time of support ranged from 8 hours to 91 days. Hemodynamic stability was achieved in all cases, but 10 patients had major complications and these precluded transplantation in 5 of them. Six patients underwent successful cardiac transplantation after a mean of 24 days of mechanical support. Five of these patients were in New York Heart Association functional class I after a mean of 14 months. One late death was due to medical noncompliance.

A pulsatile VAD can provide prolonged hemodynamic support before cardiac transplantation, with well-preserved end-organ function. Proper patient selection is critical. Renal failure is a grave prognostic sign. The Pierce-Donachy VAD is well suited for biventricular support.

Heterotopic Prosthetic Ventricles as a Bridge to Cardiac Transplantation: A Multicenter Study in 29 Patients

Farrar DJ, Hill JD, Gray LA Jr, Pennington DG, McBride LR, Pierce WS, Pae WE, Glenville B, Ross D, Galbraith TA, Zumbro GL (Pacific Presbyterian Med Center, San Francisco; Univ of Louisville–Jewish Hosp, Louisville, Ky; St Louis Univ; Pennsylvania State Univ; Harley Street Clinic, London; et al)
N Engl J Med 318:333–340, Feb 11, 1988   5–39

Many candidates for cardiac transplantation die before a donor heart is obtained. Providing complete circulatory support during the waiting period was first attempted with an orthotopic artificial heart. Alternatively, a heterotopic partial artificial heart, also called a ventricular assist device—a prosthetic left ventricle that bypasses the diseased ventricle— can be used. A multicenter experience with heterotopic prosthetic ventricles for left or biventricular support as a bridge to transplantation was reported.

Circulation was supported by heterotopic prosthetic ventricles in 29 candidates for heart transplantation who were expected to die before donor hearts could be procured. Twenty-one patients, with an average age of 36 years, underwent successful transplantation after 8 hours to 31 days of circulatory support. The other patients died because their conditions could not be stabilized for transplantation, despite blood flow restoration. Fourteen patients had biventricular support; 15 had only left ventricular support, with pharmacologic assistance of right heart function. Before transplantation, blood flow from the left prosthetic ventricle averaged 2.8 ± 0.4 L/minute/m^2 of body surface area and, from the right prosthesis, 2.4 ± 0.4 L, compared with an average flow of 1.6 ± 0.5 L/minute/m^2 before implantation. Twenty of the 21 patients who underwent transplantation were discharged from the hospital after a median of 31 days. Nineteen were alive 7 to 39 months after transplantation, and 11 of the first 12 were alive at 1 year.

Heterotopic placement of prosthetic ventricles as a bridge to transplantation is an effective method of temporarily supporting cardiac function in critically ill patients without removing the natural heart. Early survival after transplantation is comparable to that with elective cardiac transplantation.

▶ The 2 articles documenting experience with left ventricular and biventricular cardiac assist devices in terminally ill patients as a prelude to cardiac transplantation (Abstracts 5–38 and 5–39) represent both a promise and a threat. The promise, of course, is avoidance of death and terminal peripheral organ failure in otherwise acceptable candidates for cardiac transplantation when a suitable donor cannot be found at the opportune moment. The threat is the enormous cost of widespread use of artificial devices for prolongation of life which, if carried to an extreme, could ensure that the only patients receiving cardiac transplants would be those already supported by a bridging device. The very limited number of organs available and the potentially unlimited access to mechanical assist devices strongly suggests that the possibility of virtually universal preliminary support in candidates for cardiac transplantation is not unthinkable. The argument that results of cardiac transplantation in patients previously supported by an artificial left ventricular assist device are no different from those expected for patients transplanted without such intervention appears to be an accident of a small and carefully selected series. It does not seem reasonable to believe as a generality.—J.J. Collins, Jr., M.D.

Follow-up of Survivors of Mechanical Circulatory Support
Kanter KR, Ruzevich SA, Pennington DG, McBride LR, Swartz MT, Willman VL (St Louis Univ)
J Thorac Cardiovasc Surg 96:72–80, July 1988   5–40

Twenty-seven patients given mechanical circulatory assistance since 1980 were followed up after discharge. Fourteen adult patients had refractory cardiogenic shock after cardiac surgery. Eight children survived mechanical support for the same indication after repair of congenital cardiac defects. Five patients were supported while awaiting cardiac transplantation. Pulsatile ventricular assist devices, centrifugal ventricular assist pumps, and extracorporeal membrane oxygenation all were used.

The mean time of support among patients with postoperative shock was 3.5 days. Two thirds of patients had major complications, most often serious bleeding or infection. Two of 4 late deaths were cardiac-related. Of the 23 surviving patients who were followed for a mean of 29 months, 17 were in functional class I and 2 were in class II when last seen. Only 1 patient was in New York Heart Association class IV. Only 4 patients had significant cardiac disability at follow-up, and 1 of these still was working.

Considerable progress has been made in mechanical circulatory assistance. Satisfactory long-term survival now is the rule for patients who are supported in refractory postoperative cardiogenic shock. Most surviving patients are leading active and productive lives.

▶ These encouraging results from the group at St. Louis University are at least as significant as the favorable results obtained with artificial circulatory assist devices used as a bridge to transplantation. If it is possible to salvage the native heart, that is certainly a greater victory.—J.J. Collins, Jr., M.D.

Effect of Triiodothyronine (T_3) on Myocardial High Energy Phosphates and Lactate After Ischemia and Cardiopulmonary Bypass: An Experimental Study in Baboons

Novitzky D, Human PA, Cooper DKC (Univ of Cape Town, South Africa)
J Thorac Cardiovasc Surg 96:600–607, October 1988   5–41

On cardiopulmonary bypass the plasma free T_3 level declines, and T_3 administration has benefited patients in very low cardiac output states after cardiac surgery. A study in pigs has shown a marked inotropic effect and a decrease in mortality when T_3 was administered after a period of myocardial ischemia and bypass.

The effects of T_3 on high-energy phosphates and lactate in the myocardium were studied in baboons subjected to 3 hours of myocardial ischemia while on cardiopulmonary bypass. Treated animals received 6 μg of T_3 at the end of ischemia. Levels of adenosine triphosphate returned to baseline in treated animals, whereas in control animals levels remained low at 2 hours. Levels of myocardial lactate rose steadily in untreated animals, and at 2 hours there was a significant group difference.

These findings suggest that T_3 exerts an inotropic effect by rapidly replacing and maintaining high-energy phosphate stores in the myocardium. Triiodothyronine appears to activate adenosine triphosphatases, and it may increase ionized calcium within the cytosol. In addition, T_3 stimulates adenyl cyclase. Administration of T_3 may prove helpful for patients having cardiac surgery involving prolonged myocardial ischemia, or when the cardiac output is low after cardiopulmonary bypass is discontinued.

▶ This interesting animal study suggests that the acutely failing heart may be assisted in a significant way by triiodothyronine, which is both readily available and easily administered.—J.J. Collins, Jr., M.D.

Cardiac Transplantation

Orthotopic Transplantation During Early Infancy as Therapy for Incurable Congenital Heart Disease
Bailey LL, Assaad AN, Trimm RF, Nehlsen-Cannarella SL, Kanakriyeh MS, Haas GS, Jacobson JG (Loma Linda Univ, Loma Linda, Calif)
Ann Surg 208:279–286, September 1988   5–42

Fourteen neonates and young infants underwent orthotopic heart transplantation since late 1985 because of hypoplastic aortic tract complex. They were among 27 patients with variations of hypoplastic left heart syndrome. Infants aged less than 1 month who weighed more than 2,200 gm at birth were accepted (table). The metabolic and hemodynamic status must have been normal, and neurologic and renal abnormalities must have been absent. Immunosuppression was with cyclosporine, methylprednisolone, and azathioprine, and gamma globulin was given for immunoenhancement.

Eleven patients (78%) survived cardiac allotransplantation. Six of the last 8 candidates underwent the procedure, and the last 7 operated patients have survived surgery. The mean time of hypothermic circulatory

---

Recipient Inclusion Criteria

1. Gestational age greater than 36 weeks* and birth weight greater than 2200 g*
2. Age of less than 1 month*
3. Cardiac evaluation
   The diagnosis of hypoplastic left heart syndrome made by attending pediatrician or pediatric cardiologist.
   Echocardiographic confirmation of diagnosis.
4. Stable metabolic and hemodynamic status while receiving PGE-1 and other supportive measures (*e.g.,* cardiac inotrope, mechanical ventilation, parenteral nutrition)
5. Psychosocial evaluation
   The candidate should live within 60 minutes of LLUMC for a minimum of 9–12 months after transplant.
   Supportive family structure.
   The candidate's family should be capable of long-term intensive care of the child and be able to support the exceptional needs of the child.
6. No clinical suspicion of major sepsis.
7. Normal neurological evaluation.
8. Normal renal evaluation:
   If BUN > 30 and creatinine < 1.5, pediatric nephrology consultation to exclude gross renal abnormalities
   Abdominal ultrasonography study showing no significant renal malformations
9. Phenotypically normal.

*Relative criteria.
(Courtesy of Bailey LL, Assaad AN, Trimm RF, et al: *Ann Surg* 208:279–286, Sept 1988.)

---

arrest was 56 minutes. All infants but 1 were successfully treated for acute rejection. In 1 recipient, cytomegalovirus infection developed. Growth and neurologic development have generally been within the normal range. Survival now averages 12.6 months. There was no late renal dysfunction.

Orthotopic heart transplantation is an effective approach to selected neonates and young infants with surgically incurable congenital heart lesions. Rejection and infection are lesser problems when surgery is done during the first month of life. Apart from continuing efforts to increase the donor organ supply, cross-species transplantation warrants exploration.

▶ These remarkable results from cardiac transplantation in infants are a tribute to the persistence and innovation of Leonard Bailey and his associates at Loma Linda. The finding that rejection and infection seem to be less severe obstacles in these infants is obviously important. It will be interesting to see whether the long-term results in these children are significantly different from what has been observed in older children and adults.—J.J. Collins, Jr., M.D.

Accelerated Coronary Vascular Disease in the Heart Transplant Patient: Coronary Arteriographic Findings

Gao S-Z, Alderman EL, Schroeder JS, Silverman JF, Hunt SA (Stanford Univ)
J Am Coll Cardiol 12:334–340, August 1988   5–43

Yearly coronary angiograms from 81 heart transplant recipients with coronary vascular disease were compared with films from 32 nontransplant patients having coronary disease. The transplant patients had survived at least 1 year and had follow-up angiograms for a mean of 2.4 years.

All lesions in control angiograms were of the discrete or tubular type, and three fourths of them were in primary epicardial coronary vessels. More of these types of lesions in the transplant patients were in secondary branches. Diffusely concentric narrowing and narrowed irregular vessels with occluded branches also were observed in transplant recipients. These lesions were more frequent in secondary and tertiary branches than in primary vessels. Collateral vessels were poor or absent in a large majority of transplant patients with total occlusion, whereas most nontransplant patients had collateral vessels.

Heart transplant patients often have a mixture of typical atheromatous lesions and unique transplant-associated distal obliterative lesions without collateral vessel development. The primary mechanism probably is immunologic injury. Theoretically, such injury to the coronary intima could lead to platelet aggregation, intimal thickening and, eventually, obliterative arterial disease. More effective immunosuppression may lower the incidence of this disease.

▶ Development of atherosclerosis as well as immunologically mediated distal vessel obliteration provides a rapidly progressive model for coronary obstructive disease. The addition of antiplatelet agents seems to have had an ameliorating affect among transplant recipients. This is an exciting area for evaluation of preventive medication as well as determining the genesis of arteriosclerotic obstructive disease.—J.J. Collins, Jr., M.D.

OKT3 Monoclonal Antibody in Cardiac Transplantation: Experience With 102 Patients

Gay WA Jr, O'Connell JG, Burton NA, Karwande SV, Renlund DG, Bristow MR (Utah Cardiac Transplant Program, Salt Lake City)
Ann Surg 208:287–290, September 1988   5–44

The OKT3 murine monoclonal antibody, reactive against CD3 surface antigen, interferes with the ability of lymphocytes to recognize foreign antigen and thereby delays or prevents cell-mediated immune rejection. Prophylactic OKT3 was used in 102 orthotopic cardiac transplant recipients, along with azathioprine and low-dose steroids. Cyclosporine was begun on postoperative day 11, and weaning from steroid was attempted at 3 weeks.

The mean time to initial rejection was 76 days. Eighty-five percent of patients were weaned from maintenance steroids. Actuarial survival at 2 and 3 years was 90%. Four patients had a return of CD3 positivity during OKT3 prophylaxis, probably because of an existing antibody to the murine protein. Eleven patients with refractory rejection received a second course of OKT3, and 10 responded.

Prophylactic OKT3 is an attractive alternative to conventional immunosuppression for transplant recipients. Side effects form high-dose steroids and cyclosporine are avoided in the perioperative period, and patients are likely not to require long-term steroids. There may, however, be distressing side effects from OKT3. These can be lessened by premedicating patients with hydrocortisone, diphenhydramine, ranitidine, and acetaminophen before the first several treatments.

▶ Most cardiac transplant units continue to use early high-dose steroid immunosuppression. The experience of the Utah group with OKT3 in lieu of early steroid therapy certainly suggests that there may be advantages.—J.J. Collins, Jr., M.D.

Coronary Artery Spasm in a Transplant Patient

Cattan S, Drobinski G, Artigou J-Y, Grogogeat Y, Cabrol C (Univ René Descartes, Hosp Cochin, and Hosp Pitié-Salpétrière, Paris)
Eur Heart J 9:557–560, May 1988   5–45

Severe coronary spasm led to the sudden death of a cardiac transplant recipient with a denervated heart, despite treatment with a calcium channel blocker.

Man, 33, with dilated cardiomyopathy for 5 years and congestive failure resistant to medical treatment, had a global ejection fraction of only 17%. Coronary angiography was normal. Cardiac transplantation was carried out using cyclosporine and steroid therapy for immunosuppression. A low output state was controlled with isoproterenol. Grand mal seizures were ascribed to postembolic infarction in the temporal and occipital regions. A coliform infection caused transient renal failure. Only mild transplant rejection occurred.

Subsequently, more severe rejection developed. Paroxysmal atrial fibrillation was well tolerated when amiodarone was given, but episodes of transient ST elevation ensued. Angiography showed multifocal coronary spasm during a time of ST elevation, which was relieved by intracoronary nitroglycerin. Several discrete atheromatous lesions also were seen. Despite nifedipine and isosorbide dinitrate therapy the patient died suddenly 11 months after transplantation. Autopsy showed recent thrombosis at 2 coronary sites. Signs of rejection persisted.

Denervation of the transplant was confirmed by ECG monitoring, carotid sinus massage, and testing with atropine and amyl nitrite. The autonomic nervous system is involved in coronary spasm, but spasm may occur in a denervated or transplanted heart without activation of the autonomic nervous system. Circulating catecholamine and other metabolic and hormonal substances may have a role in coronary spasm in these circumstances.

▶ Demonstration of coronary artery spasm following cardiac transplantation and its relief by intracoronary nitroglycerin is a very interesting observation. Fortunately, such severe spasm seems uncommon.—J.J. Collins, Jr., M.D.

Responses of Coronary Artaries of Cardiac Transplant Patients to Acetylcholine
Fish RD, Nabel EG, Selwyn AP, Ludmer PL, Mudge GH, Kirshenbaum JM, Schoen FJ, Alexander RW, Ganz P (Brigham and Women's Hosp, Boston, Harvard Univ)
J Clin Invest 81:21–31, January 1988   5–46

Accelerated coronary atherosclerosis is a serious complication in heart transplant patients. It is a major cause of death and occurs in 40% to 50% of patients who survive the surgery for 5 years. Graft atherosclerosis is difficult to detect and is not always noted in routine coronary angiography. Endothelial dysfunction, which has been associated with atherosclerosis, could be an early indicator of graft atherosclerosis in heart transplant patients.

Thirteen transplant patients were treated for endothelial dysfunction by an infusion of acetylcholine into the left anterior descending artery. Nine of the patients had undergone transplantation a year previously, and 4 had received heart transplants 2 years previously. Quantitative angiography was used to evaluate vascular responses.

Only 1 of the 13 patients showed normal dilation to acetylcholine throughout the arterial segments. Nitroglycerine, however, dilated nearly all segments. The patients showed no clinical signs of atherosclerosis or of any altered functional response in the vessels.

Thus acetylcholine, which dilates vessels by releasing a vasorelaxant from the endothelium, points up the impairment in the coronary arteries of heart transplant patients. The assessment of endothelial dysfunction may aid in early detection of coronary artery disease in these patients.

▶ This very interesting study illustrates further the reactivity of coronary arteries in cardiac allografts. The observation of widespread endothelial dysfunction suggests the possibility that coronary artery spasm perhaps occurring diffusely may be more common than is currently suspected in cardiac transplant recipients.—J.J. Collins, Jr., M.D.

General Cardiac Surgical Problems

Successful Treatment of Right Ventricular Failure With Atrial Septostomy
Swanson MJ, Fabaz AG, Jung JY (Ingham Med Ctr, Lansing, Mich)
Chest 92:950–952, November 1987   5–47

Perioperative right ventricular failure is a difficult surgical problem and carries with it a high mortality. It is necessary to both decompress the acutely failing ventricle and improve the systemic circulation.

A patient with severe right ventricular failure after coronary revascularization was weaned from cardiopulmonary bypass after an atrial septal defect was created. The procedure shunted blood to the more compliant left ventricle, decompressing the failing right ventricle and augmenting left ventricular preload. Cardiac output increased as a result. Progressive hemodynamic improvement took place as right-to-left intracardiac shunting declined and arterial hypoxemia resolved.

Global ischemic insult may be the most frequent cause of acute right ventricular failure. It may be secondary to inadequate myocardial protection, fibrillation, embolism of the right coronary artery, acute graft occlusion volume overloading, or reperfusion injury. An interatrial septal defect can relieve experimental right ventricular strain and has been used in certain congenital cardiac disorders. A flow-directed pulmonary artery catheter may facilitate hemodynamic management. The potential risks of a residual septal defect and paradoxical embolism must be balanced against the risks of right ventricular failure.

▶ When the only other option is use of a pulmonary artery balloon, creation of an atrial septal defect for relief of right ventricular failure seems a reasonable alternative. A small atrial septal defect may be enough. The hazard of paradoxical embolization should be greatest during the first several days while right ventricular failure continues. Later, however, there may be minimal danger, and it is entirely possible that closure of the defect will not always be necessary.— J.J. Collins, Jr., M.D.

Pericardial Flap Prevents Sternal Wound Complications
Nugent WC, Maislen EL, O'Connor GT, Marrin CAS, Plume SK (Dartmouth–Hitchcock Med Ctr, Hanover, NH)
Arch Surg 123:636–639, May 1988   5–48

As proposed by Flege, interposition of vascularized tissue between the heart and sternum after cardiac operation might prevent sternal dehiscence and mediastinitis. A pericardial flap based on the right pleuroperi-cardial reflection was used for this study. The flap is draped over the right ventricle at the end of the procedure; no attempt is made to close the pericardium laterally.

Before this flap procedure was started, wound dehiscence or mediastinitis occurred in 2.7% of 952 cardiac surgery patients. When 2 surgeons subsequently used the flap technique in 226 of 270 patients, none had mediastinitis or sternal wound dehiscence. However, mediastinitis developed in 3 of 100 patients operated on conventionally. There were no specific complications from construction of the pericardial flap.

Routine use of a pericardial flap facilitates sternal healing after cardiac surgery and prevents mediastinitis. The flap protects the heart should repeat sternotomy be necessary. In addition, it facilitates use of the internal mammary artery as a bypass conduit, and it helps protect the right internal mammary artery when placed anteriorly.

▶ This relatively simple procedure may not only be efficacious in preventing sternal wound complications but may make subsequent sternotomy a safer procedure. Corroboration of the effectiveness of this procedure in preventing sternal wound complications would be valuable.—J.J. Collins, Jr., M.D.

Should the Temperature Chart Influence Management in Cardiac Operations? Result of a Prospective Study in 314 Patients
Wilson APR, Treasure T, Grüneberg RN, Sturridge MF, Burridge J (Univ College, London)
J Thorac Cardiovasc Surg 96:518–523, October 1988   5–49

The relation between infection and fever after cardiac surgery was examined by analyzing postoperative temperatures of 314 patients in a prospective trial of antibiotic prophylaxis. The drugs used were teicoplanin, tobramycin, flucloxicillin, and tobramycin. Temperatures were recorded every 6 hours for 1 week after surgery.

The duration of postoperative temperature elevation was correlated with both the length of bypass and the presence of lower respiratory tract infection. However, neither surgical sepsis nor urinary tract infection was consistently associated with the duration or degree of postoperative fever. All patients had a marked temperature rise immediately after surgery. Temperatures were higher after coronary artery surgery than after valve operations.

A rise in temperature after cardiac surgery is not a reliable sign of infection. It must be interpreted in light of the clinical findings, laboratory results, and the duration of cardiopulmonary bypass.

▶ In an era when complex postoperative monitoring is commonplace to say the least, it is refreshing to see that research continues into the significance of body temperature after operations involving cardiopulmonary bypass. The conclusion that early postoperative fever is not associated with a higher incidence of late infection is in keeping with the experience of most cardiac surgeons.—J.J. Collins, Jr., M.D.

Thoracic Surgery Manpower: The Fourth Manpower Study of Thoracic Surgery: 1985 Report of the Ad Hoc Committee on Manpower of The American Association for Thoracic Surgery and The Society of Thoracic Surgeons
Loop FD, Wilcox BR, Cunningham JN Jr, Fosburg RG, Geha AS, Laks H, Mark JBD, Badhwar K, Williams GW (Cleveland Clinic Found)
Ann Thorac Surg 44:450–461, November 1987   5–50

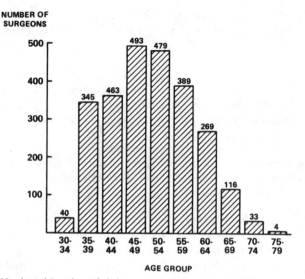

Fig 5–26.—Number of Board-certified thoracic surgeons in active practice by age group in 1985. (Courtesy of Loop FD, Wilcox BR, Cunningham JN Jr, et al: *Ann Thorac Surg* 44:450–461, November 1987.)

Responses from questionnaires given to 2,657 active, board-certified thoracic surgeons concerning their practices were compared with those obtained in manpower surveys in 1976 and 1980. The most active years were 35 to 54 in the most recent survey (Fig 5–26). Fewer thoracic surgeons were practicing alone in 1985 than in past years, and their share of cardiac operations has continued to decline. Older surgeons perform more major general thoracic operations, but the reverse is the case for cardiac operations.

There are fewer general thoracic and cardiac operations per surgeon in the western United States than in the central and eastern regions (Fig 5–27). Fewer cardiac operations per surgeon are done in smaller than in larger population areas. Nearly 1,800 heart transplantations were reported. More than half the respondents thought their level of clinical activity was about right, and only 3% responded that their workload was too heavy.

About 160 residents are trained annually. A preponderance of the program directors questioned believe that too many are being trained. They

Responses to Questions About Manpower and Education			
Question	Yes	No	Uncertain
Training too many	78	15	14
Decrease no. of trainees	74	22	11
Lengthen residency	65	38	4

(Courtesy of Loop FD, Wilcox BR, Cunningham JN Jr, et al: *Ann Thorac Surg* 44:450–461, November 1987.)

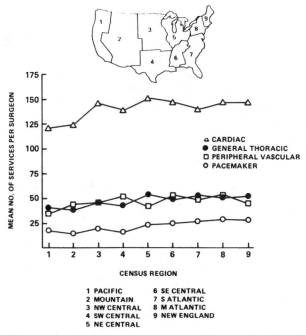

Fig 5–27.—Mean number of procedures per surgeon according to region (zip code). Included are Board-certified thoracic surgeons who reported number of operations for cardiac surgery, general thoracic surgery, peripheral vascular surgery, or pacemaker procedures. (Courtesy of Loop FD, Wilcox BR, Cunningham JN Jr, et al: *Ann Thorac Surg* 44:450–461, November 1987.)

also reported that they believe residency programs should be lengthened (table).

Predictions of thoracic surgery manpower should be made cautiously because the field is changing so rapidly. Safer treatment now is possible for elderly and high-risk patients, including those for whom reoperation is considered. Emerging technologies for valve repair and complex revascularization will ensure a continuing increase in surgical volume. In addition, coronary balloon angioplasty, alone or combined with interventions for myocardial infarction, is likely to increase the number of operations.

▶ Somewhere within this compilation of data lie significant facts and trendsupon which future plans should be based. Although some of the information is inaccurate (number of cardiac transplants performed), the numbers in general appear reasonable and defensible. The authors should be congratulated not only for accumulating the data but for their discussion of the various opinions prevalent regarding quality of training, number of trainees, and future needs for both general thoracic and cardiac surgery. It is incumbent upon leaders in the speciality, particularly those directly associated with training and certification, to recognize those changes that are inevitable and to emphasize desirable trends while attempting to suppress those that would not be in the best interest of patients. Wisdom and courage are necessary.—J.J. Collins, Jr., M.D.

6 Hypertension

Introduction

In 1988, some major changes in the way we diagnose and treat hypertension were formalized and made "official" in the publication of the Fourth Joint National Committee report, reviewed as Abstract 6–1. These changes have been slowly evolving, but their acceptance seems to have suddenly accelerated. They reflect both the availability of more knowledge and a greater willingness to make some changes in the way we manage what has become the major single indication for visits to physicians and the use of prescription drugs: the management of hypertension.

In association with these changes in clinical practice, there have been some significant advances in the basic understanding of what is responsible for the initiation of hypertension and the ways in which hypertension leads to trouble. All in all, it has been an interesting year: no major breakthroughs but lots of new insights and ideas that should translate into better care of millions of people.

To examine the 50 papers that can be included in this section. I have divided them into 5 main sections, with some subdivisions: (1) diagnosis; (2) pathophysiology; (3) nondrug therapy; (4) drug therapy; and (5) secondary forms. Before going into the specifics, let us examine the Fourth Joint National Committee report, which serves as a useful overview of the entire area.

N.M. Kaplan, M.D.

The 1988 Report of the Joint National Committee on Detection, Evaluation, and Treatment of High Blood Pressure
1988 Joint National Committee (Natl High Blood Pressure Education Program, Bethesda, Md)
Arch Intern Med 148:1023–1038, May 1988   6–1

Nearly 60 million persons in the United States have elevated blood pressure or are on antihypertensive medication. The risk of cardiovascular complications increases with the levels of both systolic and diastolic blood pressure. The goal of treatment is to maintain the arterial pressure at less than 140/90 mm Hg. Nonpharmacologic measures for lowering the blood pressure include weight reduction, the avoidance of alcohol and tobacco, and sodium restriction. Biofeedback and relaxation techniques may be helpful, as is regular aerobic exercise. The role of modifying dietary fat intake remains uncertain.

Drug therapy is warranted when the diastolic pressure is consistently greater than 94 mm Hg, or when risk factors such as male sex, smoking, or hyperlipidemia are present. Initial drug treatment is to be chosen from 4 classes of drugs: thiazide diuretic, β-blocker, calcium entry blocker, or angiotensin converting enzyme inhibitor. If necessary the dose may be raised, another type of agent may be added, or the initial choice may be replaced by a drug of another class (Fig 6–1). Drug treatment may be reduced in stepwise manner if hypertension is controlled for at least a year. Refractory hypertension due to varying causes (table) may require

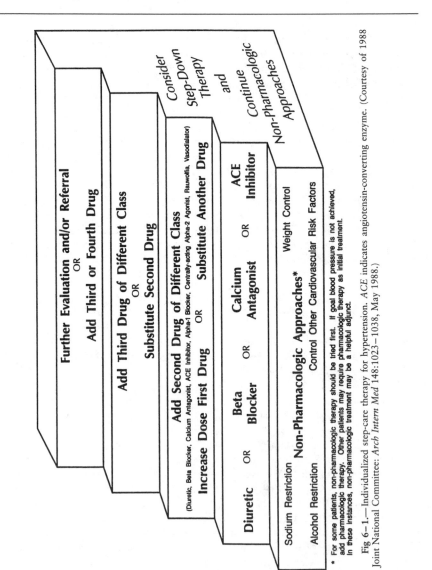

Fig 6–1.— Individualized step-care therapy for hypertension. ACE indicates angiotensin-converting enzyme. (Courtesy of 1988 Joint National Committee: *Arch Intern Med* 148:1023–1038, May 1988.)

Causes of Refractory Hypertension

```
Nonadherence to therapy
Drug-related
  Doses too low
  Inappropriate combinations (e.g., 2 centrally acting
    adrenergic inhibitors)
  Rapid inactivation (e.g., hydralazine)
  Effects of other drugs
    Sympathomimetics
    Antidepressants
    Adrenal steroids
    Nonsteroidal anti-inflammatory drugs
    Nasal decongestants
    Oral contraceptives
Associated conditions
  Increasing obesity
  Excess alcohol intake: >30 ml/day (1 oz/day)
  Renal insufficiency
  Renovascular hypertension
  Malignant or accelerated hypertension
  Other causes of hypertension
Volume overload
  Inadequate diuretic therapy
  Excess sodium intake
  Fluid retention from reduction of blood pressure
  Progressive renal damage
```

(Courtesy of 1988 Joint National Committee: *Arch Intern Med* 148:1023–1038, May 1988.)

patients to tolerate some adverse drug effects, or studies of renin may be appropriate.

The appropriate follow-up interval for treated patients should be individualized. Pressures are recorded in both the standing and the supine or sitting positions. The physician and patient should agree on a blood pressure goal. Patients should incorporate treatment into their daily life-styles and self-monitor their blood pressure. A simple treatment regimen and proper instructions will promote compliance. Relatively inexpensive treatment also is helpful.

► This fourth report of the Joint National Committee is a vast improvement over the previous 3, largely reflecting the acceptance of a broader, yet more conservative approach toward the treatment of hypertension. As a member of this and the third committee, I can attest to the thoroughness and deliberation that goes into the preparation of these reports.

My major concern is that it does not advocate as much of a change from past practice as it should. The report is the consensus of a 15-person committee and therefore must reflect a wide spectrum of beliefs. Moreover, there is a legitimate concern not to call for too many changes too quickly, lest some be upset by the call for so many moves away from current practice as to be disruptive.

Nonetheless, I would have preferred a number of additions and subtractions, including removal of the term *step care,* which not only stays in the text but is the obvious approach portrayed in the step-ladder figure (see Fig 6–1), and the use of a term such as *individualized* to describe the overall approach. Even more choices for initial therapy and a more accepting attitude toward ambulatory monitoring of the blood pressure seem appropriate. However, I do not want to sound hypercritical or too picky: this report is, overall, a sensible, reasonable, and practical guide to improved management of hypertension. It should be read by all practitioners.—N.M. Kaplan, M.D.

Diagnosis

▶ ↓ First, we will look at the current status of hypertension management in one area in the United States. Then we will explore some of the issues in diagnosis.—N.M. Kaplan, M.D.

A Community Blood Pressure Survey: Rochester, Minnesota, 1986
Phillips SJ, Whisnant JP, O'Fallon WM, Hickman RD (Mayo Clinic, Rochester, Minn; Iowa State Univ)
Mayo Clin Proc 63:691–699, July 1988   6–2

Better control of hypertension is credited with being the factor most responsible for the decrease in incidence of stroke in Rochester, Minnesota, in 1945–1979. Prevalence and control of hypertension were studied in a random sample of 2,122 subjects aged 35 and older in Rochester. Hypertension was defined as a history of hypertension, or a systolic pressure of 160 mm Hg or greater or a diastolic pressure of 95 mm Hg or greater, or both, at the time of interview.

Thirty-one percent of the subjects surveyed were hypertensive, and 12% of them had no past history of hypertension. Of those with a history, 77% were taking antihypertensive medication. More than one fifth of the patients had a systolic pressure of 160 mm Hg or more or a diastolic pressure of 95 mm Hg or more, or both. Half of the patients had systolic pressures of 140 mm Hg or greater or diastolic pressures of 90 mm Hg or greater, or both. Three fourths of treated patients with hypertension were taking a diuretic, alone or in combination with other drugs. Side effects were described by 12% of treated patients.

The findings of other community studies of blood pressure cannot be directly compared with the Rochester data. In any case, such comparisons are less informative than correlating improved blood pressure control with changes in hypertension-associated events in a given community.

▶ Statisticians and clinicians at the Mayo Clinic have an excellent handle on the health status of the residents of Rochester, Minnesota. This carefully performed survey demonstrates the excellent status of both the recognition and treatment of hypertension in this community, with 88% of those found to have hypertension already having been identified as hypertensive and 77% of them on medication.

The rest of the world likely is not doing as well as the residents of Rochester. We have long been aware of the lesser extent of detection and treatment among the economically deprived. This extends beyond African-Americans and Hispanics: Asians in California are also less aware and less treated, partly because of poverty and partly because of less availability of health care (1).

The need for greater certainty that the blood pressure is elevated at all times (except during sleep) and under most circumstances has become increasingly important as millions of people with minimally elevated pressures are being considered for lifelong therapy. In Framingham, over 80% of hypertensive men and women aged 60 to 89 were receiving antihypertensive drug therapy during 1979–1981 (2).

With the realization that antihypertensive drug therapy may be life-saving, we also need to be sure we are not exposing many people to unnecessary and potentially harmful overmedication. As will be described in Abstract 6–25, in the same Framingham population, men receiving antihypertensive therapy had more than twice the risk of sudden death than those not on therapy, a risk that could not be attributed to other predisposing factors for sudden death (3).

The need for greater care in diagnosis, then, is obvious, as further documented in the following study of "white coat hypertension."—N.M. Kaplan, M.D.

References

1. Stavig GR, Igra A, Leonard AR: Hypertension and related health issues among Asians and Pacific Islanders in California. *Public Health Rep* 103:28–37, 1988.
2. Dannenberg AL, Garrison RJ, Kannel WB: Incidence of hypertension in the Framingham study. *Am J Public Health* 78:676–679, 1988.
3. Kannel WB, Cupples LA, D'Agostino RB, et al: Hypertension, antihypertensive treatment, and sudden coronary death: The Framingham study. *Hypertension* 11(Suppl II):II-45–II-50, 1988.

How Common Is White Coat Hypertension?
Pickering TG, James GD, Boddie C, Harshfield GA, Blank S, Laragh JH (New York Hosp–Cornell Univ Med Ctr)
JAMA 259:225–228, Jan 8, 1988   6–3

A physician visit may provoke an increase in blood pressure. "White coat" hypertensives are those subjects who have elevated blood pressure at the clinic but normal pressures at other times. The authors studied 37 normotensive subjects and 292 with borderline hypertension, whose average clinic diastolic pressure was 90–104 mm Hg. Forty-two patients with established hypertension also were studied. None were on antihypertensive medication at the time of study.

Twenty-one percent of borderline hypertensive patients and 5% of those with established hypertension had ambulatory pressures in the normal range, using the 90th centile value of the awake pressure distribution in normotensive persons as a cutoff. Females, younger subjects, and those with more recent diagnoses were most likely to have "white coat" hypertension. A generalized increase in pressure lability was not evident in these subjects, nor was the pressor response while at work exaggerated.

White coat hypertension is more frequent when blood pressure is recorded by a physician than by a technician. The persistence of the phenomenon in some cases suggests that anxiety is not the sole explanation. It may be a conditioned response after initial examination reveals elevated pressure secondary to anxiety or the "orienting reflex." Sympathetic arousal increases the blood pressure on subsequent visits, and the phenomenon is reinforced as a classically conditioned response.

▶ The answer to the question raised in the title of this article is about 21%. This is a lovely demonstration of a major problem in clinical practice: the overdiagnosis of hypertension by dependency upon only office readings of the blood pressure, particularly when they are taken by a white-coated physician. Note that the problem is not that of first or second readings, which are almost always higher than subsequent ones and which, for most patients, mandate multiple sets of readings over at least a 3-month period before deciding upon the diagnosis and the need for therapy. The patients in this study had been found to have persistent office hypertension over an average duration of 6 years.

The solution to the problem: have your patient take home readings with one or another of the inexpensive ($50–$75) semiautomatic devices that do not require use of a stethoscope or reading of a gauge. Automatic monitoring over a single 24-hour interval (as used by Pickering et al.) may also give good information more quickly.

There is an obvious need for 24-hour monitoring in assessing the response to antihypertensive therapy both for the degree and the duration. Weber et al. (1) found that 6 of 15 patients chosen for a trial of a calcium-entry blocker on the basis of office diastolic readings greater than 95 mm Hg were not hypertensive during 24-hour monitoring. Not surprising, they showed almost no response to the drug. The technique will find increasing use both for diagnosis and for assessing therapy. Another special need for a device that is not dependent on the loudness of Korotkoff sounds is the recognition of pseudohypertension in the elderly.— N.M. Kaplan, M.D.

Reference

1. Weber MA, Cheung DG, Graettinger WF, et al: Characterization of antihypertensive therapy by whole day blood pressure monitoring. *JAMA* 259:3281–3285, 1988.

Screening for Pseudohypertension: A Quantitative, Noninvasive Approach
Hla KM, Feussner JR (Duke Univ; VA Med Ctr, Durham, NC)
Arch Intern Med 148:673–676, March 1988   6–4

Cuff blood pressure measurements may overestimate true pressure in some elderly patients, leading to unneeded or excessive treatment. Direct intra-arterial diastolic pressure measurements were compared with both indirect cuff estimates and automatic infrasonic recorder (IR) blood pressure measurements in 36 hypertensive men aged 60 and older. A receiver operating characteristic curve was used to determine whether a difference between cuff and IR diastolic pressures identified patients likely to have pseudohypertension, defined by a cuff–intra-arterial pressure difference of at least 10 mm Hg.

Mean diastolic blood pressure was 85 mm Hg by cuff; 80 mm Hg by the IR method; and 76.5 mm Hg intra-arterially. A cuff–IR difference cutoff of 4 mm Hg, derived from the receiver operating characteristic curve, correctly identified 13 of the 14 patients with pseudohypertension. Of 22 patients having a cuff–intra-arterial difference of less than 10 mm Hg, 14 were correctly identified using the 4-mm Hg cutoff. This cutoff value was 93% sensitive and 64% specific for pseudohypertension and had positive and negative predictive values of 62% and 93%, respectively.

The IR is an accurate noninvasive substitute for intra-arterial pressure measurements. A difference of 4 mm Hg or more between cuff and IR diastolic pressure estimates identifies a majority of patients with pseudohypertension. The IR may be the best means of screening elderly patients and of monitoring their response to antihypertensive therapy.

▶ The stiffer vessels in older people are responsible for a greater amount of blood pressure variability (1). And the stiffness may become so great within atherosclerotic, calcified arteries that the pressure in the balloon simply is not transmitted to the inside of the vessels; thus, the not uncommon finding of higher routine cuff readings in the elderly, i.e., pseudohypertension. Until now, the only way to exclude pseudohypertension has been with invasive intra-arterial measurements. The study by Hla and Feussner shows that a device, the Infrasonde, which infrasonically measures the subaudible oscillations in the arterial wall under the cuff will give readings as accurate as intra-arterial measurements.

For most situations wherein multiple readings are needed over a short interval, either to establish the level of blood pressure under usual life circumstances or to assess the efficacy and duration of therapy, an automatic ambulatory blood pressure monitor will increasingly be used. As shown in the next abstract, the technique, when used appropriately, is cost-effective.—N.M. Kaplan, M.D.

Effect of Ambulatory Blood Pressure Monitoring on the Diagnosis and Cost of Treatment for Mild Hypertension
Krakoff LR, Eison H, Phillips RH, Leiman SJ, Lev S (City Univ of New York)
Am Heart J 116:1152–1154, October 1988 6–5

Clinical trials of therapy for mild hypertension identified in screening programs have demonstrated that the average blood pressure (BP) in a substantial number of patients is actually not elevated. This finding underlines the need for more precise early identification of persons whose BPs are likely to remain elevated after the initial screening period.

In this study, noninvasive ambulatory BP monitoring was used to evaluate 60 patients, aged 18 to 68 years, in whom mild hypertension had been detected on 2 or more occasions and who had been advised to start antihypertensive drug treatment. In each patient, ambulatory monitoring was performed either before treatment or at least 2 months after withdrawal of drug therapy, on a day of typical activity. Blood pressure measurements were made every 20 to 30 minutes from 6:00 A.M. to midnight, and every 60 minutes from midnight to 6:00 A.M.

Average ambulatory systolic and diastolic pressures were significantly lower in the entire study group than were casual pressures. Of the 60 evaluated patients, 45% had average ambulatory systolic pressures of less than 130 mm Hg, 60% had average diastolic pressures of less than 85 mm Hg, and 38% had average systolic and diastolic pressures of less than 130/85 mm Hg. There was no significant correlation between casual and average ambulatory pressures.

A preliminary evaluation of the cost-effectiveness of ambulatory BP monitoring showed that nearly 38% of those initially labeled as hypertensive had average ambulatory pressures low enough to permit observation without drug treatment. Thus, the cost of ambulatory monitoring would be largely offset by the cost savings of not providing antihypertensive treatment (Fig 6–2).

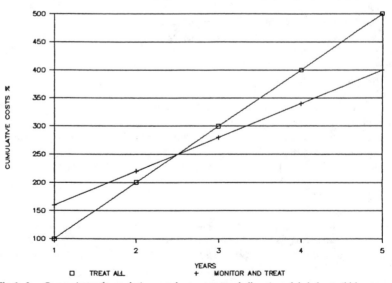

Fig 6–2.—Comparison of cumulative cost for treatment of all patients labeled as mild hypertensive to cost for initial ambulatory blood pressure monitoring and treatment of those persons whose blood pressure is no greater than 130/85 mm Hg (60%). Results are expressed as percentage of cumulative costs at end of each year of treatment. (Courtesy of Krakoff LR, Eison H, Phillips RH, et al: *Am Heart J* 116:1152–1154, October 1988.)

Ambulatory BP monitoring may direct antihypertensive therapy to patients with confirmed elevated average BP measurements and eliminate those with confirmed normal average BP. Aggressive treatment of patients with true hypertension might more effectively reduce long-term cardiovascular morbidity than large-scale treatment of all patients identified as hypertensive in casual screening programs.

▶ Legitimate concern has been expressed over the costs of promiscuous use of automatic ambulatory blood pressure monitoring. But, as analyzed by Krakoff et al., when it is done in patients with fairly mild hypertension, enough of them will be found not to be hypertensive—and thereby be saved perhaps from lifelong expenses of therapy—that it clearly can save overall costs.

Beyond the need to ensure accuracy in detecting hypertension, there is an even greater need to prevent it. This must start in childhood wherein the pathophysiology has its beginning.—N.M. Kaplan, M.D.

Pathophysiology

Persistent Elevation of Blood Pressure Among Children With a Family History of Hypertension: The Minneapolis Children's Blood Pressure Study
Munger RG, Prineas RJ, Gomez-Marin O (Univ of Minnesota)
J Hypertens 6:647–653, August 1988   6–6

The clustering of hypertension in families is a well-known phenomenon of which the causes are not well understood. Although genetic factors are often cited as important to familial aggregation of high blood pressure, environmental factors are considered to be a major contributing factor. However, most studies of risk factors among children in familial hypertension have been cross-sectional, and the emergence of hypertension in children with or without a positive family history has not been studied. This longitudinal study examined and tracked the systolic blood pressure levels of children with and without a family history of hypertension.

Of 10,423 school-age children who underwent blood pressure screening in 1978, 2,641 children aged 6–8 years were selected for this study. Home interviews were conducted with 1,509 children and their parents during which supine blood pressure, anthropometric measurements, and overnight urine samples were obtained. All parents completed demographic, medical history, socioeconomic, recent life-event, and psychologic questionnaires. Supine blood pressure levels were measured in the children on 9 more occasions over an 8-year study period.

Children with a family history of hypertension had a higher mean systolic blood pressure at the first screening than children without such a family history. This difference persisted at each of the succeeding 9 school visits. In hypertensive families, the parents had a lower income and greater body weight, were less well-educated, and were more likely to be black than parents in families without a family history of hypertension. The blood pressure correlations between mothers and their children

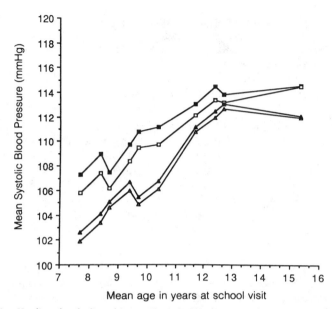

Fig 6–3.—Unadjusted and adjusted means of systolic blood pressure of girls in hypertensive and normotensive families, measured over 10 school visits. ■, hypertensive families, unadjusted means; □, hypertensive families, adjusted means; ▲, normotensive families, adjusted means; △, normotensive families, unadjusted means. (Courtesy of Munger RG, Prineas RJ, Gomez-Marin O: *J Hypertension* 6:647–653, August 1988.)

were generally greater than between fathers and their children. After 12 years of age, the pattern of increase in adjusted mean systolic blood pressure with age differed for boys and girls. Boys showed a continuous linear increase in systolic blood pressure between the ages of 8 and 16 years, whereas the rate of increase in systolic blood pressure among girls lessened between the ages of 13 and 16 years (Fig 6–3).

Elevation in systolic blood pressure of children from hypertensive families is apparent well before puberty and is continued during adolescent growth spurt. The family environment appears to play an important role in the development of familial hypertension.

▶ As seen in Figure 6–3, even very young daughters of hypertensive parents have higher pressures than do children of normotensive patients. Even greater differences were seen in boys. Obviously, children of hypertensive parents need to be advised of the need to avoid obesity and high sodium intake and to keep under appropriate surveillance.

The need for preventive measures and surveillance apparently extend beyond the children of hypertensive parents: an increased risk of hypertension was noted among a group of young men whose weight at birth was small for their gestational ages (1). So it appears that the sins of the parents are passed on to the child.

Beyond being born small or to a hypertensive parent, there are a number of other predictors for the development of hypertension. One may be an exaggerated pressor response to exercise.—N.M. Kaplan, M.D.

Reference

1. Gennser G, Rymark P, Isberg PE: Low birth weight and risk of high blood pressure in adulthood. *Br Med J* 296:1498–1500, 1988.

Exaggerated Systolic Blood Pressure Response to Exercise: A Normal Variant or Hyperdynamic Phase of Essential Hypertension?
Iskandrian AS, Heo J (Hahnemann Univ)
Int J Cardiol 18:207–217, 1988   6–7

Some patients without a history of hypertension and with resting normotension have an exaggerated systolic pressure response to exercise. It is not clear whether this is caused by high cardiac output or to excessively increased total vascular resistance. Left ventricular function was studied by first-pass nuclide angiography at rest and on symptom-limited exercise in 27 normal subjects, in 25 subjects with a systolic pressure exceeding 200 mm Hg on exercise, and in 25 patients with essential hypertension and no coronary artery disease.

The subjects with exercise hypertension had a higher exercise cardiac index than the control normotensive subjects, but there were no differences in vascular resistance, left ventricular ejection fraction, end-systolic volume, or heart rate. Exercise tolerance was similar in the 2 groups. Compared with patients having essential hypertension, the exercise responders had a higher exercise heart rate, cardiac index, systolic pressure, and left ventricular ejection fraction. Total vascular resistance and end-systolic volume on exercise were lower in the exercise responders.

Subjects with an exaggerated systolic blood pressure response to exercise differ hemodynamically from patients having essential hypertension. The response therefore may reflect a supernormal adaptation to exercise. These subjects may pursue a normal life-style, including competitive activities, and need not be given antihypertensive drugs. Follow-up is warranted to determine whether left ventricular hypertrophy develops in these subjects.

▶ This study examines a phenomenon that is being increasingly recognized as more and more healthy people are having exercise stress tests: an exaggerated rise in blood pressure despite normal blood pressure at rest. Hypertension appears to develop in more of such people than in those who do not have exercise-induced rises, as reviewed by Jetté et al. (1). Moreover, an exaggerated blood pressure response to exercise has been seen more commonly among normotensive adolescents with a family history of hypertension, who are at increased risk of hypertension (2), so it really may turn out to have significant predictive value. Nonetheless, most with such a response have not yet been noted to have hypertension, so my advice is: first, do not do stress tests on asymptomatic people; second, as Iskandrian and Heo state, do not restrict such people from exercise or call them "prehypertensive." The better course would be to encourage a regular aerobic exercise program that will likely reduce the blood pressure.

The next abstract examines others potential predictors.—N.M. Kaplan, M.D.

References

1. Jette M, Landry F, Sidney K, et al: Exaggerated blood pressure response to exercise in the detection of hypertension. *J Cardiopulmonary Rehabil* 8:171–177, 1988.
2. Molineux D, Steptoe A: Exaggerated blood pressure responses to submaximal exercise in normotensive adolescents with a family history of hypertension. *J Hypertension* 6:361–365, 1988.

Race and Sex Differences in the Correlates of Blood Pressure Change
Daniels SR, Heiss G, Davis CE, Hames CG, Tyroler HA (Univ of North Carolina; Children's Hosp Med Ctr, Cincinnati)
Hypertension 11:249–255, March 1988   6–8

Previous longitudinal studies have shown that the initial level of blood pressure, baseline weight, change in weight, baseline skinfold thickness, body mass index, baseline hematocrit, and age are correlated with changes in blood pressure over time. However, these studies were done in white men who were normotensive at the beginning of the study. In the present longitudinal study the differences in the correlates of changes in blood pressure were measured among the 4 major race-sex groups, with patients representing the entire range of blood pressure at inifiation of the study.

Between 1960 and 1962, 3,102 individuals drawn from a biracial community in Evans County, Georgia, received a complete medical examination. Between 1967 and 1969, 2,530 (81%) of these were reexamined. Data obtained at both survey points included systolic and diastolic blood pressure, age, height, weight, hematocrit, serum level of cholesterol, and socioeconomic status. The Quetelet index of body mass was determined in both phases of the study for each subject. Socioeconomic status was measured with the McGuire-White index.

In white men the level of systolic blood pressure, age, and change in Quetelet index were significant correlates for systolic change, whereas age, change in hematocrit, and change in Quetelet index were significant correlates for diastolic change. In white women the level and change in socioeconomic status, change in Quetelet index and change in cholesterol were significant correlates for systolic change, whereas age, level and change in socioeconomic status, level and change in Quetelet index and change in hematocrit were significant correlates for diastolic change. The level of Quetelet index was of only borderline significance when the other significant variables were included in the model for white women.

In black men the change in Quetelet index and age were the only significant correlates for systolic change. In black women only age was a significant correlate for diastolic change.

The results indicate there may be important differences in these correlates between race-sex groups and thus in the mechanism of blood pressure change for different race-sex groups.

▶ Although fewer of these features were correlated with a rise in blood pressure in blacks, the blacks started with significantly higher blood pressures so that they could have already experienced the deleterious effects of weight gain, rise in serum cholesterol, etc.

Regardless, blacks have more hypertension than whites of comparable age, sex, weight, etc. And, as nicely reviewed by Gillum (1), they suffer from strokes at a rate 2.5 times greater than that for whites. Fortunately, improved control of hypertension has reduced their stroke mortality.

Part of the greater propensity for hypertension to develop in blacks may be related to a heightened level of stress and suppressed anger invoked by the discriminations they suffer as a minority group that has long been denied equal access. Blacks or nonblacks who cope with anger by conscious inhibition of its expression tend to have more hypertension (2). Blacks put through stresses in a laboratory have greater rises in blood pressure than do nonblacks (3), and blacks are more sensitive to the pressor effects of infused norepinephrine (4).

In a more obvious manner, people who suffer from severe anxiety attacks may have striking rises in blood pressure.—N.M. Kaplan, M.D.

References

1. Gillum RF: Stroke in blacks. *Stroke* 19:1−9, 1988.
2. Goldstein HS, Edelberg R, Meier CF, et al: Relationship of resting blood pressure and heart rate to experienced anger and expressed anger. *Psychosom Med* 50:321−329, 1988.
3. Light KC, Obrist PA, Sherwood A, et al: Effects of race and marginally elevated blood pressure on responses to stress. *Hypertension* 10:555−563, 1987.
4. Dimsdale JE, Graham RM, Ziegler MG, et al: Age, race, diagnosis, and sodium effects on the pressor response to infused norepinephrine. *Hypertension* 10:564−569, 1987.

Heart Rate and Blood Pressure During Placebo-Associated Panic Attacks
Balon R, Ortiz A, Pohl R, Yeragani VK (Lafayette Clinic, Detroit; Wayne State Univ; St Joseph Hosp, Mt Clemens, Mich)
Psychosom Med 50:434−438, 1988   6−9

The heart rate increases during spontaneous panic attacks. Heart rate and blood pressure also change in lactate-induced attacks, but these changes are influenced by the cardiovascular effects of lactate. Sodium lactate, isoproterenol, or dextrose was infused into each of 86 patients with panic disorder. Fourteen patients panicked during the dextrose infusion. All the patients were actively symptomatic, averaging 1 or more panic attacks a week.

Patients who panicked had higher baseline Panic Disorder Scale (PDS) scores. They also had higher heart rate and higher systolic blood pressure measurements than patients who did not panic. Baseline and peak PDS scores were correlated significantly in nonpanickers but not in patients who panicked.

Significant increases in heart rate and blood pressure are observed in patients with panic disorder during a dextrose-associated panic attack. However, these effects do not reliably reflect the increase in anxiety as measured by the PDS.

▶ The blood pressure usually rises during anxiety-induced hyperventilation episodes and, to an even greater degree, overt panic attacks. Clinicians often do not recognize the multiple manifestations of acute hyperventilation, including headaches, dizziness, chest pain, and paresthesias, along with tachycardia and an elevated blood pressure.

Panic attacks should be easier to recognize but, here again, we often fail to recognize their effect on the blood pressure. This study examines the mechanisms involved.

Another common problem may also be a common precursor of hypertension: sleep apnea. Among 372 snorers, obesity, obstructive sleep apnea, and nocturnal hypoxia were more common and these, in turn, were associated with more hypertension (1).

Heredity, stress, and obesity are 3 of the more obvious factors involved in the propensity toward hypertension. Another than keeps recurring is high sodium intake.—N.M. Kaplan, M.D.

Reference

1. Hoffstein V, Mateika S, Rubinstein I, et al: Determinants of blood pressure in snorers. *Lancet* 2:992–994, 1988.

Intersalt: An International Study of Electrolyte Excretion and Blood Pressure: Results for 24 Hour Urinary Sodium and Potassium Excretion
Intersalt Cooperative Research Group
Br Med J 297:319–328, July 30, 1988   6–10

Studies of isolated populations generally have shown a linear relation between sodium intake and blood pressure. Urinary electrolyte excretion was related to blood pressure in 10,079 men and women aged 20–59 years at 52 centers worldwide. Observers were centrally trained, and a central laboratory was utilized. The results of regression analyses done at each center were pooled.

Sodium excretion varied widely from 0.2 mM/24 hours in Brazil to 242 mM/24 hours in China. Urinary sodium excretion was correlated significantly with blood pressure in individual subjects within centers. At 4 centers there was very low sodium excretion as well as low blood pressure and little or no upward slope of blood pressure on age. At the other 48 centers, sodium excretion was significantly related to the slope of

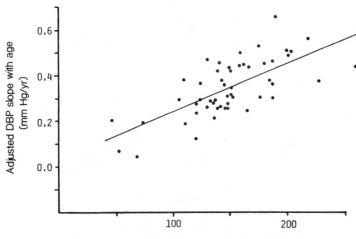

Fig 6–4.—Cross center plot of diastolic blood pressure slope with age and median sodium excretion and fitted regression lines also adjusted for body mass index and alcohol intake (52 centers). (Courtesy of Intersalt Cooperative Research Group: *Br Med J* 297:319–328, July 30, 1988.)

blood pressure with age but not to median blood pressure or the prevalence of elevated blood pressure (Fig 6–4). Potassium excretion was correlated negatively with blood pressure in individual subjects, but across centers there was no consistent association. In individual subjects, body mass index and heavy alcohol use had strong and independent associations with blood pressure.

Sodium excretion is related significantly to blood pressure in individual subjects in the Intersalt study. The relationship is at least partly independent of body mass and alcohol intake. A lower sodium intake may favorably influence blood pressure, change in blood pressure with age, and cardiovascular mortality.

▶ The results of this massive study have been used as evidence both for and against a causal connection between high sodium intake (reflected by 24-hour sodium excretion) and hypertension. Those who use it "against" quote the lack of association between current sodium intake and current blood pressure or the prevalence of hypertension. Those who use it "for" quote the significant association between sodium intake and the rising slope of blood pressure with age as shown in Figure 6–4. I am more impressed by the latter, but then I have been a believer in the role of sodium for a long time.

The relationship is complicated in that only part of the population is "sodium-sensitive," and this appears to be a familial characteristic, supporting a genetic mechanism (1). Moreover, it may be that the chloride portion of sodium chloride is the culprit. At least in rats, NaCl raises blood pressure but $NaHCO_3$ does not (2).

Equally involved in the pathophysiology of hypertension, if not more so, is dyslipidemia.—N.M. Kaplan, M.D.

References

1. Luft FC, Miller JZ, Weinberger MH, et al: Influence of genetic variance on sodium sensitivity of blood pressure. *Klin Wochenschr* 65:101–109, 1987.
2. Luft FC, Steinberg H, Ganten U, et al: Effect of sodium chloride and sodium bicarbonate on blood pressure in stroke-prone spontaneously hypertensive rats. *Clin Sci* 74:577–585, 1988.

Familial Dyslipidemic Hypertension: Evidence From 58 Utah Families for a Syndrome Present in Approximately 12% of Patients With Essential Hypertension

Williams RR, Hunt SC, Hopkins PN, Stults BM, Wu LL, Hasstedt SJ, Barlow GK, Stephenson SH, Lalouel J-M, Kuida H (Univ of Utah)
JAMA 259:3579–3586, June 24, 1988   6–11

Epidemiologic studies have found that essential hypertension (EH) clusters in families. Therefore, pathophysiologic syndromes leading to EH may involve shared genes, shared environmental factors, or a combination of both. The initial data of an ongoing study in Utah of population-based sets of hypertensive siblings whose EH was diagnosed before age 60 are presented.

Of 222,546 living adults for whom detailed histories were collected, 24,569 (11%) had diagnoses of EH, including 12,610 (51%) whose diagnoses were made before age 60. Of these, 6,128 had at least 1 sibling who also had EH before age 60, representing 25% of all adults identified with EH. From this group, 131 subjects with EH in 58 sibships were identified as having concordant abnormalities in fasting serum lipid concentrations in 2 or more siblings. The lipid profiles of these 131 subjects were then studied in detail.

After adjusting for the effects of antihypertensive medications, lipid abnormalities in the most extreme tenth percentile were observed 3.9 times more often than expected for high-density lipoprotein cholesterol, 3.0 times more often for triglycerides, 1.9 times more often for low-density lipoprotein cholesterol, and 2.4 times more often for any of the 3 abnormalities in any given hypertensive patient. Seven sibships had abnormalities in all 3 lipid parameters, 8 sibships had abnormalities in 2 of the 3 lipid levels, and only 2 sibships were concordant for isolated high-density lipoprotein abnormalities. At least 2 sibships had concordant morbid obesity.

These data suggest an association between hypertension and a syndrome of mixed lipid abnormalities, probably familial combined hyperlipidemia. It is concluded that familial dyslipidemic hypertension may be a specific syndrome with lipid abnormalities that are more severe than the blood pressure elevations.

▶ Hypertension and hyperlipidemia are 2 of the 3 major risks factors for premature cardiovascular disease. Surveys estimate that at least 40 million Americans have hypertension, and about the same number are hypercholesterolemic. With so many having each, the coexistence of both is expected to be fairly common.

As others have suggested, the 2 coexist even more frequently than expected by chance alone. Such coexistence could reflect the contribution of obesity, diabetes, or alcohol abuse. But, as demonstrated in this lovely study from Utah, patients with elevated blood pressure who have a strong family history of hypertension and are therefore more likely to share genetic disorders, have more than twice the frequency of significant lipid abnormalities. That is more reason to be concerned about the potential hyperlipidemic effects of diuretics and some β-blockers.

The association between dyslipidemia and hypertension is so striking that there must be an explanation. There is no certainty as to what explains the association, but 1 possibility that must be strongly considered is hyperinsulinemia.—N.M. Kaplan, M.D.

Altered Erythrocyte and Plasma Sodium and Potassium in Hypertension, a Facet of Hyperinsulinemia

Halkin H, Modan M, Shefi M, Almog S (Chaim Sheba Med Ctr, Tel Hashomer, Israel)
Hypertension 11:71–77, January 1988   6–12

Because insulin mediates cell membrane cation transport, hyperinsulinemia and insulin resistance may underlie the altered internal cation distribution that characterizes the glucose intolerance, obesity, and hypertension (GOH) conditions. Red cell cations, plasma potassium, and glucose and insulin responses to oral glucose were studied in 30 nonobese normotensive subjects having normal glucose tolerance and 59 others with GOH abnormalities. In addition, serum urate and plasma triglycerides were estimated.

Internal cation imbalance was found in 88% of the patients with GOH abnormalities and 40% of controls. Insulin levels, triglycerides, and uric acid were shifted toward higher values in the GOH group. Rates of cation imbalance increased with the insulin response. Correlations with triglycerides and uric acid also were evident. Among untreated hypertensives, there were higher degrees of correlation between cation imbalance, glucose intolerance, and obesity.

Internal cation imbalance, with increased red cell sodium and decreased potassium, is associated with hyperinsulinemia in the presence or absence of GOH conditions. The findings implicate hyperinsulinemia in the cation transport abnormalities typical of these conditions. It is not clear whether this association reflects a direct role of insulin in the regulation of internal cation balance in humans.

▶ The evidence for a pivotal role of hyperinsulinemia in hypertension continues to grow. This article focuses upon the relationships between hypertension, obesity, and glucose intolerance, an area this Israeli group has explored carefully. There is increasing evidence that hyperinsulinemia is also present, along with peripheral insulin resistance, in *nonobese* hypertensives as well (1, 2). And assuming that hyperinsulinemia is contributing to the hypertension (and likely to the other complications of those with upper body obesity), there is more disturbing information from Reaven's group at Stanford: a high carbohydrate, low fat diet, as typically used to reduce caloric intake in the treatment of obesity, may further increase plasma insulin levels.—N.M. Kaplan, M.D.

References

1. Ferrannini E, Buzzigoli G, Bonadonna R, et al: Insulin resistance in essential hypertension. *N Engl J Med* 317:350–357, Aug 6, 1987.
2. Shen D-C, Shieh S-M, Fuh MM-T, et al: Resistance to insulin-stimulated-glucose uptake in patients with hypertension. *J Clin Endocrinol Metab* 66:580–583, March 1988.

Effect of a Low Fat Diet on Carbohydrate Metabolism in Patients With Hypertension
Parillo M, Coulston A, Hollenbeck C, Reaven G (Stanford Univ; VA Med Ctr, Palo Alto, Calif)
Hypertension 11:244–248, March 1988   6–13

There is increasing evidence that hypertensive patients have associated abnormalities of carbohydrate metabolism. Previous studies have shown that obesity is associated with insulin resistance and hyperinsulinemia. Lowering the blood pressure in obese individuals by physical training was correlated with associated reductions in plasma levels of insulin rather than with weight loss. Moreover, only hyperinsulinemic obese subjects showed a decrease in blood pressure after physical training. Other studies also support the view that hypertension and hyperinsulinemia are probably related.

To assess the effect of low fat, high carbohydrate diets on carbohydrate metabolism in hypertensive patients, the plasma levels of glucose and insulin were measured in 8 patients with medication-controlled hypertension and 8 normotensive volunteers during a standard 75-gm oral glucose tolerance test. In addition, plasma levels of glucose and insulin were measured at hourly intervals in response to a conventional diet that contained 40% carbohydrate. The effect of increased dietary intake of carbohydrates on ambient plasma levels of glucose and insulin was then studied in the 8 hypertensive patients by using a 2-period crossover design for a total of 30 days.

The hypertensive patients had significantly higher than normal plasma levels of glucose and insulin, compared with controls, both in response to the oral glucose challenge and after a diet that contained 40% carbohydrates. When dietary carbohydrate was further increased by 16% to 56% with a reciprocal reduction in dietary fat from 41% to 25% of total calories, the hyperglycemia and hyperinsulinemia in the hypertensive patients was exacerbated even further (Fig 6–5).

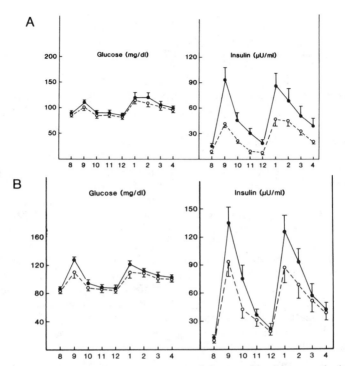

Fig 6-5.—**A,** mean (± SEM) plasma concentrations of glucose and insulin in normal subjects *(open circles)* and subjects with hypertension *(solid circles)* from 0800 to 1600 hours in response to control diet containing 19% protein, 41% fat, and 40% carbohydrate. Breakfast was eaten at 0800 (20% of daily calories) and lunch was eaten at 1200 (40% of total calories). Blood was drawn before breakfast and every hour thereafter until 1600. **B,** mean (± SEM) plasma concentrations of glucose and insulin in hypertensive subjects after 14 days of consuming either control diet *(open circles)* or low fat-high carbohydrate diet *(solid circles)* containing 19% protein, 25% fat, and 56% carbohydrate. Breakfast and lunch were eaten at same time as in **A** and percentage of calories consumed at each meal was also same. Blood was drawn at same time as in **A.** (Courtesy of Parillo M, Coulston A, Hollenbeck C, et al: *Hypertension* 11:244-248, March 1988.)

Because of the low fat, high carbohydrate diets that are commonly recommended to hypertensive patients, the associated abnormal glucose and insulin metabolism would be aggravated further. Because hyperglycemia and hyperinsulinema are risk factors for coronary heart disease, it may be prudent to reassess the clinical advisability of low fat, high carbohydrate diets in the management of hypertension.

► In view of the evidence that hyperinsulinemia may be the unifying and causal connection between obesity (in particular upper body obesity), dyslipidemia, and glucose intolerance, we do need to be careful not to inadvertently aggravate the situation further. Whatever serves as the trigger to start the hypertensive process likely causes it to persist by stimulating hypertrophy of the smooth muscle of the arterioles (1). Moreover, the thin endothelial lining of the vessels, long considered just a passive envelope, has now been recognized to play an important role.—N.M. Kaplan, M.D.

Reference

1. Heagerty AM, Izzard AS, Ollerenshaw JD, et al: Blood vessels and human essential hypertension. *Int J Cardiol* 20:15–28, 1988.

Endothelium-Dependent and Endothelium-Independent Vasodilation in Resistance Arteries From Hypertensive Rats

Tesfamariam B, Halpern W (Univ of Vermont)
Hypertension 11:440–444, May 1988   6–14

Essential hypertension has been characterized by increased peripheral vascular resistance after morphological or functional changes in the arterial wall. Whether these changes also include the endothelium and the functional coupling between endothelial and smooth muscle cells in resistance arteries has not yet been confirmed.

Acetylcholine, an endothelium-dependent vasodilator, and sodium nitroprusside, a presumed endothelium-independent vasodilator, were used to characterize relaxation responses of mesenteric resistance arteries obtained from normotensive Wistar-Kyoto rats and stroke-prone spontaneously hypertensive rats. The mesenteric arteries were preconstricted with norepinephrine or 5-hydroxytryptamine, which reduced the vessel diameters by 50% to 60%. Relaxation responses in the preconstricted arteries were obtained with a pressurized vessel technique that maintains the shape of the wall, applies a true transmural pressure to the vessel wall, and does not damage the endothelium.

Mesenteric resistance arteries from hypertensive rats were significantly less responsive to the endothelium-dependent vasodilator acetylcholine at low concentration ranges, compared with segments from normotensive control rats, but these segments relaxed to a greater extent than did vessel segments from normotensive rats at all concentrations of sodium nitroprusside. Removal of endothelium significantly enhanced sodium nitroprusside-induced dilations in each rat strain. Functional alterations in the endothelium may well play a role in hypertensive disease.

▶ This is one of a large number of recent papers attesting to an active role of the endothelium, both in dilation and constriction of the vascular bed. Of these, perhaps the most significant is the identification and complete characterization of a potent, slow-acting powerful pressor peptide, called endothelin (1).

A host of substances beyond the traditional circulating hormones (endocrines) are being recognized to exert significant roles in circulatory dynamics. These include some that act on surrounding cells (paracrines) and others that act within the cell of origin (autocrine). One of the more important of these substances is angiotensin, an old hormone that is receiving new attention.—N.M. Kaplan, M.D.

Reference

1. Yanagisawa M, Kurihara H, Kimura S, et al: A novel potent vasoconstrictor peptide produced by vascular endothelial cells. *Nature* 332:411–415, 1988.

Circulating Versus Local Renin-Angiotensin System in Cardiovascular Homeostasis

Dzau VJ (Brigham and Women's Hosp, Boston)
Circulation 77(Suppl I):I-4–I-13, June 1988   6–15

The contributions of the circulating renin-angiotensin system to cardiovascular homeostasis have been well studied. Experimental and clinical studies have shown that long-term administration of these inhibitors is effective in the treatment of hypertension and heart failure.

A concept has recently emerged that proposes that the renin-angiotensin system is not solely an endocrine system, but that endogenous renin-angiotensin systems are present in many local tissues, exerting autocrine and paracrine influences on local tissue function. Such potential autocrine-paracrine systems may be important in the regulation of functions of local tissue. For example, locally produced vascular angiotensin may influence the contractile state of blood vessels (Fig 6–6).

Recent experimental studies have already confirmed that renin and angiotensinogen genes and their products are expressed at many local tissue sites of the major organs, including the kidneys, adrenals, brain, heart, and blood vessels, which play important roles in cardiorenal homeostasis. Under different circumstances the activity of these tissue systems can influence the pharmacologic response to inhibitors of the renin-angiotensin system.

There is some evidence to suggest that the tissue angiotensin-converting enzyme (ACE) may be the primary site of action of ACE in-

ENDOTHELIAL – SMOOTH MUSCLE CELL INTERACTION

A.

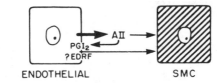

ENDOTHELIAL   SMC

SMOOTH MUSCLE CELL – CELL INTERACTION

B.

SMC   SMC

Fig 6–6.—Possible mechanisms of action of vascular renin angiotensin. **A,** endothelial cells release angiotensin II *(AII)*, which stimulates autocrine secretion of prostacyclin *(PGI₂)* and possibly endothelial-derived relaxant factor *(EDRF)*. These vasoactive agents influence contractile state of vascular smooth muscle. **B,** smooth muscle cell *(SMC)* releases AII, which stimulates autocrine contraction. Angiotensin II may also produce paracrine influence on smooth muscle tone by activating AII receptors on adjacent smooth muscle cell or by facilitating norepinephrine *(NE)* release by sympathetic nerve endings. (Courtesy of Dau VJ: *Circulation* 77(Suppl I): I-4–I-13, June 1988.)

hibitors. Consequently, the duration of action of an ACE inhibitor may well be dependent more on the duration of tissue ACE inhibition than on the drug's serum half-life. The importance of tissue ACE rather than its serum counterpart in determining the response to ACE inhibitors was demonstrated in several experimental studies in which the magnitude and duration of the reduction in blood pressure appeared to be correlated better with the inhibition of ACE activity in certain critical tissues than with the inhibition of serum enzyme activity.

Further studies are needed to determine the clinical significance of the differential effects of pharmacologic ACE inhibitors on tissue renin-angiotensin systems.

▶ Figure 6–6 shows how the autocrine and paracrine functions of angiotensin (and many other substances) can be involved. There is no doubt about the local generation and release of angiotensin II within peripheral vascular tissue (1). When the therapeutic efficacy of angiotensin-converting enzyme inhibitors is discussed later in this chapter, remember that they may act largely by blocking the production of intravascular angiotensin II (2).

Yet another new hormone that has circulatory effects is atrial natriuretic factor, or atriopeptin.—N.M. Kaplan, M.D.

References

1. Mizuno K, Nakamaru M, Higashimori K, et al: Local generation and release of angiotension II in peripheral vascular tissue. Hypertension 11:223–229, 1988.
2. Sakaguchi K, Chai SY, Jackson B, et al: Inhibition of tissue angiotensin-converting enzyme: Quantitation by autoradiography. *Hypertension* 11:230–238, 1988.

Is Atriopeptin a Physiological or Pathophysiological Substance? Studies in the Autoimmune Rat
Greenwald JE, Sakata M, Michener ML, Sides SD, Needleman P (Washington Univ, St Louis)
J Clin Invest 81:1036–1041, April 1988   6–16

Atriopeptin (AP) is a recently identified natriuretic-diuretic and vasodilatory peptide that is synthesized and secreted from mammalian atria. It has been shown to be intimately involved in intravascular volume and blood pressure homeostasis. However, it is not yet known whether AP is truly a physiologic substance, because plasma AP levels do not always correlate with diuresis or natriuresis. A population of autoimmune rats sensitized against their own AP was developed and used, together with nonimmunized rats, in a series of experiments to assess the consequences of prolonged AP deficiency on physiologic and pathophysiologic processes.

In the autoimmune rat, natriuresis in response to acute intravascular volume expansion was inhibited, but natriuresis produced by chronic oral salt loading was not suppressed. Apparently, natriuresis that occurs in response to acute volume expansion is dependent on AP, but natriuresis produced by chronic salt loading is not.

When evaluated as a function of blood pressure in the spontaneously hypertensive nonimmunized rat, plasma AP was increased by a factor of 3. Prior immunization against AP did not affect the rate of development, extent of development of hypertension, or daily sodium excretion of the autoimmune rats when compared with the nonimmunized spontaneously hypertensive controls.

In nonimmunized rats, subcutaneous injection of the mineralocorticoid desoxycorticosterone acetate led to an initial period of sodium retention, followed by natriuresis. Mineralocorticoid escape was not affected by prior immunization against AP.

Atriopeptin is an important natriuretic substance in response to acute intravascular volume loading. However, AP does not seem to be involved in the natriuretic response to chronic intravascular volume loading, blood pressure regulation, or mineralocorticoid escape.

▶ Despite the tremendous amount of investigation performed on the atrial natriuretic factor in the past 5 years, it likely is not a major player in cardiovascular hemodynamics. This ingenious study suggests its role is as a natriuretic hormone that helps to excrete acute volume loads, not an unimportant function but not a major one in long-term volume control. Nonetheless, atrial natriuretic factor may be somehow involved in primary hypertension: plasma levels have been found to be elevated by some (but not all) and in one study were correlated with various evidences of left ventricular involvement (1). It may act only as a biologic furosemide, but it certainly has excited a great deal of research interest. It may not save many lives but sure has kept a lot of investigators off the street.

The possible involvement of atrial natriuretic factor in left ventricular hypertrophy leads us to the final area of intense work on the pathophysiology of hypertension: the response of the heart to the afterload, which translates into left ventricular hypertrophy.—N.M. Kaplan, M.D.

Reference

1. Wambach G, Bunner G, Stimpel M, et al: Relationship between plasma atrial natriuretic peptide and left atrial and left ventricular involvement is essential hypertension. *J Hypertension* 6:573–577, 1988.

Supernormal Contractility in Primary Hypertension Without Left Ventricular Hypertrophy
de Simone G, Di Lorenzo L, Costantino G, Moccia D, Buonissimo S, de Divitiis O (Univ of Naples; La Sapienza Univ, Rome)
Hypertension 11:457–463, May 1988   6–17

Various explanations have been offered of why patients with hypertension sometimes show an increase in cardiac performance. The links between systolic function and the development of left ventricular hypertrophy in hypertensive patients, as well as the presence of supernormal left ventricular function, have been the subject of a number of studies with contradictory results. A homogeneous group of 43 patients with uncomplicated primary hypertension without echocardiographic left ventricular hypertrophy were selected for study to avoid the inconsistencies found in studies of patients with different levels of wall stress and contractility.

The 43 previously untreated hypertensive patients were matched with 54 volunteers who did not have hypertension or a family history of hypertensive disease. All of the subjects had similar diets and were matched for age, sex, and size. Hypertension was defined as diastolic blood pressure of 99 mm Hg or greater. Readings were taken on 5 different days.

Echocardiography showed normal systolic function in spite of increased wall stress in hypertensive patients. Supernormal performance was found in 11 of these patients, and this finding was linked to an improved inotropic state, associated with the highest level of wall stress and inadequate left ventricular hypertrophy. In contrast, hypertensive patients with normal performance showed evidence of a normal inotropic state and lower wall stress. Supernormal performance appears to be an adaptation to high wall stress in order to maintain systolic ventricular performance; however, the therapeutic significance of this pattern is not clear.

▶ As no surprise, this study shows that the heart works harder in the face of high systemic resistance. What it does show nicely is that, in the absence of overt hypertrophy, it may have to work even harder, which is another way of saying that some hypertrophy is a good thing.

On the other hand, even a good thing can be overdone.—N.M. Kaplan, M.D.

Left Ventricular Hypertrophy: Its Prime Importance as a Controllable Risk Factor
Weber JR (Univ of Pennsylvania)
Am Heart J 116:272–279, July 1988   6–18

About half of all patients with hypertension have echographic evidence of left ventricular hypertrophy (LVH). Although some physicians view LVH as an adaptation to chronic pressure overload of the ventricle, hypertrophy is an independent risk factor for adverse cardiac events, including congestive heart failure and sudden death. Coronary insufficiency syndrome also is associated with LVH; the incidence of myocardial infarction is increased. Echocardiography is preferable to the ECG for determining LVH. An increased left ventricular mass on echocardiography is a predictor of cardiac risk.

While diuretic therapy alone may not lead to regression of left ventricular mass, α-methyldopa has significantly reduced left ventricular mass even if blood pressure lowering is minimal. β-Blockers also have reduced left ventricular mass. Metoprolol therapy increases stroke volume and may decrease systemic vascular resistance. In addition to lowering diastolic pressure to the lowest safe level, it may also be appropriate to alter antihypertensive therapy to be sure that LVH is minimized.

▶ One of the more important new players in the field of clinical hypertension is left ventricular hypertrophy (LVH). Long recognized in its more flagrant degrees by electrocardiography to be an independent risk factor for premature coronary disease and sudden death, LVH is now much easier to recognize in an earlier and milder form by echocardiography. In Framingham, the prevalence of LVH by echo is closely associated with higher systolic pressure, progressively increasing with increments from 110 upward (1). Not unexpectedly, echocardiography can also detect left atrial enlargement in hypertensive patients as well (2).

Now that we can find hypertrophy more easily, there is only naturally a great deal of interest to reverse it with appropriate antihypertensive therapy. As the review by Weber documents, most drugs except diuretics and direct vasodilators (hydralazine and minoxidil) have been found to reverse LVH. What effect that will have on the long-term cardiac consequences of hypertension remains to be seen.—N.M. Kaplan, M.D.

References

1. Levy D, Anderson KM, Savage DD, et al: Echocardiographically detected left ventricular hypertrophy: Prevalence and risk factors. *Ann Intern Med* 108:7–13, 1988.
2. Miller JT, O'Rourke RA, Crawford MH: Left atrial enlargement: An early sign of hypertensive heart disease. *Am Heart J* 116:1048–1051, 1988.

Nondrug Therapy

▶ ↓ The list of effective nondrug therapies for hypertension has not expanded, but there is more evidence for the effectiveness of some of them. Weight loss, regular aerobic exercise, and moderation of alcohol have the most solid support. Moderation of sodium intake, increased potassium (and some would say calcium and magnesium) intake, and one form of relaxation or another also seem to be worthwhile.

Not only may these help lower pressures that are high but they also may prevent the pressure from becoming elevated. At least weight gain, alcohol intake beyond 2 drinks a day, and heavy sodium intake are associated with the development of hypertension (1).—N.M. Kaplan, M.D.

Reference

1. Friedman GD, Selby JV, Quesenberry CP Jr, et al: Precursors of essential hypertension: Body weight, alcohol and salt use, and parental history of hypertension. *Prev Med* 17:387–402, 1988.

Effects of Weight Loss on Clinic and Ambulatory Blood Pressure in Normotensive Men
Fortmann SP, Haskell WL, Wood PD, Stanford Weight Control Project Team (Stanford Univ)
Am J Cardiol 62:89–93, July 1, 1988   6–19

It is known that obesity and physical inactivity are associated with both increased cardiovascular risk and elevated blood pressure, but the interrelation of exercise, blood pressure, and weight loss is not well defined. The independent effects of weight loss and exercise on blood pressure were measured in 115 sedentary, overweight, normotensive men who were randomly assigned to a control group, a group to lose weight over 1 year by moderate dieting, or a group to lose weight by increased caloric expenditure through exercise. Median daytime and evening blood pressures were obtained from measurements made every 20 minutes while subjects were awake.

Daily calorie intake decreased over the year in all 3 groups, but only the intake of the diet group changed significantly more than that of the control group. Total fat intake decreased significantly in both dieters and exercisers, compared with controls. Maximal oxygen uptake increased significantly in exercisers, but it decreased slightly in the other 2 groups. Exercisers did not achieve the desired total body-fat loss, but they were not far behind dieters.

Clinic blood pressure decreased similarly in all 3 groups, but daytime and evening ambulatory pressure decreased in both intervention groups and increased in controls.

Weight loss achieved through dieting or exercise may cause important decreases in blood pressure in normotensive men. There appears to be no unique benefit to exercise. These results, if confirmed, may have important implications for the prevention of cardiovascular disease.

▶ Presumably, the same subjects were also shown in other papers to lower their serum triglycerides and raise their high-density lipoprotein-cholesterol levels almost equally by weight loss achieved by either diet or exercise (1). Exercise is almost certainly effective in reducing the risk of dying from coronary heart disease in a manner that is independent of conventional coronary risk factors (2). Let us hear it then for joggers: losing weight, lowering blood pressure, preventing heart attacks, and according to some of my friends, even enjoying the torture. I just hope that my stationary bike works as well.

There is an easier way to lower the blood pressure, at least for about half of hypertensive people (see Abstract 6–20).—N.M. Kaplan, M.D.

References

1. Wood PD, Stefanick ML, Dreon DM, et al: Changes in plasma lipids and lipoproteins in overweight men during weight loss through dieting as compared with exercise. *N Engl J Med* 319:1173–1179, 1988.
2. Ekelund L-G, Haskell WL, Johnson JL, et al: Physical fitness as a predictor of cardiovascular mortality in asymptomatic North American men. *N Engl J Med* 319:1379–1384, 1988.

Review of Salt Restriction and the Response to Antihypertensive Drugs: Satellite Symposium on Calcium Antagonists
Luft FC, Weinberger MH (Indiana Univ)
Hypertension 11(Suppl I):I-229–I-232, February 1988

6–20

A high salt intake disposes to essential hypertension by mechanisms that remain unclear. In some patients, a lowered salt intake fails to decrease the blood pressure. Salt reduction has been proposed as an adjunct to drug treatment of hypertension and is especially indicated when drugs promoting salt retention are employed. Salt restriction augments the effects of β-blockers and thiazide diuretics on blood pressure. The variable results obtained may be related to differing numbers of salt-sensitive and salt-resistant subjects in different trials.

Converting enzyme inhibitors affect the circulating and tissue renin-angiotensin system and also impede the degradation of bradykinin, which influences renal sodium homeostasis. Some of these drugs influence the production of E prostaglandins, which may be important in the hypotensive response, especially during high salt intake. The actions of converting enzyme inhibitors on renal function and blood pressure likely are affected by dietary salt intake.

The action of calcium blockers on blood pressure apparently is not enhanced by dietary salt restriction, perhaps because these drugs are themselves natriuretic. If salt-sensitive hypertension is mediated by an inhibitor of sodium transport that leads to increased cytosolic calcium, calcium blockers should be most effective with a salt-rich diet, which promotes high levels of such an inhibitor.

▶ Sodium restriction may be helpful in reducing the blood pressure of only the half of hypertensives who are "sodium-sensitive," a distinction explored very nicely by these same Indiana investigators (e.g., Miller et al: *J Chron Dis* 40:245–250, 1987). However, as this review demonstrates, there is considerable evidence that moderate sodium restriction to half of usual current intake is helpful in augmenting antihypertensive efficacy of most drugs used to treat hypertension. As the authors emphasize, the only class of drugs for which that may not be true is the calcium entry blockers, perhaps because they themselves are natriuretic. However, as we shall see later in this chapter, not all agree, as an additive effect of either dietary sodium restriction or diuretics is found with these agents as well.

Beyond the possible therapeutic effect, moderate restriction of sodium intake rather surprisingly might be helpful in reducing the degree of left ventricular hypertrophy that we have noted to be a major risk for sudden death.—N.M. Kaplan, M.D.

Dietary Salt Intake: A Determinant of Cardiac Involvement in Essential Hypertension
Schmieder RE, Messerli FH, Garavaglia GE, Nunez BD (Ochsner Clinic, New Orleans)
Circulation 78:951–956, October 1988   6–21

A given increase in afterload does not always produce the same degree of left ventricular hypertrophy. An attempt was made to learn whether dietary salt intake influences structural adaptation of the left ventricle and the development of hypertrophy. Dietary salt intake by 42 patients with essential hypertension was assessed via 24-hour sodium excretion. Hemodynamic and echocardiographic studies were done simultaneously.

Sodium excretion was the strongest predictor of posterior wall and relative wall thicknesses, greater thickness correlating with higher sodium excretion. Sodium excretion was not correlated with end-diastolic volume. Correlation with septal weakness was only modest. Among endocrine parameters, only plasma epinephrine was correlated weakly with posterior wall thickness. Diastolic blood pressure and body mass index were low-grade determinants of posterior wall thickness.

Dietary salt intake is a strong determinant of cardiac structural adaptation in hypertensive subjects. It could act in conjunction with the renin-angiotensin-aldosterone system, the sympathetic nervous system, or fluid volume homeostasis. There is preliminary evidence that strict sodium depletion might reduce left ventricular mass in persons with essential hypertension.

▶ These findings are surprising but not unexpected. As the authors note, high dietary sodium intake may expand fluid volume and increase preload to the left ventricle. Other mechanisms may be involved, but this seems another reason to at least hold back on the salt shaker.

At the same time, replacing processed food (high sodium, low potassium) with more fresh food (low sodium, high potassium) will also provide more potassium intake, which is associated with less hypertension in large-population studies (1) and less endothelial cell damage in experimental studies (2).

In addition to the likely roles of too much sodium and too little potassium, 2 other major minerals in the body composition may also be involved in hypertension and may be in need of manipulation.—N.M. Kaplan, M.D.

References

1. Khaw K-T, Barrett-Connor E: The association between blood pressure, age, and dietary sodium and potassium: A population study. *Circulation* 77:53–61, 1988.
2. Sugimoto T, Tobian L, Ganguli MC: High potassium diets protect against dysfunction of endothelial cells in stroke-prone spontaneously hypertensive rats. *Hypertension* 11:579–585, 1988.

Calcium and Magnesium in Essential Hypertension
Tillman DM, Semple PF (Western Infirmary, Glasgow, Scotland)
Clin Sci 75:395–402, October 1988   6–22

A prospective study of calcium and magnesium metabolism was carried out in 38 patients with untreated essential hypertension, who had an outpatient diastolic pressure greater than 95 mm Hg, and in age- and sex-matched controls. Nine persons with borderline hypertension also were studied.

Total serum calcium was insignificantly higher in hypertensive persons than in controls. Serum magnesium levels were comparable in the 2 groups. There were no important differences in serum or plasma ionized calcium, even after correcting for pH. Urinary calcium was significantly higher in hypertensive persons, but not after correction for sodium excretion. Urinary potassium and magnesium were lower in hypertensive subjects than in controls. Parathyroid hormone levels were normal in all subjects. On regression analysis, magnesium excretion was correlated inversely and significantly with systolic and diastolic blood pressure in both the supine and upright positions. This relationship persisted after correcting for age and calcium excretion.

There is no convincing evidence that the calcium ion concentration is increased in the blood of hypertensive patients. Magnesium excretion is correlated inversely with blood pressure, and this may not be totally explained by differences in extracellular fluid volume.

▶ This is one of the more complete and carefully done studies, comparing untreated hypertensives to age- and sex-matched normotensive subjects with measurements of all the important components of calcium and magnesium, except for their intracellular concentration. As amply shown by others, hypertensives tend to excrete more calcium, but this seems mainly attributable to their higher sodium intake (and excretion). Unlike Tillman and Semple, others have noted slightly lower ionized calcium and higher parathyroid hormone levels in some hypertensives, changes that could easily go along with excess calcium excretion (1–3). It all may be a matter of degree or methodology, but at least the scenario of increased calcium excretion → lower serum ionized calcium → increased parathyroid hormone → a rise in blood pressure could explain the apparent fall in blood pressure that is seen in perhaps 25% of hypertensives given supplemental calcium (4).

Increased amounts of free calcium within smooth muscle cells have been widely incriminated as responsible for the increased vascular resistance of hypertension. The evidence remains questionable (Haller H, Phillip T: Intrazelluläres freies kalzium und plasma-kalzium bei patienten mit essentieller hypertonie. *Klin Wochenschr* 66:455–461, 1988).

The lower urinary magnesium excretion noted by Tillman and Semple remains unexplained, but there is no good evidence that magnesium supplements will lower blood pressure.

Let us go on to other components of the nondrug prescription, including (would you believe?) the laying on of hands.—N.M. Kaplan, M.D.

References

1. McCarron DA, Pingree PA, Rubin RJ, et al: Enhanced parathyroid function in essential hypertension: A homeostatic response to a urinary calcium leak. *Hypertension* 2:162–168, 1980.
2. Strazzullo P, Nunziata V, Cirillo M, et al: Abnormalities of calcium metabolism in essential hypertension. *Clin Sci* 65:137–141, 1983.
3. Hvarfner A, Bergström R, Mörlin C, et al: Relationship between calcium metabolic indices and blood pressure in patients with essential hypertension as compared with a healthy population. *J Hypertens* 5:451–456, 1987.

4. Kaplan NM: Calcium and potassium in the treatment of essential hypertension. *Sem Nephrol* 8:176–184, 1988.

Paranormal Healing and Hypertension

Beutler JJ, Attevelt JTM, Schouten SA, Faber JAJ, Mees EJD, Geijskes GG
(Univ Hosp, State Univ, Utrecht, the Netherlands)
Br Med J 296:1491–1494, May 28, 1988   6–23

Paranormal healing has become increasingly popular in the Netherlands. In 1986 some 65,000 patients visited 600 healers, which resulted in 2 million patient consultations. Paranormal healing is performed either by laying on of hands or by healing at a distance, in which case healing occurs by thought projection.

To determine whether paranormal healing might reduce blood pressure in essential hypertension and whether such an effect might be the result of a paranormal, psychological, or placebo factor, a prospective study was conducted of 115 patients with documented essential hypertension randomly assigned to 3 study groups. Forty patients were treated by laying on of hands, 37 were treated by paranormal healing at a distance, and 38 patients had no paranormal healing. Treatment consisted of a 20-minute session 1 morning each week for 15 weeks. Twelve well-known healers acquainted with both forms of paranormal healing were selected from among members of several Dutch societies of paranormal healing and were assigned to the 77 study participants. The 3 groups were similar in baseline characteristics.

At the end of the 15-week study period, systolic and diastolic blood pressures were significantly reduced in all 3 groups, but patients who were treated by healing at a distance had consistently lower weekly diastolic pressure, compared with that of controls. However, the differences did not reach statistical significance.

Because no treatment was consistently better than another, the data cannot be taken as evidence of a paranormal effect on blood pressure. It is assumed that the fall in pressure in all 3 groups was caused either by the psychosocial interaction with the patient or was a placebo effect of the trial itself.

▶ Laying on of hands is amazingly popular in the Netherlands, likely to compensate for their not having as many TV faith healers. This study confirms what is obvious from every well-designed study of any and every therapy for hypertension: just repeatedly taking the blood pressure, particularly with a placebo but not requiring one, will result in lowering of the blood pressure in most people over at least a few months' time. Hands or no hands, the psyche is a powerful determinant of blood pressure, and getting comfortable with the measurement or the investigator, or whatever is going on, over time will result in a fall in blood pressure. Those who claim a blood pressure effect without a proper placebo-controlled study are just kidding themselves and, more dangerous, a lot of gullible people as well.

Last, the most important nondrug therapy for hypertension will not lower the blood pressure but will do more to reduce cardiovascular mortality than any other.—N.M. Kaplan, M.D.

Impact of Smoking on Heart Attacks, Strokes, Blood Pressure Control, Drug Dose, and Quality of Life Aspects in the International Prospective Primary Prevention Study in Hypertension
Bühler FR, Vesanen K, Watters JT, Bolli P (Univ Hosp, Ciba-Geigy Ltd, Basel Switzerland)
Am Heart J 115(suppl):282–288, January 1988   6–24

Smoking is a major risk factor for cardiovascular morbidity and mortality. To determine the effects of smoking on cardiac and cerebrovascular event rates, blood pressure control, drug use, and quality of life, the data from the International Prospective Primary Prevention Study in Hypertension (IPPPSH) was analyzed with regard to smoking status.

Of the 6,357 persons included in this study, 37% of the men and 23% of the women were smokers. During the course of the study, 537 individuals changed their smoking status. Smoking doubled the occurrence of cardiac and cerebrovascular events. Smoking status did not affect blood pressure control or the type of drugs used. However, smokers were given higher doses of oxprenolol, a β-blocker. Heart rates were higher in smokers than in nonsmokers. Smoking increased hematocrit in a dose-dependent manner. Dyspnea and cold extremities were more common among smokers.

Smoking appears to interfere with quality of life by increasing the cardiovascular complication rate. Smokers were given higher doses of β-blocker, but did not appear to receive any benefit from this. Therefore, antihypertensive treatment with β-blockers will be successful only if the smoking status of the patient is considered.

▶ Not only is smoking evil for what it does itself, it also interferes with the effectiveness of most β-blockers. As we will see (Abstract 6–28), this may not apply to all of this class of drugs, but it is another reason to do everything you can to get your hypertensive patients to quit smoking.

One more habit that some find almost as pleasurable as smoking is drinking coffee. Although the large-scale evidence does not show either a cardiovascular or a hypertensive risk from coffee, there is little question that caffeine will cause a transient rise in blood pressure that potentiates the pressor response to stressful circumstances (1). Moreover, increasing coffee consumption has been noted to be associated, independently of other variables, with higher serum cholesterol levels (2). The effect was minimal with 1–2 cups per day and really only clinically significant with about 6. So, we need not give up this pleasure, just keep it within bounds.—N.M. Kaplan, M.D.

References

1. Pincomb GW, Lovallo WR, Passey RB, et al: Effect of behavior state on caffeine's ability to alter blood pressure. *Am J Cardiol* 61:798–802, 1988.

2. Davis BR, Cub JD, Borhani NO, et al: Coffee consumption and serum cholesterol in the hypertension detection and follow-up program. *Am J Epidemiol* 128:124–136, 1988.

Drug Therapy

▶ ↓ Once the various nondrug modalities are given a fair chance, most truly hypertensive people are likely going to need antihypertensive drugs to reduce their pressures to safe levels. But there is increasing evidence of dangers from the use of drugs, not only from their undesirable side effects but also from their presumably desirable efficacy in lowering the blood pressure.

The latter point deserves emphasis: in 8 separate studies, wherein reduction of elevated blood pressure to a level of 90 mm Hg was shown to be associated with a decrease in coronary mortality, when blood pressure was lowered to less than 90 mm Hg (and even more strikingly when it was lowered to less than 85 mm Hg), coronary mortality bounced back up. This "J-curve" was mainly seen in patients with preexisting coronary disease, who have a "poor coronary flow reserve," which makes the myocardium vulnerable to lower coronary perfusion pressures that can be tolerated by patients without stenotic coronary arteries (1). The presence of left ventricular hypertrophy may add to the danger (2).

The evidence is clear: too much of a good thing may be deadly. We need to lower pressures gently and to no lower than 85 mm Hg. For many, a diastolic level of 90 mm Hg will be safer, although the risk for stroke is greater at that level. It likely does not matter how the pressure is lowered, but the studies, until now, have all used diuretics or β-blockers or both. Other drugs may be less likely to cause hypoperfusion, but I will bet it is not a specific drug effect. Rather, any drug that lowers pressure may be harmful to some people with poor autoregulatory ability to increase blood flow as blood pressure is lowered.

The problem is most serious in the coronary circulation. But, as will be noted at the end of this section, it likely is responsible for another consequence of the reduction of blood pressure: impotence. Even if the heart is beating, one of life's pleasures may thereby be lost.

One more general word: as noted in the review of the 1988 Joint National Committee report (Abstract 6–1), more choices of initial and subsequent therapies are being advocated on an individualized basis with the hope of providing better and less bothersome control of the blood pressure with drugs that are most appropriate for each patient. The aim is laudable, but targeted, individualized therapy is not yet feasible for all patients. For example, the responses of a group of middle-aged white patients to either an angiotensin-converting enzyme inhibitor or a calcium entry blocker were totally unpredictable (1). Some responded to only one, some to neither, others to both. What is required is an open mind and the willingness to change courses if needed.

Before considering various specific drugs, let us review some of the general information about the benefits and costs of therapy.—N.M. Kaplan, M.D.

Reference

1. Bidiville J, Nussberger J, Waeber G, et al: Individual responses to converting enzyme inhibitors and calcium antagonists. *Hypertension* 11:166–173, 1988.

Hypertension, Antihypertensive Treatment, and Sudden Coronary Death: The Framingham Study

Kannel WB, Cupples LA, D'Agostino RB, Stokes J III (Boston Univ Med Ctr)

Hypertension 11(Suppl II):II-45–II-50, March 1988   6–25

Blood pressure reduction slows lipid-induced atherogenesis, but the efficacy of treatment in avoiding coronary heart disease is less clear. Review was made of 183 sudden deaths of males and 77 of females in the Framingham cohort of 5,209 subjects aged 30–62 years who entered the study from 1948 to 1952. In 118 sudden deaths there was past evidence of coronary heart disease. Sudden deaths increased with advancing age in both sexes.

The risk of sudden death and other initial manifestations of coronary heart disease increased with the severity of hypertension. In patients with past coronary disease, however, the risk of sudden death was not significantly related to hypertensive status. Antihypertensive treatment contributed independently to the risk of sudden death in men, and marginally in women. There was no evidence that the excess mortality was confined to subjects with ECG abnormalities. In women with past heart disease, antihypertensive therapy strongly disposed to sudden death if coexisting diabetes was present.

These data indicate a persistently increased risk of sudden death associated with antihypertensive therapy. As deaths from heart failure, renal failure, and stroke diminish, more emphasis will be placed on lowering coronary mortality and sudden deaths. Antihypertensive therapy will be tailored so that it is more effective against atherogenesis and less likely to promote myocardial irritability. Diuretic treatment tends to worsen the lipid profile and to decrease the serum potassium level and glucose tolerance.

▶ This is another piece of disturbing evidence about the potential hazards of currently used antihypertensive therapy. The increase in sudden deaths is frightening and must give further pause for those who wish to treat everyone with any degree of elevated blood pressure.

This article unfortunately does not detail the drugs being given to those who died suddenly. Because Framingham is presumably like the rest of the United States, most were probably on a diuretic. The danger of diuretic-induced hypokalemia for inducing ventricular ectopy, I believe, has been amply documented, more reason for everyone to read the 1988 Joint National Committee report (Abstract 6–1) and minimize the hazards.

Despite the potential hazards, the evidence that reducing the blood pressure will reduce the incidence of and mortality from stroke and, likely, congestive heart failure is clear. For those with fairly mild hypertension, the benefit, using either a diuretic or a β-blocker, as seen in the massive Medical Research Council of England trial, was to reduce the number of strokes by about one half while having little effect on coronary events (1).

The overall protection seen in a less well controlled study of English patients was noted to reflect the treated blood pressure and not the level present before treatment.—N.M. Kaplan, M.D.

Reference

1. Medical Research Council Working Party: Stroke and coronary heart disease in mild hypertension: Risk factors and the value of treatment. *Br Med J* 296:1565–1570, 1988.

Treated Blood Pressure, Rather Than Pretreatment, Predicts Survival in Hypertensive Patients: A Report From the DHSS Hypertension Care Computing Project (DHCCP)
Bulpitt CJ, Beevers DG, Butler A, Coles EC, Fletcher AE, Hunt D, Munro-Faure AD, Newson R, O'Riordan PW, Petrie JC, Rajagopalan B, Rylance PB, Twallin G, Webster J, Dollery CT (Hammersmith Hosp, London; John Radcliffe Infirmary, Oxford, England; King's College Hosp, London; Aberdeen Royal Infirmary, Aberdeen, Scotland; Dudley Royal Hosp, Birmingham, England; et al)
J Hypertens 6:627–632, August 1988   6–26

The Department of Health and Social Security Hypertension Care Computing Project (DHCCP) was initiated in England in 1971 to determine the causes of deaths of patients with hypertension and to identify the risk factors for death in these patients as determined at entry into the study and during follow-up. Data on 2,855 hypertensive patients for whom pretreatment systolic blood pressure and diastolic blood pressure levels were known and whose untreated diastolic blood pressure was at least 90 mm Hg are reported. Although the DHCCP collects much information on its enrolled patients, this report deals only with the prediction of death and survival based on a subset of data that includes sex and age at entry and systolic blood pressure and diastolic blood pressure before treatment and during 0–3, 3–12, 12–24, and 24–36 months of follow-up. Survival was assessed in relation to pretreatment blood pressure levels and blood pressure levels achieved during treatment.

After a maximum follow-up of 126 months and an average follow-up of 51 months, 191 of the 2,855 study patients had died. This included 62 men and 23 women who had died of ischemic heart disease, and 22 men and 22 women who had died of cerebrovascular disease. For the patients who had died, the average untreated systolic blood pressure was 180 mm Hg in men and 184 mm Hg in women. The average untreated diastolic blood pressure was 113 mm Hg in men and 111 mm Hg in women.

In contrast with other epidemiologic studies, which reported that increased levels of untreated blood pressure adversely affected survival, pretreatment blood pressure levels in this study were not useful predictors of mortality. However, both blood pressure level measurements taken during treatment were useful predictors of mortality. The strongest association between blood pressure and total mortality was for the diastolic blood pressure during the second year of treatment. The relative hazard rate for elevated diastolic blood pressure at 12–24 months in this study was higher than that of the Hypertension Detection and Follow-up Program in the United States.

▶ This is not too surprising, but it is nice to know that, however high the pressure is before therapy, if it is reduced effectively, mortality will be lowered. And, according to the results of 1 large trial, the impact on coronary mortality may be far better than seen in all diuretic-based and most β-blocker-based trials by use of a specific β-blocker.—N.M. Kaplan, M.D.

Primary Prevention With Metoprolol in Patients With Hypertension: Mortality Results From the MAPHY Study
Wikstrand J, Warnold I, Olsson G, Tuomilehto J, Elmfeldt D, Berglund G on behalf of the Advisory Committee (Sahlgrenska Univ Hosp, Gothenburg, Sweden; AB Hässle, Mölndal, Sweden; Karolinska Inst, Stockholm; Natl Public Health Inst, Helsinki)
JAMA 259:1976–1982, Apr 1, 1988   6–27

The value of metoprolol, a relatively β_1-selective β-blocker, as initial antihypertensive therapy was studied in white men aged 40 to 64 years, some with newly detected and some with previously treated hypertension. The sitting blood pressure was 100 to 130 mm Hg at randomization. Metoprolol was given in a dose of 200 mg daily to 1,609 patients, whereas 1,625 received 50 mg of hydrochlorothiazide or 5 mg of bendroflumethiazide daily. The median follow-up was 4.2 years.

Mortality was significantly lower in patients randomized to metoprolol than in the diuretic group. The benefit was not concentrated in a single geographic region. Cardiovascular mortality and deaths from coronary heart disease and stroke all were lower in the metoprolol group. Total mortality was significantly lower among smokers randomized to metoprolol than among those given diuretic therapy.

Cardiovascular mortality is lowered among men with mild to moderate hypertension who are begun on metoprolol therapy rather than a thiazide diuretic. The effect is due chiefly to decreases in fatal coronary heart disease and fatal stroke. The effect of metoprolol is important because of the high prevalence of hypertension and the increased risk in the hypertensive population.

▶ Because of the overall inability of diuretic-based therapy to reduce coronary heart disease (CHD) mortality, there has been a great hope that β-blockers would do better, particularly because they have been shown to provide secondary protection for those who have already had an acute myocardial infarction. Unfortunately, they did not reduce CHD morbidity or mortality below that seen with diuretics in 3 previously reported large trials: Medical Research Council: *Lancet* 2:539–543, 1981; IPPSH: *J Hypertens* 3:379–392, 1985; HAPPHY: *J Hypertens* 5:561–572, 1987.

This study is the first to report a significantly lower CHD mortality with β-blocker therapy. The patients were the half of those in the HAPPHY trial who were on metoprolol; the other half took atenolol. It looks like metoprolol may be special, but I am still not convinced. Nonetheless, as the next abstract shows, it will largely overcome the structural changes of hypertension.—N.M. Kaplan, M.D.

Cardiovascular and Renal Effects of Long-term Antihypertensive Treatment

Hartford M, Wendelhag I, Berglund G, Wallentin I, Ljungman S, Wikstrand J (Univ of Gothenburg, Sweden)
JAMA 259:2553–2557, May 6, 1988   6–28

The extent to which long-term antihypertensive therapy can restore the cardiovascular and renal systems to those found in normotensives of similar age is unknown. Thirteen hypertensive men aged 56 years and 37 normotensive control subjects of the samge age were studied. The mean diastolic blood pressure was 105 mm Hg or higher, and there were signs of hypertensive cardiac involvement. Combination drug therapy was preferred to high doses of a single drug. Primary treatment was with the cardioselective β-blocker metoprolol.

Central and peripheral hemodynamics were normal after 7 years of antihypertensive treatment. Left ventricular (LV) hypertrophy was resolved in proportion to the quality of blood pressure control. Systolic wall stress also normalized, and systolic LV function was well preserved at follow-up, as was diastolic LV function. Microalbuminuria was resolved, and renal vascular resistance was decreased. There was no change in glomerular filtration rate.

Cardiovascular abnormalities characteristic of hypertension can be substantially reduced by long-term antihypertensive therapy. Both cardiac hypertrophy and structural vascular changes regress. The increased microalbuminuria seen in hypertensive subjects can be normalized by long-term treatment, starting with the β-blocker metoprolol.

▶ This is a nicely performed study of the long-term (7-year) effects of the therapy of hypertension with the β-blocker metoprolol. Others have reported improvements in hemodynamics after shorter-term therapy with various drugs, but this study also is strengthened by the comparison against normotensive controls followed over the same period.

Now if we could only get good data on the reduction of coronary disease beyond that reported in the previous abstract. Until more definite evidence is available, we can only choose between the available drugs and hope that, by avoiding side effects and carefully lowering pressure, we can protect our patients.

Abstracts 6–29 through 6–31 examine the effects of what is still far and away the most popular form of therapy: diuretics.—N.M. Kaplan, M.D.

Reduced Concentrations of Potassium, Magnesium, and Sodium-Potassium Pumps in Human Skeletal Muscle During Treatment With Diuretics

Dørup I, Skajaa K, Clausen T, Kjeldsen K (Odder Hosp, Odder, Denmark; Univ of Åarhus, Denmark)
Br Med J 296:455–458, Feb 13, 1988   6–29

Diuretics induce loss of potassium and magnesium. Potassium deficiency is associated with a selective loss of sodium-potassium pumps from skeletal muscle in animals. To determine the incidence of potassium deficiency among patients receiving long-term diuretic therapy and potassium supplements, skeletal muscle needle biopsy specimens were taken from 25 patients aged 44–83 years, who had taken diuretics for 2–14 years, and the potassium, magnesium, and sodium-potassium pump levels of the specimens were measured.

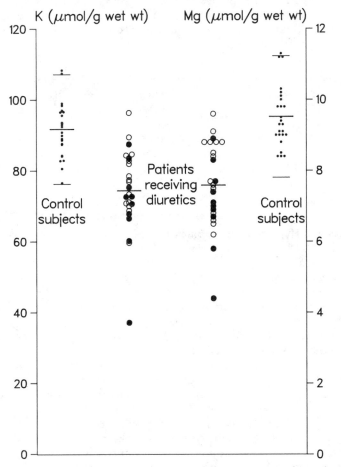

Fig 6–7.—Concentrations of potassium and magnesium in biopsy specimens of vastus lateralis muscle from 25 patients receiving diuretics and 25 age-matched controls. Mean value for each group is marked by *horizontal bar*, as are 95% confidence intervals for controls (●). ○ = patients with hypertension; ● = those with congestive heart failure. (Courtesy of Dørup I, Skajaa K, Clausen T, et al: *Br Med J* 296:455–458, Feb 13, 1988.)

The potassium, magnesium, and sodium-potassium pump levels in these patients were significantly lower than that of age-matched controls (Fig 6–7). However, in only 1 of these patients was the serum potassium level depressed. Mean muscle magnesium and potassium concentrations were linearly related. The concentration of ^{3}H-ouabain binding sites was assayed in samples from 12 patients with mean muscle potassium concentrations below 80 μmole/gm. In these patients there was a linear correlation between the cellular potassium:sodium ratio and the concentration of ^{3}H-ouabain binding sites. This indicated that potassium deficiency led to down-regulation of sodium-potassium pumps in the skeletal muscle of these patients.

Despite the use of potassium supplements, long-term use of diuretics may be associated with potassium and magnesium deficiency in skeletal muscle. This deficiency may occur even when serum electrolyte levels appear normal. The use of skeletal muscle needle biopsy allows these deficiencies to be detected.

▶ The point made in Figure 6–7 is important: concentrations of K+ and Mg++ within muscles were often reduced in association with chronic diuretic therapy even though plasma levels were normal. The possibility of tissue depletion of electrolytes must be considered whenever diuretics are used.

One way to limit the problems is to reduce the dose. First, there is evidence that when 50 mg of hydrochlorothiazide does not work adequately, the better course is to add another drug, not to increase the diuretic dose.—N.M. Kaplan, M.D.

Diuretics and Hypertension in Black Adults
Hawkins DW, Dieckmann MR, Horner RD (Univ of Georgia; Med College of Georgia; East Carolina Univ)
Arch Intern Med 148:803–805, April 1988   6–30

Clinical trials have demonstrated that thiazide diuretics are more effective than β-blockers in the treatment of hypertension in black adults. To determine the correct treatment for blacks whose hypertension was not controlled by standard diuretic dosages, a randomized controlled trial of high-dose thiazide diuretic versus usual-dose thiazide diuretic plus metaprolol, a selective $β_1$-antagonist, was conducted in 38 black hypertensive patients who did not respond sufficiently to usual-dose diuretic alone.

At the end of the 8-week treatment period, patients in the combined therapy group had significantly lower diastolic blood pressure than those in the high-dose diuretic group. Plasma renin status did not appear to affect the outcome of either treatment regimen.

The combination of metoprolol and thiazide diuretic appears to be effective in controlling blood pressure in black adult hypertensives who do not respond to diuretic alone. In those black hypertensives with low plasma renin activity, the combined therapy was more effective than higher doses of diuretic.

▶ Although β-blockers do not work as well in blacks as do diuretics, they are effective particularly when added as a second agent. The main message of this study, however, is that 50 mg of hydrochlorothiazide is about at the top of the dose-response curve. Even better evidence that 50 mg may be much more than needed is available.—N.M. Kaplan, M.D.

The Case for Low Dose Diuretics in Hypertension: Comparison of Low and Conventional Doses of Cyclopenthiazide
McVeigh G, Galloway D, Johnston D (Queen's Univ of Belfast; Napp Research Ctr, Cambridge, England)
Br Med J 297:95–98, July 9, 1988   6–31

Because many adverse effects, including hypokalemia, are associated with thiazide diuretics, the lowest effective dose of cyclopenthiazide was sought in a study of newly diagnosed hypertensive patients receiving a single drug who were willing to change treatment. Patients were assigned on a double-blind basis to treatment with 50, 125, or 500 μg of cyclopenthiazide or a placebo. Fifty-three patients with mild essential hypertension entered the study.

Systolic and diastolic blood pressure was significantly lower after 8 weeks in patients given the 2 higher doses of diuretic; the lowest dose exhibited no significant activity. The fall in serum potassium was most evident with the 500-μg dose, as was the change in serum urate. There was no dose-related change in 24-hour urinary sodium excretion. Plasma renin activity rose significantly with the highest drug dose. Side effects were comparably frequent in all groups and generally were minor.

A 125-μg dose of cyclopenthiazide is an effective and safe treatment for mild essential hypertension. Use of the lowest effective dose of diuretic can lower blood pressure with minimal metabolic disturbance, and this is especially helpful in managing elderly patients, who are vulnerable to the effects of conventional diuretic doses.

▶ Most of the "experts" have been telling you to cut down on the dosage of diuretics, if not to cut them out completely, because their use in high doses has not been shown to reduce the coronary morbidity and mortality of hypertension, likely because of their adverse biochemical effects.

This long-needed study shows that what many have thought to be "low-dose" is really much more than needed. The most popular diuretic used in England, cyclopenthiazide, is about 70 times more potent than our most popular one, hydrochlorothiazide (HCTZ). These results show that one quarter of the usual dose gave all of the antihypertensive effect and less of the metabolic problems of the full amount. That translates to about 9 mg of HCTZ. Now that is a low dose!

After diuretics, β-blockers are the second most widely used antihypertensive drugs. Their chronic use may be especially effective in patients with ischemic heart disease, as reflected in what can be seen acutely under the stress of anesthesia.—N.M. Kaplan, M.D.

Myocardial Ischemia in Untreated Hypertensive Patients: Effect of a Single Small Oral Dose of a Beta-Adrenergic Blocking Agent
Stone JG, Foëx P, Sear JW, Johnson LL, Khambatta HJ, Triner L (Columbia Univ; Oxford Univ)
Anesthesiology 68:495–500, April 1988   6–32

Myocardial ischemia may occur in untreated hypertensive patients during anesthesia. Intraoperative ECGs of 128 mildly hypertensive surgical patients were reviewed. None of the patients was on chronic antihypertensive therapy. However, 89 received a single small oral dose of labetalol, atenolol, or oxprenolol along with premedication. The dose of labetalol was 100 mg, that of atenolol was 50 mg, and that of oxprenolol was 20 mg.

Myocardial ischemia was observed in 13 patients. The incidence was 28% in untreated patients and 2% in those given a β-blocker. The abnormalities occurred during tracheal intubation or during emergence from anesthesia or during both. Tachycardia consistently occurred during ischemia, but there was no substantial rise in blood pressure (table).

Even mildly hypertensive patients may have a brief hyperdynamic stress response to anesthesia, accompanied by myocardial ischemia. The risk of myocardial ischemia is reduced by giving a single small oral dose of a β-blocker at the time of premedication. Prophylaxis is as effective at the end of anesthesia as during induction. Patients with ischemic heart disease also may benefit from pretreatment with a β-blocker.

▶ This study may not reflect what β-blockers can do chronically but Abstracts 6–27 and 6–28 suggest that coronary protection might be provided, at least by some. At the same time, β-blockers may cause some bothersome side effects. Some are a result of known pharmacologic consequences of β-receptor block-

	Mean Arterial Pressure (mm Hg)			
	Day Before Surgery	Pre-induction	Intubation (Peak)	Emergence (Peak)
Untreated	116 ± 1	112 ± 2*	125 ± 3†	127 ± 2†
Labetalol	115 ± 2	98 ± 2*	92 ± 3	101 ± 4
Atenolol	117 ± 2	100 ± 3*	106 ± 5	107 ± 3
Oxprenolol	119 ± 2	108 ± 2*	118 ± 4†	119 ± 3†

Mean ± SEM.
*Significant difference from day before surgery.
†Significant difference from preinduction.
(Courtesy of Stone JG, Foëx P, Sear JW, et al: *Anesthesiology* 68:495–500, April 1988.)

ade, e.g., interference with exercise ability; others are more nonspecific, e.g.,sleep disturbances (1). The former may be lessened by use of β_1-selective agents as shown in the next abstract; the latter, by agents that are less lipid (brain) soluble (2).—N.M. Kaplan, M.D.

References

1. Frishman WH: Beta-adrenergic receptor blockers: Adverse effects and drug interactions. *Hypertension* 11(Suppl II):II-21–II-29, 1988.
2. Kales A, Bixler EO, Vela-Bueno A, et al: Effects of nadolol on blood pressure, sleep efficiency, and sleep stages. *Clin Pharmacol Ther* 43:655–662, 1988.

Hypertension, Exercise, and Beta-Adrenergic Blockade
Ades PA, Gunther PGS, Meacham CP, Handy MA, LeWinter MM (Univ of Vermont)
Ann Intern Med 109:629–634, Oct 15, 1988   6–33

The interaction of aerobic conditioning and β-blocker therapy was examined in 30 sedentary hypertensive patients with a mean age of 46.5 years. The mean diastolic pressure was 95 mm Hg or greater but was less than 105 mm Hg. A 10-week conditioning program was based on walking and jogging, cycling, rowing, and trampolining. Some patients received 100 mg of metoprolol twice daily or 80 mg of propranolol twice daily.

The 2-β-blockers produced equivalent blockade before conditioning. Maximal oxygen uptake was reduced by 13% with propranolol, and exercise duration also was decreased with this drug. Peak oxygen uptake rose with training. The resting systolic blood pressure was markedly lower after conditioning in placebo and metoprolol recipients, but not in patients given propranolol. Peak oxygen uptake increased 24% in response to training in those given placebo and 8% in those given metoprolol. In propranolol-treated patients it did not increase.

Nonselective β-blockade prevents the blood pressure-lowering effects of aerobic conditioning in hypertensive patients. It also adversely affects the exercise response acutely and chronically. If a selective β-blocker is used and the patient complies with an aerobic exercise program, treatment often can be tapered or withdrawn.

▶ Some people have a major problem in maintaining their desired level of physical activity while taking a β-blocker. If it is a problem and a β-blocker is deemed the best choice for therapy, a more cardioselective one may be better. Others have found that conditioning can be accomplished with either selective or nonselective agents (1).

After β-blockers, centrally acting α-agonists have been the third most popular class of drugs. They tend to cause sedation and dry mouth, but cardiac side effects have not been prominent. However, both clonidine and another, not yet available α_2-agonist were found to depress sinus and atrioventricular nodal function (2).

Meanwhile, 2 newer classes, angiotensin-converting enzyme inhibitors and calcium-entry blockers, have begun to be more widely used, joining with α_1-blockers (prazosin, terazosin) as vasodilators that do not suppress cardiac output and do not have an adverse impact on lipid levels.

Calcium-entry blockers have a modest natriuretic effect of their own (3). There have been reports that they may not have an additive antihypertensive effect when added to a diuretic.—N.M. Kaplan, M.D.

References

1. Madden DJ, Blumenthal JA, Ekelund L-G: Effects of beta-blockade and exercise on cardiovascular and cognitive functioning. *Hypertension* 11:470–476, 1988.
2. Roden DM, Nadeau JHJ, Primm RK: Electrophysiologic and hemodynamic effects of chronic oral therapy with the alpha$_2$-agonists clonidine and tiamenidine in hypertensive volunteers. *Clin Pharmacol Ther* 43:648–654, 1988.
3. Graves J, Kenamond TG, Whittier FC: Acute effects of nifedipine on renal electrolyte excretion in normal and hypertensive subjects. *Am J Med Sci* 296:114–118, 1988.

Verapamil and Bendrofluazide in the Treatment of Hypertension: A Controlled Study of Effectiveness Alone and in Combination
Benjamin N, Phillips RJW, Robinson BF (St George's Hosp, London)
Eur J Clin Pharmacol 34:249–253, April 1988   6–34

Two drugs used to treat hypertension, verapamil and bendrofluazide, were compared by administering them alone and together in a 12-week randomized, patient-blind study. Twenty patients completed the trial. All had primary hypertension and were previously untreated or were scheduled to start a new medication.

Each of the patients received a placebo identical to either verapamil or bendrofluazide during the first 4 weeks. For the second 4 weeks, patients were given either verapamil (160 mg twice daily) and bendrofluazide placebo or bendrofluazide (5 mg once a day) and placebo verapamil. All patients received both drugs in the previous dosage for the final 4 weeks. Blood pressure, heart rate, and blood and urine biochemistry were measured before treatment and after each 4-week period.

Placebo treatment caused a fall in mean blood pressure of less than 1 mm Hg supine and 2 mm Hg standing. Verapamil resulted in a significantly greater fall in mean blood pressure than did bendrofluazide in the second 4 weeks. Adding bendrofluazide to verapamil caused no significant change in blood pressure, whereas adding verapamil to bendrofluazide brought about an added reduction in pressure of 18 mm Hg, both supine and standing. Heart rate was appreciably lowered by verapamil alone. Bendrofluazide caused a lowering of plasma potassium concentration and urinary calcium excretion and an increase in plasma urate concentration. Verapamil caused no significant changes in plasma or urine.

Doses of 160 mg of verapamil twice daily are more effective against hypertension than is a daily dose of 5 mg of bendrofluazide. There were more side effects noted with verapamil, but none were serious.

▶ When a diuretic was added to the calcium entry blocker (CEB), no greater fall in blood pressure occurred. When the CEB was added to the diuretic, the blood pressure fell further. The data suggest that the CEB accomplished all of the blood pressure effect that could be achieved with any drug, whereas the diuretic lowered the blood pressure only part of the way, so the addition of the CEB caused a further fall. Whatever the explanation, the data support an additive effect when a CEB is added to a diuretic, unlike that reported by others.

Another probable misconception about CEBs is that they are less effective in patients who are younger or who have higher levels of plasma renin activity and more effective in older and lower-renin patients. As reviewed by Shepherd (1), these differences have not been substantiated and the responses to CEBs are determined only by the dose of the drug and the initial level of blood pressure, not unlike other antihypertensive agents.

CEBs work as well as or better than other antihypertensives and tend to cause few bothersome side effects.— N.M. Kaplan, M.D.

Reference

1. Shepherd AMM: Determinants of antihypertensive response to calcium antagonists in systemic hypertension. *Am J Cardiol* 62:92G–96G, 1988.

Nifedipine and Atenolol Singly and Combined for Treatment of Essential Hypertension: Comparative Multicentre Study in General Practice in the United Kingdom
Nifedipine-Atenolol Study Review Committee
Br Med J 296:468–472, Feb 13, 1988   6–35

A randomized, double-blind comparison of the calcium channel antagonist nifedipine and the β-adrenergic blocker atenolol for the treatment of essential hypertension was performed with 410 patients.

Both nifedipine and atenolol significantly reduced blood pressure. Reduction of blood pressure to less than 95 mm Hg was achieved in 65% of the 410 patients. Nifedipine reduced blood pressure more than did atenolol. The 149 patients who did not respond to either drug were given a combination of the 2 drugs for 8 weeks. All of these patients responded to the combined regimen. Adverse effects severe enough to necessitate withdrawal of medication occurred in 12% of those taking nifedipine and 19% of those taking atenolol. The most common side effects of nifedipine were flushing and edema. The most common side effects of atenolol were diarrhea and dyspepsia.

Nifedipine and atenolol were both effective in controlling blood pressure in 65% of the subjects with essential hypertension. However, nefedipine was more effective than was atenolol. A combined regimen provided the best control of blood pressure, while requiring lower dosages of each drug.

▶ Calcium entry blockers appear to have some special effects on renal function.—N.M. Kaplan, M.D.

Effect of Nifedipine on Renal Function in Patients With Essential Hypertension

Reams GP, Hamory A, Lau A, Bauer JH (Univ of Missouri–Columbia)
Hypertension 11:452–456, May 1988   6–36

Although the systemic effects of calcium channel antagonists have been well studied, their effect on renal function is not yet fully understood. Results from earlier studies with diltiazem and amlodipine suggest that calcium antagonists have the potential to enhance effective renal plasma flow and renal blood flow, to preserve or improve glomerular filtration rate, and to lower renal vascular resistance. A clinical study was done to assess the short-term effects of nifedipine on renal function.

Twenty-six patients aged 32–70 years with essential hypertension for a mean duration of 9.4 years were treated for 4 weeks with nifedipine alone, 30–120 mg/day, taken in 3 divided doses. Included were patients with a mean 5-minute recumbent diastolic blood pressure of 95–114 mm Hg after a run-in period of 2–4 weeks with placebo. Excluded were those who had moderate to severe cardiomegaly, congestive heart failure, recent myocardial infarction, heart block, or overt diabetes mellitus. Renal function studies were performed after the placebo run-in period and at the end of the 4-week drug treatment period. No other drugs were administered. Patients were instructed to follow a no-added-salt diet.

Nifedipine monotherapy effectively lowered blood pressure in 19 (73%) of the 26 patients. No significant postural changes in blood pressure occurred in any of the patients, and the heart rate was not increased. After 4 weeks of nifedipine therapy there were no significant differences in the urinary excretion of sodium, potassium, and creatinine. Serum sodium and potassium levels were also unchanged. At the end of the study period a 13.3% increase in glomerular filtration rate and a 19.6% increase in effective renal plasma flow/renal blood flow were observed, whereas the renal vascular resistance had been reduced by 25.2%. The filtration fraction and urinary albumin excretion did not change. Changes in renal function were independent of patients' initial glomerular filtration rate. No correlation was found between systemic and renal effects of nifedipine monotherapy.

Nifedipine monotherapy appears to have the potential to improve renal function abnormalities associated with essential hypertension. Its effect on renal function seems independent of its effect on blood pressure.

▶ These increases in glomerular filtration and renal blood flow presumably reflect a preferential vasodilatory effect of calcium entry blockers on renal afferent arterioles. The results look beneficial, but there is a nagging concern about whether such presumed increases in perfusion through the renal glomeruli might cause further glomerulosclerosis. On the other hand, angiotensin-converting enzyme inhibitors preferentially dilate renal efferent arterioles and may reduce intraglomerular pressure. This, in turn, may be responsible for a special ability of these drugs to protect renal function.—N.M. Kaplan, M.D.

Prevention of Diabetic Nephropathy with Enalapril in Normotensive Diabetics with Microalbuminuria
Marre M, Chatellier G, Leblanc H, Guyene TT, Menard J, Passa P (Hôpital Saint-Louis, Hôpital de la Pitié-Salpêtrière, INSERM, Paris)
Br Med J 297:1092–1095, Oct 29, 1988   6–37

The large-scale treatment of insulin-dependent diabetic patients with the portable insulin pump is not practical. Because inhibition of angiotensin-converting enzyme lowers albumin excretion in normotensive diabetic patients with persistent microalbuminuria, the long-term effects were studied with ambulatory patients who had had diabetes for 5 years or longer. The albumin excretion rate exceeded 30 mg per 24 hours. Patients were assigned to receive 20 mg of enalapril daily or a matched placebo for 1 year. There were 10 patients in each group.

Enalapril significantly lowered albumin excretion (Fig 6–8). No treated patient had persistent macroalbuminuria. Mean arterial pressure was lower during enalapril therapy, and treatment duration was a significant factor. Arterial pressure rose linearly during administration of placebo and did not change significantly in patients receiving enalapril. Glomerular filtration rate declined in placebo recipients. Effective renal plasma flow increased during enalapril therapy, and the filtration fraction decreased.

Long-term inhibition of angiotensin-converting enzyme in normotensive diabetic patients with persistent microalbuminuria can prevent diabetic nephropathy. It is not clear whether reduced albumin excretion is related to a systemic fall in blood pressure or a reduction within the glomeruli specifically caused by converting enzyme inhibition.

▶ Note that this study was performed in *normotensive* diabetic patients with albuminuria. Similar decreases in proteinuria have previously been reported with angiotensin-converting enzyme (ACE) inhibitors in hypertensive diabetic patients with nephropathy. Whether the protective effect reflects a fall in blood pressure, as seen in both the normotensive and hypertensive subjects, or is some special effect of these drugs on renal function remains to be seen in human subjects. In rats, the ACE inhibitors appear to provide special renal protection, beyond their antihypertensive effects (1). The best currently available data show that traditional antihypertensive drugs (diuretics, β-blockers, and hydralazine) protect as well as ACE inhibitors, but no direct comparisons have been made in humans.

Regardless, ACE inhibitors are becoming major players in the antihyperten-

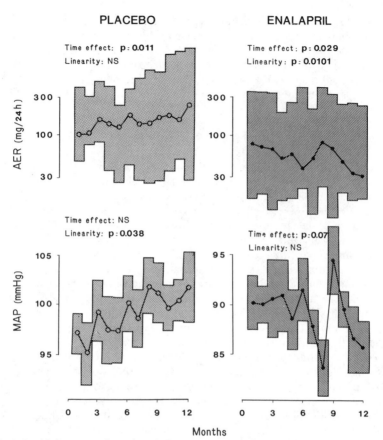

PLACEBO   ENALAPRIL

Fig 6–8.—Median (range) logarithm of albumin excretion (**upper panels**) and mean (SEM) arterial pressure (**lower panels**) in 10 patients treated with placebo (**left panels**) and 10 treated with enalapril (**right panels**). *Shaded areas* correspond to range and SEM values, respectively. (Courtesy of Marre M, Chatellier G, Leblanc H, et al: *Br Med J* 297:1092–1095, Oct 29, 1988.)

sive field. Part of this reflects their apparent benign side effect profile when compared with β-blocker (propranolol) or a central α-agonist (methyldopa). The better "quality of life" with the ACE inhibitor (captopril) was partially negated when a diuretic had to be added for antihypertensive efficacy as was needed more with captopril than with either of the other drugs (2). Nonetheless, captopril caused fewer side effects, including sexual dysfunction.

One could argue that the Croog study was stacked, comparing captopril against 2 other drugs with fairly high side effect profiles. Regardless, captopril is now being compared with other ACE inhibitors, mainly enalapril, which has been used for more than 3 years. As might be expected, the captopril manufacturer (Squibb) says theirs is best, whereas the enalapril maker (Merck) says theirs is best. In fact, there seems little difference between them, and both are quite safe (3). The only serious risk seems to be in patients with significant renal ischemia, in whom removal of angiotensin II support of renal perfusion may lead to a rapid loss of function (4).—N.M. Kaplan, M.D.

References

1. Zatz R, Dunn BR, Meyer TW, et al: Prevention of diabetic glomerulopathy by pharmacological amelioration of glomerular capillary hypertension. *J Clin Invest* 77:1925–1930, June 1986.
2. Croog SH, Levine S, Sudilovsky A, et al: Sexual symptoms in hypertensive patients: A clinical trial of antihypertensive medications. *Arch Intern Med* 148:788–794, 1988.
3. Inman WHW, Rawson NSB, Wilton LY, et al: Postmarketing surveillance of enalapril. I: Results of prescription-event monitoring. *Br Med J* 297:826–829, 1988.
4. Speirs CJ, Dollery CT, Inman WHW, et al: Postmarketing surveillance of enalapril. II: Investigation of the potential role of enalapril in deaths with renal failure. *Br Med J* 297:830–832, 1988.

Safety Issues During Antihypertensive Treatment With Angiotensin Converting Enzyme Inhibitors
Weber MA (VA Med Ctr, Long Beach, Calif)
Am J Med 84(Suppl 4A):16–23, April 15, 1988   6–38

Captopril was the first of the presently available angiotensin-converting enzyme (ACE) inhibitors, and most therapeutic trials have been carried out using this agent. When captopril was first tested clinically, it was used in high doses in the treatment of severe hypertension, often in the presence of renal insufficiency. Numerous side effects of captopril were reported with these early trials, including headache, dizziness, nausea, diarrhea, weakness, proteinuria, rash, neutropenia, and altered taste sensation, but these complications usually disappeared rapidly upon discontinuation of the drug.

Meanwhile, other ACE inhibitors such as enalapril have become available, and today captopril and enalapril are widely used in the treatment of mild to moderate hypertension. The trend to using lower doses has eliminated most of the adverse effects reported with the higher doses used in the earlier studies. The most common adverse effect seen with low-dose ACE inhibitors is a skin rash that often responds to a further reduction of the dosage. Cough and rare occurrences of angioedema have also been reported. Rash and taste disturbance may occur more commonly with captopril than with enalapril

Low doses of ACE inhibitors are safe and effective in the treatment of uncomplicated mild to moderate hypertension. Adverse renal effects have been reported in very few patients, and some patients with underlying renal disease may actually attain an improved renal status during treatment with these agents. Angiotensin-converting enzyme inhibitors do not adversely affect either the central nervous system or biochemical parameters.

A review of the data on ACE inhibitors shows that these compounds offer potential advantages over previously available antihypertensive agents.

▶ One side effect that is being noted with surprisingly high frequency with all ACE inhibitors is a dry, hacking cough. It appears to reflect an increased sensitivity of the cough reflex (1), perhaps from increased levels of bradykinin, which are present because the same ACE enzyme that is inhibited by these drugs both converts angiotensin I to II and is responsible for the breakdown of bradykinin.

Before subjecting any patient on an ACE inhibitor to a work-up for a prolonged, resistant cough, stop the drug. The cough will likely disappear.

As we have noted, there are now lots of options for initial and subsequent therapy. In the desire to choose the most appropriate one, certain features may be helpful.—N.M. Kaplan, M.D.

Reference

1. Morice AH, Brown MJ, Lowry R, et al: Angiotensin-converting enzyme and the cough reflex. *Lancet* 2:1116–1118, 1987.

Age and Antihypertensive Drugs: Hydrochlorothiazide, Bendroflumethiazide, Nadolol, and Captopril
Freis ED, VA Cooperative Study Group on Antihypertensive Agents (VA, Washington, DC)
Am J Cardiol 61:117–121, Jan 1, 1988   6–39

Elderly hypertensive patients usually have higher systolic blood pressure in relation to diastolic blood pressure than younger hypertensive patients. Thus, elderly and younger patients may respond differently to antihypertensive drugs. To determine age-related changes in response to antihypertensive agents, data from 3 double-blind studies conducted by the VA Cooperative Study Group were reviewed. (For this review age 55 years was taken as the dividing point between young and old age.)

In the first study drug responses in 121 patients aged 55–65 years and 191 patients aged younger than 55 years who were treated with hydrochlorothiazide were compared with those in 107 patients aged 55–65 years and 191 patients aged younger than 55 years who were treated with propranolol.

Hydrochlorothiazide reduced both systolic and diastolic blood pressure significantly more in older white patients than in younger ones. Age-related reductions in black patients for both age groups were greater only with regard to systolic pressure. Responses to propranolol did not significantly vary with age except for white patients aged older than 60 years who showed significantly smaller reductions in systolic pressure than younger patients.

In the second study drug responses were compared in 365 patients aged 20–69 years who were randomly assigned to treatment with nadolol, bendroflumethiazide, or a combination of both drugs. There was no difference in the degree of blood pressure reduction between the 2 age groups for nadolol alone. However, the combination of both drugs decreased the systolic blood pressure more in older than in younger patients.

In the third study drug responses were compared in 255 patients aged

55−69 years and in 166 patients aged younger than 55 years who were randomly assigned to treatment with captopril alone or with hydrochlorothiazide. No age-related difference in blood pressure response was observed for captopril alone, but the addition of hydrochlorothiazide tended to result in greater blood pressure reductions in the older patients.

The response to treatment with antihypertensive agents in older hypertensive patients varies with the type of drug administered. Age appears to increase the antihypertensive response to thiazide diuretics, but not to β-adrenergic blockers or captopril.

▶ The differences are not absolute, but they do confirm the impression that elderly and black patients respond particularly well to diuretics and that black patients respond less well to β-blockers. Others have claimed that angiotension-converting enzyme (ACE) inhibitors work less well in the elderly, but the next abstract agrees with the previous one: ACE inhibitors work quite well in the elderly.—N.M. Kaplan, M.D.

Efficacy and Safety of Lisinopril in Older Patients With Essential Hypertension

Gomez HJ, Smith SG III, Moncloa F (Merck Sharp & Dohme Research Labs, Rahway, NJ)
Am J Med 85(Suppl 3B):35−37, Sept 23, 1988   6−40

Angiotensin-converting enzyme inhibitors are thought to be more effective in the treatment of hypertension in patients with normal and elevated renin levels, whereas diuretics or calcium-channel blockers are recommended for patients with low renin-angiotensin system activity. However, several recent studies have demonstrated that angiotensin-converting enzyme inhibitors also effectively reduce hypertension in older patients with low levels of plasma renin activity. The efficacy and safety of lisinopril, a long-acting, angiotensin-converting enzyme inhibitor, were assessed in patients with normal or low levels of plasma renin activity.

The study population consisted of 97 older patients with essential hypertension, aged older than 65 years, and 710 younger hypertensive patients, aged younger than 65 years, who were enrolled in 1 of 4 multicenter monotherapy trials of 8 to 12 weeks' duration. Doses of lisinopril were titrated until a diastolic pressure of less than 90 mm Hg was attained, or to a maximal dose of 80 mg/day. The efficacy of lisinopril monotherapy was evaluated in terms of the magnitude of the blood pressure reduction.

Lisinopril, 20 mg per day, was the most commonly used dose in each of the 4 trials. In general, the blood pressure responses achieved in older patients were equal to or greater than those achieved in younger patients (table). Lisinopril was generally well tolerated. The most commonly reported side effects reported by older patients were headache (8.3%), cough (6.2%), and rash (3.1%), whereas dizziness (5.9%), headache (5.5%), and cough (4.1%) were the most common side effects among

Mean Blood Pressure Changes Produced by Lisinopril (20 mg per day) in Mild-to-Moderate Hypertensive Patients by Age

		<45 Years (n = 68)	45–54 Years (n = 72)	55–64 Years (n = 73)	≥65 Years (n = 27)
				Age Group	
Baseline, in mm Hg	Systolic	148	155	159	169
	Diastolic	100	102	100	101
Change in mm Hg	Systolic	−17	−24	−25	−26
	Diastolic	−16	−17	−17	−17

(Courtesy of Gomez HJ, Smith SG III, Moncloa F: *Am J Med* 85(Suppl 3B):35–37, Sept 23, 1988.)

younger patients. Only 5 of the 97 older patients experienced hypotension-related undesirable effects. Laboratory changes were mild and did not necessitate the withdrawal of any patients.

Lisinopril is safe and effective in the treatment of essential hypertension, including in older patients with low levels of plasma renin activity.

▶ It turns out that age is less important a determinant of the response to various antihypertensive drugs than some have claimed. Race is more so, with blacks responding somewhat less than nonblacks to β-blockers and ACE inhibitors.

The propensity to various side effects may also be considered in making the choice. One that has been claimed to be more or less common with one or another type of drug likely is not.—N.M. Kaplan, M.D.

Sexual Dysfunction in Hypertensive Men: A Critical Review of the Literature
Bansal S (Brown Univ)
Hypertension 12:1–10, July 1988   6–41

Sexual dysfunction is frequent in hypertensive men; about one tenth of even normotensive men aged younger than 40 have sexual problems at a given time. There is no definite evidence of a higher prevalence of dysfunction in treated patients compared with untreated patients. Nevertheless, hypotensive therapy is considered an important cause of sexual dysfunction. There is clinical evidence that drug treatment may raise the frequency of erectile failure in hypertensive patients. The factors most important in sexual dysfunction in this setting remain to be identified, but vascular, neurogenic, and psychogenic factors all may be involved.

When sexual potency returns after treatment is withdrawn but the blood pressure rises, or if withdrawal is contraindicated, another hypotensive agent having a different mechanism of action may be tried. The distinction between organic and psychogenic dysfunction is very important. Patients with abnormal nocturnal penile tumescence and normal hormone levels should have penile blood flow studies. Some patients with nonendocrine organic dysfunction respond to the α_2-adrenergic antagonist yohimbine or to papaverine hydrochloride, alone or combined with phentolamine. A penile prosthesis may provide rigidity. When patients refuse to take drugs because of sexual dysfunction, close assessment of all risk factors is essential.

▶ Impotence is one of the more common and bothersome side effects of antihypertensive drug therapy. As this review documents, sexual dysfunction is fairly common even without therapy and much of what is ascribed to the drugs may have been present but unrecognized.

Nonetheless, too much and too fast a reduction in pressure may reduce blood flow through the penis enough to precipitate erectile impotence, particularly in men with preexisting atherosclerotic vascular disease in the genital vessels. It is likely not related so much to the type of drug as to its effect. Better to go slow and careful.

A more serious but less obvious problem with some antihypertensive drugs is their adverse effect on blood lipids.—N.M. Kaplan, M.D.

Are Effects of Antihypertensive Treatment on Lipoproteins Merely "Side-Effects"? A Comparison of Prazosin and Metoprolol

Lithell H, Haglund K, Granath F, Östman J (Uppsala Univ, Uppsala, Sweden; Huddinge Hosp, Huddinge, Sweden; Univ of Stockholm)
Acta Med Scand 223:531–536, 1988   6–42

Many antihypertensive agents cause undesirable alterations in lipoprotein and glucose metabolism and in electrolyte balance. Even when relatively slight metabolic alterations result from drug treatment they may counteract the effect of decreased blood pressure. The lipid and lipoprotein responses to prazosin, an α_1-receptor-blocking agent, were compared to those of metoprolol in a group of hypertensive patients.

Twenty previously untreated patients and 17 who were previously treated with β-blocking agents were randomly assigned to receive either metoprolol or prazosin twice daily, with the dose being titrated according to the blood pressure response. Doses were adjusted until a supine systolic blood pressure of less than 160 mm Hg and a diastolic blood pressure of less than 90 mm Hg were achieved. At 6 months the patients switched to the alternative treatment for 6 months.

The same blood pressure level was attainable with both drugs. The differences in serum level of cholesterol after treatment were a decrease of 0.22 mmole/L (8.4 mg/dl) with prazosin and a rise of 0.19 mmole/L (7.2 mg/dl) with metoprolol. High-density lipoprotein cholesterol rose slightly with prazosin and fell with metoprolol.

This difference in metabolic response to prazosin and metoprolol at the same blood pressure level may be important in long-term prevention of ischemic heart disease. Monitoring the metabolic effects of antihypertensive treatment seems advisable. In the event of a pronounced metabolic effect, a change in therapy may be indicated.

▶ The rise in cholesterol and triglycerides and fall in high-density lipoprotein cholesterol with the β-blocker have been repeatedly shown with all of these agents except for pindolol, which has a high degree of intrinsic sympathomimetic activity. These effects may be meaningful, particularly in patients already at high risk for coronary disease such as diabetics.

These and other problems with various drugs have led to a move to discontinue therapy after a prolonged period of good control.—N.M. Kaplan, M.D.

The Effect of Withdrawing Antihypertensive Therapy: A Review

Fletcher AE, Franks PJ, Bulpitt CJ (Hammersmith Hosp, London)
J Hypertens 6:431–436, June 1988   6–43

Hypertensive therapy may be withdrawn to avoid side effects if blood pressure is well controlled and if normotension is maintained. Few randomized controlled trials have been done on the effects of withdrawal. In reported trials, from 15% to more than 50% of patients have remained normotensive after discontinuance of medication. A high pretreatment blood pressure and marked obesity predict the return of high blood pressure after withdrawal, as do a short treatment time and left ventricular hypertrophy. In addition, males are more likely than females to have recurrent high blood pressure. Little is known of the effect of the type of treatment on the response to withdrawal in man.

The serum potassium increases when thiazide and related diuretics are withdrawn. The serum uric acid also declines. The effects of withdrawal on glucose tolerance require further study. In community studies, many persons will not be suitable candidates for withdrawal of antihypertensive therapy because of preexisting high blood pressure or obesity. Experience in the Netherlands suggests that the impact of withdrawal on health resources is not likely to be marked.

▶ As more and more patients with milder hypertension are being treated, and as more and more concern about the adverse effects of therapy has been expressed, there is increasing interest in withdrawing therapy, if not permanently, at least for a little vacation.

As documented in this review, from 15% to more than 50% of successfully treated patients will remain normotensive for up to 1 year after therapy is withdrawn. Some of these patients may never have been truly hypertensive before they were put on therapy (remember the 20% prevalence of "white-coat" hypertension). Others likely corrected aggravating factors such as obesity, alcohol abuse, and too much sodium.

Is it worth the effort to withdraw therapy? For some, yes, but for most, probably not. At least, reduction of dosage should always be considered in those who are well controlled.—N.M. Kaplan, M.D.

Secondary Forms

▶ ↓ Another important way to avoid the problems of lifelong therapy is to cure the hypertension by relief of a secondary cause: greatly to be desired but not often possible. Nonetheless, the search may be useful, particularly for renovascular hypertension.—N.M. Kaplan, M.D.

Captopril Scintigraphy in the Diagnosis of Renovascular Hypertension
Sfakianakis GN, Jaffe DJ, Bourgoignie JJ (Univ of Miami)
Kidney Int 34(Suppl 25):S-142–S-144, September 1988   6–44

Conventional radionuclide renal scanning is not useful in the diagnosis of renovascular hypertension. The diagnostic accuracy of renograms have been shown to be improved by performing the tests after pretreatment with captopril. However, it is not known whether renograms using different radiopharmaceuticals are equally useful. In this study, renograms using sodium-I-131-o-iodohippurate (HIP) and Tc-99m-diethylene-triamine-pentaacetic acid (DTPA) were obtained before and after single-dose administration of captopril.

The study population included 31 patients who underwent baseline and postcaptopril scintigraphic studies of 61 kidneys with both radio-

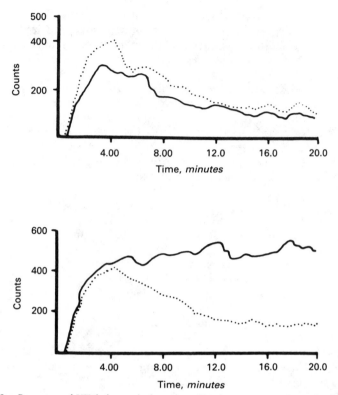

Fig 6–9.—Renogram of HIP before and after captopril treatment in a patient with 70% to 80% occlusion of the main right renal artery. **Top,** baseline renogram does not indicate renovascular hypertension. **Bottom,** captopril had little effect on HIP in left kidney (••••) but induced changes typical of renovascular hypertension in the right kidney (——). (Courtesy of Sfakianakis GN, Jaffe DJ, Bourgoignie JJ: *Kidney Int* 34(Suppl 25):S-142–S-144, September 1988.)

pharmaceuticals. Sixteen of the 31 patients were hypertensive and had stenotic lesions of the renal arteries that were responsible for renovascular hypertension. Of the other 15 patients, 6 were normotensive and 9 were hypertensive with normal renal angiograms and/or renal vein renin studies.

In 9 kidneys with intrinsic disease and marked decreases in glomerular filtration rate, baseline HIP and DPTA renograms were abnormal, with poor isotope uptake. Captopril had no effect on either HIP or DTPA studies. Three kidneys with completely occluded renal arteries could not be visualized on HIP renograms and could be visualized only faintly on DTPA renograms. Captopril had no effect on either HIP or DTPA studies. Four kidneys with more than 95% of arterial occlusion and greater than 80% decrease in function had abnormal baseline studies that did not improve with captopril. However, the HIP study showed continuous isotope accumulation in the renal cortex that was indicative of renovascular hypertension; the DTPA study showed only unilateral decrease in function. Seven of 14 kidneys with 60% to 95% arterial occlusion had normal baseline HIP and DTPA studies. However, both HIP and DTPA renograms became abnormal after captopril administration (Fig 6–9). The remaining 7 kidneys had poor function and abnormal baseline HIP and DTPA renograms, but neither were characteristic of renovascular disease. After captopril, the HIP renogram became positive for renovascular disease in all 7 kidneys, whereas 4 of the 7 DTPA studies remained unchanged.

Conventional renal scintigraphy has limited sensitivity for diagnosing renovascular hypertension. However, pretreatment with captopril increases the sensitivity and specificity of DTPA and HIP scintigraphies for the diagnosis of renovascular hypertension. The sensitivity of HIP scintigraphy was superior to that of DTPA scintigraphy for diagnosing renovascular hypertension.

▶ The search will likely be easier with noninvasive scintigraphy after a single dose of captopril. However, if there is a strong suspicion that renovascular hypertension is present, renal arteriography is still the diagnostic procedure of choice.

Once the diagnosis is made, there may be a need to ascertain the likelihood of a response to angioplasty or surgery before these procedures are performed (see Abstract 6–45). The need is probably less for angioplasty, but the patient should be capable of withstanding surgery if complications occur.—N.M. Kaplan, M.D.

Blood Pressure During Long-Term Converting-Enzyme Inhibition Predicts the Curability of Renovascular Hypertension by Angioplasty
Staessen J, Wilms G, Baert A, Fagard R, Lijnen P, Suy R, Amery A (Univ Hosp Sint Rafaël-Gasthuisberg, Katholieke Univ, Leuven, Belgium)
Am J Hypertens 1:208–214, April 1988   6–45

Percutaneous transluminal renal angioplasty (PTRA) is used in the treatment of patients with suspected renovascular hypertension. A diagnosis of renovascular hypertension is often made on the basis of renin concentrations in the venous blood of both kidneys, which requires selective renal vein catheterization, an invasive procedure that prolongs hospitalization. Recently, the blood pressure level during long-term converting-enzyme inhibition (CEI) therapy was shown to predict the outcome blood pressure after renovascular surgery or nephrectomy.

In a prospective study a comparison was made of the extent to which systolic and diastolic blood pressure during long-term CEI therapy and the ipsilateral to contralateral renal vein ratio could predict the success of PTRA. Success was defined as a systolic blood pressure of less than 160 mm Hg and a diastolic blood pressure of less than 95 mm Hg. The study was done in 28 hypertensive patients, 13 men and 15 women, with unilateral renal artery stenosis of at least 50%. Eleven patients were treated with captopril, and 17 received enalapril. Percutaneous transluminal re-

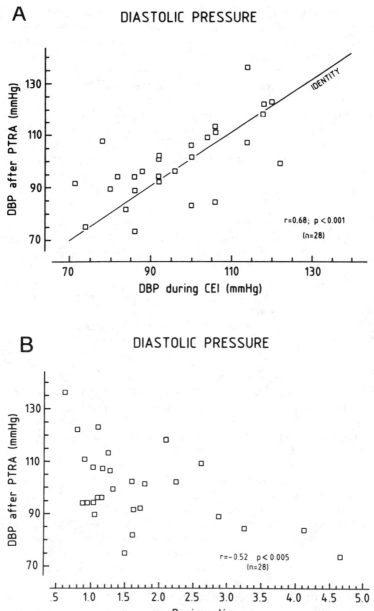

Fig 6–10.—A, diastolic blood pressure after PTRA plotted against blood pressure observed at second visit during CEI. **B,** diastolic blood pressure after PTRA plotted against ipsilateral to contralateral renal vein renin ratio. (Courtesy of Staessen J, Wilms G, Baert A, et al: *Am J Hypertens* 1:208–214, April 1988.)

nal angioplasty was performed irrespective of the patients' blood pressure response to CEI and irrespective of their renal vein renin measurements.

The outcome blood pressure after PTRA was positively related to the blood pressure during CEI and negatively related to the renal vein renin ratio (Fig 6–10). These associations were independent and statistically significant. Thus, blood pressure measurements during long-term CEI predict the curability of renovascular hypertension by PTRA and may be used either alone or in association with the renal vein renin ratio.

▶ Long-term medical therapy is not usually indicated, unless the patient is unable to withstand angioplasty and, with that, the possibility of surgery. Clearly the response to angiotensin-converting enzyme inhibitor therapy is as good a predictor for the response to angioplasty as the renal vein renin ratio.

Other secondary causes are less common than renovascular disease. Pheochromocytomas are rare but can be relatively easily diagnosed and managed (see Abstract 6–46).—N.M. Kaplan, M.D.

Advances in the Diagnosis and Treatment of Pheochromocytoma
Havlik RJ, Cahow CE, Kinder BK (Yale Univ)
Arch Surg 123:626–630, May 1988   6–46

The diagnosis and treatment of pheochromocytomas have improved dramatically in recent years as the result of advances in imaging techniques, assay methods, and drug therapy. Surgical excision remains the definitive treatment for these rare tumors which affect fewer than 1% of all hypertensive patients. Significant therapeutic refinements have been developed in preparing the patient for surgery, in the intraoperative management of the erratic hypertension and arrhythmias that may occur when the tumor is manipulated, and in the management of the severe hypotension that may follow excision. The impact of these developments was retrospectively reviewed.

During a 10-year period 9 female and 9 male patients aged 18 to 51 years had 19 operations for 20 pheochromocytomas. One patient had metachronous pheochromocytomas. Two patients had MEN IIA syndrome, 1 had neurofibromatosis, and 1 had von Hippel-Lindau syndrome. In all cases a biochemical diagnosis was confirmed either by measurement of 24-hour urinary excretion of catecholamines or by epinephrine-norepinephrine fractionation. Two patients had normal levels of catecholamines.

Clinical symptoms included sustained and paroxysmal hypertension in 11 patients and paroxysmal hypertension alone in 2. Five patients were normotensive. Fourteen patients had headaches, 12 had palpitations, and 12 experienced diaphoresis.

Preoperative localization of the pheochromocytoma in the most recently treated patients was accomplished by ultrasound, computed tomography, and ^{131}I-iobenguane scanning. Hypertension was controlled before operation with total α-adrenergic blockade by using phenoxybenzamine in 9 patients and with selective blockade by using prazosin in 6.

Phenoxybenzamine offered no advantage over prazosin with regard to perioperative fluid requirements or intraoperative hemodynamic stability. β-Adrenergic blockade was added before surgery in patients with arrhythmias or predominantly epinephrine-secreting tumors.

Recent developments in biomedical science have simplified the diagnosis and treatment of pheochromocytoma.

▶ A form of secondary hypertension that is seldom considered is hypothyroidism (see Abstract 6–47).—N.M. Kaplan, M.D.

Effects of Thyroid Function on Blood Pressure: Recognition of Hypothyroid Hypertension

Streeten DHP, Anderson GH Jr, Howland T, Chiang R, Smulyan H (State Univ of New York Health Science Ctr, Syracuse)
Hypertension 11:78–83, January 1988   6–47

Hypothyroidism has been associated with diastolic hypertension. To determine the strength of this association, blood pressure was monitored in 40 patients during radioiodine therapy. The induction of hypothyroidism in these patients significantly increased diastolic blood pressure. In 16 of these patients, blood pressure exceeded 90 mm Hg. In 9 of the 16 patients, thyroxine administration reduced diastolic blood pressure to less than 90 mm Hg.

To determine the frequency of the association between hypothyroidism and diastolic blood pressure, serum thyroxine and thyrotropin were measured in 688 hypertensive patients. Of the 688 patients, 25 were determined to be hypothyroid. After thyroid hormone replacement therapy, 32% of these 25 patients had their blood pressure reduced to less than 90 mm Hg.

Hypothyroidism appears to cause hypertension. Hypothyroid diastolic hypertension occurred in 1.2% of this series of hypertensive patients. Therefore, it should be considered in all cases of hypertension.

▶ The finding of previously unrecognized hypothyroidism in 3.6% of these patients seems a bit high but certainly suggests that thyroid function tests be more frequently performed as part of the work-up.

Another common form of secondary hypertension is that seen during pregnancy: preeclampsia or pregnancy-induced hypertension or gestational hypertension (see Abstract 6–48).—N.M. Kaplan, M.D.

Blood Pressure in the Midtrimester and Future Eclampsia

Chesley LC, Sibai BM (State Univ of New York Downstate Med Ctr; Univ of Tennessee, Memphis)
Am J Obstet Gynecol 157:1258–1261, November 1987   6–48

Several investigators have suggested that blood pressure levels during the second trimester might have prognostic significance for the later development of toxemia. To investigate whether blood pressure readings during the second trimester are indeed predictive of the subsequent development of eclampsia, the records of 207 nulliparas and 20 multiparas in whom eclampsia developed and for whom accurate serial blood pressure readings had been recorded were retrospectively reviewed. Mean arterial pressures were calculated by adding one third of the pulse pressure to the diastolic reading.

Only 22% of the nulliparas and 30% of the multiparas had a mean arterial pressure of 90 mm Hg or more during the second trimester before the development of eclampsia, and only 34% of the nulliparas and 35% of the multiparas had a maximal mean arterial pressure of 90 mm Hg or more during that period. Only 8.2% of the nulliparas had a maximal diastolic pressure of 80 mm Hg or more and none had a diastolic pressure of 90 mm Hg or more during the second trimester.

There was no correlation in these data between increased blood pressure levels during the second semester and the subsequent development of eclampsia. Increased blood pressure levels during the second trimester may at most be predictors of transient hypertension.

▶ This study discounts the prior claim that higher blood pressure during the midportion of pregnancy can predict the development of later preeclampsia. The majority of those who have the classical form of gestational hypertension have an elevated blood pressure (and usually proteinuria) only during the last few weeks.

The cause of gestational hypertension remains unknown, with increasing evidence for a prostaglandin deficiency (1). As seen with essential hypertension, hyperinsulinemia has been noted (see Abstract 6–49).—N.M. Kaplan, M.D.

Reference

1. Friedman SA: Preeclampsia: A review of the role of prostaglandins. *Obstet Gynecol* 71:122–137, 1988.

An Association Between Hyperinsulinemia and Hypertension During the Third Trimester of Pregnancy
Bauman WA, Maimen M, Langer O (VA Med Ctr, Bronx, NY; Albert Einstein College of Medicine)
Am J Obstet Gynecol 159:446–450, August 1988   6–49

Hypertension predisposes pregnant women to several complications. Plasma levels of insulin have recently been associated with hypertension, suggesting that insulin may be a regulator of blood pressure during pregnancy.

The serum glucose and plasma insulin response to oral glucose was studied in 27 normotensive and 16 hypertensive nondiabetic women during the third trimester of pregnancy. Several women were drug abusers or

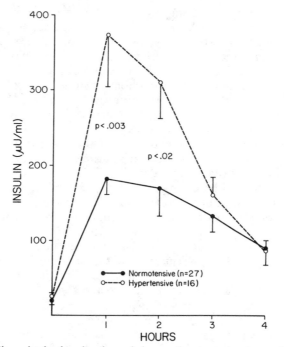

Fig 6–11.—Plasma levels of insulin after oral glucose tolerance test in normotensive and hypertensive women. (Courtesy of Bauman WA, Maimen M, Langer O: *Am J Obstet Gynecol* 159:446–450, August 1988.)

cigarette smokers, or both, during pregnancy. All received a 100-gm glucose load.

The mean plasma level of insulin in normotensive and hypertensive women after a glucose tolerance test is shown in Fig 6–11. Glucose tolerance in hypertensive women was not significantly different from that in normotensive women. In a subgroup of 8 hypertensive hyperinsulinemic women, glucose tolerance did not differ from that in women with normal insulin responses. Five of 16 hypertensive women, 3 of whom were hyperinsulinemic, delivered low birth weight infants. Nine of 27 normotensive women delivered offspring of low birth weight. There were no significant differences in human placental lactogen values among the groups.

Hypertension alone appears to increase the risk for intrauterine growth regardation. Low birth weight in neonates delivered by hypertensive women, with or without hyperinsulinemia, probably results from placental vasculopathy with an associated reduced microvascular circulation. Although glucose tolerance was similar in all groups, it can be inferred that peripheral insulin resistance must have been markedly increased in the subgroup with hyperinsulinemia and hypertension.

▶ The mechanism for hyperinsulinemia with gestational hypertension is as obscure as for the hyperinsulinemia noted in essential hypertension. The mechanism is now unknown but hopefully will be recognized and thereby provide some important information about their pathogenesis.

Lastly, severe hypertension can complicate the postoperative period (see Abstract 6–50).—N.M. Kaplan, M.D.

Postoperative Hypertension: A Comparison of Diltiazem, Nifedipine, and Nitroprusside
Mullen JC, Miller DR, Weisel RD, Birnbaum PL, Teoh KH, Madonik MM, Ivanov J, Laidley DT, Liu P, Teasdale SJ (Toronto Gen Hosp)
J Thorac Cardiovasc Surg 96:122–132, July 1988   6–50

Many patients become hypertensive after coronary bypass surgery, at a time when functional and metabolic recovery is incomplete. The efficacy of various treatments was studied in a randomized trial of 62 patients whose mean arterial pressure exceeded 95 mm Hg postoperatively. All drugs were titrated to maintain a mean arterial pressure of about 90 mm Hg.

All 3 drugs lowered arterial pressure to a similar degree. Heart rate was lowered most during diltiazem therapy, whereas it increased with nitroprusside and nifedipine therapy. Cardiac index responses were similar in all treatment groups. Myocardial performance was depressed by diltiazem and nifedipine; left ventricular strokework indices were lower than at baseline. Systolic function was better after nitroprusside than with diltiazem. Myocardial oxygen consumption was similar in all groups.

Nitroprusside is the most convenient means of controlling postoperative hypertension, but it may not improve metabolism. Nifedipine and diltiazem may be useful adjuncts when increased contractility accompanies postoperative hypertension. Calcium antagonists also may improve myocardial metabolism. However, these drugs must be used cautiously in patients with poor ventricular function.

▶ A common problem in every surgical suite is postoperative hypertension. The problem is particularly common after coronary bypass surgery, with some reporting a 33% to 50% prevalence. The control of postoperative hypertension may be critical, and nitroprusside is the "gold standard." Here is evidence that calcium entry blockers may be equally effective in lowering the blood pressure and even more cardioprotective.

This seems an appropriate way to end the 1988 literature coverage of hypertension: newer agents can provide more effective control of even life-threatening rises in pressure.—N.M. Kaplan, M.D.

Subject Index

A

Ablation
  catheter, of accessory pathways, results, 150
Abnormality (*see* Anomalies)
Abscess
  aortic root, of cavity, with aortic valve endocarditis, 246
  periannular, aortic valve replacement in, sutureless, 244
Accessory pathways
  catheter ablation of, results, 150
Acetylcholine
  coronary artery response to, after heart transplant, 271
Acquired immunodeficiency syndrome
  myocarditis at necropsy in, 135
Addiction, drug
  with endocarditis, infective, 164
  Staphylococcus aureus endocarditis in, 165
Adolescence
  arrhythmia during, with hypertrophic cardiomyopathy, 62
α_2-Adrenergic receptor blockade
  intracoronary, attenuating ischemia during exercise (in dog), 32
β-Adrenergic (*see* Beta-adrenergic blocker)
Afterload
  resistance and end-systolic pressure-thickness relationship, 20
Age
  antihypertensives and, 324
  myocardial adaptation to volume overload and (in rat), 12
Aged
  aortic valve selection in, 237
  lisinopril for, in essential hypertension, 325
AIDS
  myocarditis at necropsy in, 135
Amiodarone
  in cardiac dysrhythmia, growth after, in children, 109
  in coronary artery disease, ventricle after, 218
Ammonia
  positron tomography, nitrogen-13, 49
Anastomosis
  aortic, growth of, sutures for (in pig), 252
  pulmonary artery-to-aorta, pulmonary valve after, 83

Aneurysm
  aortic, new multiple-stage approach, 255
  coronary artery, prevention in Kawasaki disease with gamma globulin, 65
  ventricular, closure with pericardium, 229
Angina
  pectoris
    with aortic regurgitation, 125
    with coronary artery disease, in aortic regurgitation, 124
    with coronary artery disease, in aortic stenosis, 123
    mental stress in, and ST segment depression, 142
    mild, medical vs. early surgical therapy, 223
    ventricular plication in, 228
    severe, and time to first new myocardial infarction, 222
    unstable, acute, aspirin and heparin in, 212
Angiography
  exercise radionuclide, after coronary artery disease treatment, 214
Angioplasty
  balloon, in coarctation of aorta
    native, 101
    results, 104
  coronary
    in acute myocardial infarction with t-PA, 176, 177
    with aortic valvuloplasty in aortic stenosis and coronary artery disease, 114
    coronary atherosclerosis progression after, 195
    coronary flow reserve after, 199
    guidelines for, of task force, 201
    ISFC/WHO Task Force Report, 198
    multiple, model of factors in restenosis, 200
    in myocardial infarction (*see under* Myocardial infarction, acute)
    in 1985–1986 and 1977–1981, 199
    restenosis after (*see* Restenosis after coronary angioplasty)
    in myocardial infarction, acute, TAMI I trial results, 182
    in renovascular hypertension, 331
    after thrombolysis for acute myocardial infarction, TIMI II A results, 180
Angiotension
  converting enzyme inhibitors in hypertension, 323
  -renin system in cardiovascular homeostasis, 297

Author Index

A

Abascal, V.M., 116
Abastado, P., 235
Abelmann, W.H., 134, 137
Abottsmith, C., 182, 183, 184
Abry, B., 262
Acampora, D., 191
Ades, P.A., 317
Aglira, B.A., 83
Ahnve, S., 155
Akasaka, T., 130
Akimoto, K., 69
Al-Aska, A.K., 66
Alboliras, E.T., 83, 84
Alderman, E.L., 132, 198, 269
Aldridge, H.T., 196
Alexander, R.W., 271
Al-Fagih, M., 82
Alheid, U., 27
Allan, L.D., 97, 98
Allen, H.D., 95
Allen, M.D., 229
Almog, S., 293
Al-Nozha, M., 66
Al-Orainey, I., 66
Amery, A., 331
Anderson, D.W., 135
Anderson, G.H., Jr., 334
Anderson, J.L., 187
Anderson, R.H., 69, 90
Antony, I., 125
Appleton, C.P., 18, 127, 131
Arcidi, J.M., Jr., 227
Ardura, J., 109
Aretz, T., 33
Armstrong, B.E., 107
Arnold, A.E.R., 177
Aronson, L., 183
Artigou, J.-Y., 270
Ashton, J.H., 42
Assaad, A.N., 267
Attevelt, J.T.M., 306
Atwood, J.E., 145
Aversano, T., 20
Aylward, P.E.G., 199

B

Bache, R.J., 4
Badhwar, K., 273
Baert, A., 331
Bahr, R.D., 176
Bailey, K.R., 120
Bailey, L.L., 267
Baim, D.S., 114
Bairey, C.N., 203
Baker, E.J., 90
Baldet, P., 136
Balon, R., 289
Bansal, S., 327

Barber, G., 83
Bareiss, P., 136
Bargeron, L.M, Jr., 77, 99
Barker, G.A., 259
Barlow, G.K., 292
Barr Taylor, C., 188
Barry, J., 142
Barry, W.H., 187
Bashey, R.I., 14
Bassenge, E., 28
Batisse, A., 78
Bauer, J.H., 320
Baughman, K.L., 237
Bauman, W.A., 335
Baumgartner, W.A., 237
Beatie, D., 108
Beck, G.J., 226
Becker, A.E., 143
Becker, L.C., 20, 35, 50, 176
Becker, T.M., 204
Bedotto, J.B., 21
Beekman, R.H., 101
Beevers, D.G., 310
Behar, V.S., 185, 186
Beiser, A., 204
Bell, W.R., 176
Beller, G.A., 190
Bellocq, J.P., 136
Benjamin, N., 318
Berglund, G., 311, 312
Berman, A.D., 112, 114, 115
Berman, D.S., 203
Bermejo, J., 109
Berry, T.E., 80
Bertrand, M., 198
Betriu, A., 177
Beumann, F.G., 234
Beutler, J.J., 306
Bietendorf, J., 203
Billhardt, R.A., 152
Billman, G.E., 56
Bircks, W., 263
Birnbaum, P.L., 337
Bishop, V.S., 6, 8
Bittner, V., 68
Blackstone, E.H., 77, 99, 241, 258, 263
Blair, R.W., 6
Blanchet, F., 125
Blanchot, P., 150
Blank, S., 281
Bloch, K.D., 3
Block, E.H., 204
Block, P.C., 116, 204
Boddie, C., 281
Bodnar, E., 243
Bodvarsson, M., 25
Boku, H., 69
Bolens, M., 91
Bolger, A., 127
Bolli, P., 307
Bolman, R.M., 67
Bologna-Campeanu, M., 108
Bonan, R., 195, 196, 200

Bonchek, L.I., 229
Booth, D.C., 29
Borbola, J., 145
Borggrefe, M., 263
Borkon, A.M., 237
Borromée, L., 78
Borst, H.G., 255
Boswick, J.M., 182, 184
Böthig, S., 198
Boucher, C.A., 33
Bouhour, J.B., 136
Bourassa, M.G., 196, 198
Bourgoignie, J.J., 329
Bowman, F.O., Jr., 96
Boyle, W., 162
Brand, D.A., 191
Brandt, A.A., 191
Braunwald, E., 156
Breatnach, E.S., 68
Breithardt, G., 263
Brenowitz, J.B., 231
Brezinski, D.A., 202
Brinker, J.A., 176
Bristow, J.D., 124
Bristow, M.R., 269
Brown, J., 147
Brown, J.W., 73
Brown, M.L., 213
Browne, K.F., 187
Bruch, P., 52
Buckley, M.J., 146
Bühler, F.R., 307
Buja, L.M., 42
Bull, C., 105
Bulpitt, C.J., 310, 328
Buonissimo, S., 299
Burek, K., 184
Burlingame, M.W., 229
Burns, J., 259
Burridge, J., 273
Burrows, F.A., 259
Burton, N.A., 269
Bush, D.E., 176
Butler, A., 310
Butterfly, J., 204

C

Cabrol, C., 270
Cahill, P.D., 236
Cahow, C.E., 333
Caldwell, R.A., 73
Califf, R.M., 182, 183, 184, 185, 186
Callahan, P., 145
Cameron, A., 215
Camilleri, J.-P., 40
Campbell, S., 142
Campbell, W.B., 197
Candela, R., 184
Candela, R.J., 182, 183
Candell-Riera, J., 129